Living Longer
With Heart Disease

Howard H. Wayne, M.D.

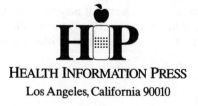

HEALTH INFORMATION PRESS
Los Angeles, California 90010

Health Information Press, Los Angeles,CA
Library of Congress Cataloging-in-Publication Data

Wayne, Howard H.
    Living longer with heart disease: the noninvasive approach that will
save your life / Howard H. Wayne
        p.   cm.
    Includes bibliographical references and index.
    ISBN 1-885987-12-9 (hardcover)
    1. Heart--Diseases--Popular works. 2. Medical misconceptions
I. Title.
RC682.W33 1998
616.1'2--dc21   98-14179
                                                                          CIP

ISBN: 1-885987-12-9

Printed in the United States of America

Health Information Press
4727 Wilshire Blvd., Suite 300
Los Angeles, CA 90010
1-800-MED-SHOP
email: MEDICALBOOKSTORE.COM

DEDICATION

This book is dedicated to my wife, Gypsy, and to my children Michael, Michelle and Bradley.

DISCLAIMER

The information presented in this book is based on the experience and interpretation of the author. Although the information has been carefully researched and checked for accuracy, currency and completeness, neither the author nor the publisher accept any responsibility or liability with regard to errors, omissions, misuse or misinterpretation.

TABLE OF CONTENTS

INTRODUCTION

PUT THE FIRE OUT!

T reating heart disease is like putting out a fire: the earlier it is discovered and extinguished, the less damage it will cause. In the same way, if heart disease is detected and properly treated, the patient's injury will be less severe, complications will be fewer, and it will be less likely to progress to end stage heart disease with heart failure. In addition, if heart disease is discovered early, the patient will probably not require treatment with heroic measures such as coronary artery bypass surgery, angioplasty, the insertion of stents, and cardiac transplantation. While these "technological triumphs" may be touted as examples of great medical successes; they are actually glaring examples of medical failures.

When we talk of treating a disease, we intuitively assume that it will be made better, or cured. Although they might temporarily relieve symptoms, surgical procedures such as bypass surgery and angioplasty do nothing to improve or cure coronary artery disease, and for this reason they are not really treatments at all. In fact, before the introduction of coronary artery bypass surgery in 1968, if someone developed heart disease, it would take many years before that person became disabled or died. Doctors have progressed, however. They have speeded up the process.

The magnitude of the failure of most doctors to diagnose heart disease early in patients without symptoms is reflected in the numbers: 10,000 victims die and 20,000 victims have heart attacks *each week* in this country. Sadly, two-thirds of them actually see a physician shortly before their catastrophic event, and are reassured that their hearts are all right. In contrast, the immense popularity of coronary artery bypass surgery, angioplasty, and the insertion of stents in patients with symptoms underscores the lack of understanding by most doctors of the fundamentals involved in the treatment of heart disease. These procedures treat the symptoms, but they do nothing to prevent its complications or its progression. Predictably, the results are less than satisfactory, and ultimately end in failure. Indeed, instead of being dramatically reduced with modern drug therapy, the frequency of heart failure, the end stage of obstructive coronary artery disease, has doubled in the past two decades from 200,000 to 400,000 patients a year. In fact, it has become the number one discharge diagnosis of hospitalized patients.

Somehow, it just doesn't seem right. The doctor fails to diagnose the patient's impending heart attack and then, provided the patient survives, he or she is told that heart surgery is imperative. In the process, the doctor is rewarded with a very handsome fee for his or her initial incompetence!

To avoid heart attacks and premature death, the heart disease patient will need to know the following important facts: the disease can progress in the complete absence of symptoms; the routine tests doctors use to detect heart disease are hopelessly antiquated and insensitive, but newer tests can detect heart disease or its progression at an early stage; and modern medications are highly effective in treating the disease, provided they are administered in adequate numbers and dosages. Every patient needs to know which tests and medications are best, as well as what tests and drugs are not effective. In addition, patients should understand that the mere presence of chest pain is not a "green light" for the cardiologist to perform immediate surgery, but it is rather a signal calling for prolonged and careful investigation of the many other conditions that may cause chest pain.

This book will arm you with this important knowledge, so that you may successfully fight heart disease. As you will see in the pages that follow, the great majority of patients who have heart disease with mild or no symptoms are grossly undertreated. However, when symptoms are present, the patient is usually overtreated. In either case, the treatment delivered is inappropriate and the patient becomes a victim of his or her doctor rather than a victim of the disease.

By learning as much about the disease as possible, the patient with heart disease will greatly increase his or her chances of achieving a normal life span with little or no disability. Heart disease often is deadly and, in fact, it is the number one cause of death in industrialized nations. However, like arthritis, it can be managed. While the disease may bother a patient at times, it should not shorten a patient's life. Heart disease can be transformed into a relatively benign illness. After reading this book, you will be much better prepared to make this transformation.

GLOSSARY

ACE inhibitors: (a.k.a. angiotensin converting enzyme inhibitors) a class of drugs used to treat hypertension and congestive heart failure. It works by interfering with the conversion of angiotensin I to angiotensin II, the latter of which is a powerful constrictor of blood vessels. Angiotensin is produced by a complex hormonal system involving the kidney, adrenal glands and liver known as the renin-angiotensin system.

agglutinate: clump together

aminophylline: substance used as a diuretic, vasodilator and cardiac stimulant

angina: severe pain, usually referring to angina pectoris

angina pectoris: the name given by doctors to a distinctive type of chest discomfort in patients with coronary heart disease when the muscle becomes ischemic. Patients describe the discomfort as if their chest were in a vise, or someone were sitting on their chest. It usually radiates across the upper and mid portion of the chest.

angiogenesis: the formation of new blood vessels

angiogram: see also *coronary angiogram*. An invasive test in which x-ray opaque dye is injected directly into an artery. As the dye passes down the artery, high-speed x-rays and/or video images are obtained. If the artery is narrowed, the obstruction will be visualized.

angiotensin II: a substance that causes vessels to constrict

antecubital fossa: the place on the forearm opposite the elbow where the stethoscope head is placed to take the blood pressure

antioxidant: an agent (such as a vitamin) that inhibits oxidation

aorta: large, main artery of the trunk; it comes from the base of the left ventricle and ends on the left side of the whole body

apexcardiogram: test that records the movement of the chest wall from the heart beat. Includes reading of the relative changes in volume and pressure inside of the heart.

arrhythmia: irregularity of the heart beat

arteriosclerosis: hardening of the arteries

arteriosclerotic plaque: A metamorphosis of the arterial wall initially caused by traumatic injury from the impact of blood as it flows through the artery. Layer after layer of clot-like material is deposited over the site of the injury. An inflammatory response follows, cellular debris, white blood cells and fat are deposited in the area, it becomes thicker and eventually can obstruct the artery. Alternatively, the plaque may rupture and cause a clot to form that obstructs the artery.

atherectomy: refers to the use of a rotor rooter type of catheter that is inserted into a coronary artery and used to cut up and scoop out any arteriosclerotic plaque

atrium: upper chamber of each half of the heart; the left atrium receives the blood from the pulmonary veins; the right atrium receives blood from the venae cavae and the coronary sinus

benzothiazepine: a class of calcium channel blocker used for treating high blood pressure

beta blockers: a class of heart drugs that suppress the effect of adrenaline on the heart. Therefore the heart rate will not increase during stress, and the work load of the heart will be reduced. They help to prevent blood pressure from increasing.

brachial artery: the main artery that carries blood from the arm to the forearm and hand

bypass surgery: (a.k.a. coronary bypass surgery) involves surgery directly to the surface of the heart. The internal mammary artery that runs along the inside of the sternum (breastbone), or a section of the saphenous vein from the inside of the thigh is used as a conduit to bypass an obstructed coronary artery. One end of the artery or vein is connected to the aorta, and the other end is inserted into the obstructed artery downstream from the obstruction so that blood may flow around the obstruction. If the patient is to receive two or more bypasses, then both the internal mammary artery and multiple sections of veins have to be used. Such bypass grafts, as they are called, only partially restore blood flow. If there is additional obstruction to blood flow downstream from where it is inserted, blood flow may not be restored at all. Bypass grafts become obstructed just like arteries, but in a much shorter time —sometimes within a few weeks or months.

cachexia: weight loss and wasting secondary to chronic disease

calcification: process by which plaques become hardened by deposits of insoluble salts of calcium or phosphate

calcium channel blocker: a class of drugs that is used to treat hypertension, angina pectoris and cardiac arrhythmias. They have the ability to block the movement of calcium into both cardiac muscle cells and the smooth muscle cells that make up the muscular wall of arteries, thereby causing them to relax. As a result, the main effect is the dilation of coronary arteries, causing an increase in blood flow and a decrease in blood pressure.

cardiologist: physician who specializes in the diagnosis and treatment of heart disease

cardiomyopathy: disease of the heart muscle, or myocardium, when underlying etiology is unknown

catecholamine: one of the hormones released under stress or fear that is responsible for increased heart rate and blood pressure. They may cause extreme constriction of blood vessels throughout the body and result in an increased tendency for the blood to clot, reduced blood flow to the heart muscle, and an increase in cardiac arrhythmias and death.

catheter: flexible plastic tube that allows passage of fluid or blood from or into a body cavity hollow organ or blood vessel

cholesterol: a steroid found in animal tissues and food, especially animal fats, and also manufactured by the liver

cholesterol-lowering drug: class of drug that claims to decrease the amount of cholesterol in the bloodstream, and to fight atherosclerosis

collateral vessels: new blood vessels that bud out upstream from an obstructed artery, and then connect up again to either a nearby healthy artery or with the same artery downstream from the obstruction, thereby preserving the flow of blood

computed tomography (CT): imaging technique that uses a computer to synthesize data from x-rays of cross-sections of soft tissue and bone

congestive heart failure: condition where the heart is unable to pump an adequate supply of blood. Clinical symptoms include congestion in the lungs and edema in the tissues.

coronary angiogram: an invasive test in which a plastic tube called a catheter is inserted into the main artery in the thigh (femoral artery) and pushed up the aorta until it reaches the heart. The catheter is then inserted into the coronary arteries as the aorta exits from the heart. X-ray opaque dye is injected under high pressure, and high-speed x-rays are taken. The artery and its branches can then be imaged. If the artery is narrowed or obstructed, its location can be identified.

coronary angioplasty: a catheter with a balloon at the tip is passed into a coronary artery to where it is narrowed and the balloon is inflated with 2 to 15 atmospheres of pressure (you have 2 atmospheres of pressure in your automobile tires). The hope is that the artery will be expanded where it is narrowed. In the process, the arterial wall is often damaged and it is sometimes perforated.

coronary arteries: the arteries on the surface of the heart that supply blood to the muscle. They arise from the aorta as soon as it exits from the heart.

coronary artery disease: the buildup of arteriosclerotic plaque in the arteries serving the heart. When the artery is sufficiently narrowed, blood flow to the heart muscle is reduced, and the muscle is said to become ischemic.

coronary artery dissection: a complication of angioplasty. When an artery is stretched, the inside lining of the artery may tear. Blood enters the wall of the torn artery and causes its muscular layers to separate. As a result, the artery may rupture, or the lumen of the artery may collapse and block the passage of blood, causing a heart attack.

coronary artery restenosis: when a section of a coronary artery that was treated with balloon angioplasty becomes narrowed or obstructed again

coronary heart disease: Coronary heart disease is the direct result of advanced obstruction of the coronary arteries. The formation of arteriosclerotic plaque along the walls of the coronary arteries is merely known as coronary artery disease. Coronary heart disease does not develop until the coronary arteries become so obstructed that adequate amounts of blood cannot reach the heart muscle. As a result, the heart muscle is permanently injured or scarred and cannot function in a normal manner. Such obstruction to blood flow may take place gradually over a period of years, or abruptly if an arteriosclerotic plaque ruptures and a clot forms that obstructs the flow of blood.

cortisol: hormone secreted by the adrenal gland and released during stress that increases heart rate and blood pressure

diabetes (or diabetes mellitus [DM]): a metabolic disease in which carbohydrate utilization is reduced; caused by a deficiency of insulin and characterized by chronic hyperglycemia, glycosuria, water and electrolyte loss, ketoacidosis and coma

diastolic pressure: intracardiac pressure during the relaxation or filling phase of a heart's cycle. It is the bottom number in the blood pressure reading. A diastolic pressure greater than 85 is abnormal.

digitalis: (a.k.a. foxglove) one of a genus of flowering plants that are the main sources of cardioactive steroid glycosides that are used in the treatment of certain heart diseases, especially congestive heart failure

dihydropyridines: part of the family of calcium channel blockers

diuretic: agent that increases the amount of urine excreted and helps to lower blood pressure

Doppler color flow imaging: imaging technique using ultrasound where different directions of flow are represented by different colors

ECG stress test: recording the electrocardiogram while exercising on a treadmill or bicycle ergometer. Based upon the principle that with only moderate narrowing of a coronary artery, blood flow to the heart muscle at rest is adequate. During exercise, the heart muscle requires much more oxygen but the blood cannot get through in sufficient amounts. The heart muscle then becomes ischemic and the electrocardiogram will usually show evidence of that ischemia.

echocardiogram: a noninvasive imaging technique based upon the principles of sonar or radar. High frequency sound waves are transmitted to the inside of the heart. The sound waves reflected back allow one to see moving images of the inside of the heart, including the magnitude and direction of thickening of the heart muscle, the pattern of motion of the muscular walls of the heart, the structure and function of all four heart valves, the thickness of the heart muscle, the dimensions and geometry of the heart's chambers, the velocity and direction of blood flow within the heart's chambers, the flow of blood within the heart muscle and many other measurements. Thus, echocardiography provides an extensive array of structural and functional information.

edema: fluid in the tissues creating a swelling

ejection fraction: the ejection fraction represents the percentage of blood ejected from the heart with each heart beat. It is a measure of how well the heart functions. Patients with normal cardiac function have ejections fractions of 60% to 75%. Moderate impairment of cardiac function is usually associated with an ejection fraction of 40% to 60%. Patients with ejection fractions of less than 20% to 30% have severe heart disease.

electrocardiogram: graphic record of the heart's electrical activity due to the currents that travel through the heart and initiate its contraction; abbreviated ECG or EKG

endothelial cells: the cells that make up the lining of all blood vessels

epinephrine: chief neurohormone that stimulates adrenergic receptors, resulting in increased heart rate and force of contraction, vaso-constriction or vasodilation and other metabolic effects

estrogen: one of a group of sex hormones; used in certain treatments of coronary disorders in women

fibrinogen: protein in the blood produced by platelets that is converted into fibrin which causes the blood to clot

flavonoids: substances of plant origin containing flavone, a plant pigment. It has been suggested the presence of flavonoid in red wine and champagne work somehow to reduce the risk of coronary artery disease

gastroesophageal reflux disease: (a.k.a. GERD) disease where the contents of the stomach are regurgitated into the esophagus causing esophagitis

heart attack: sudden insufficiency of blood supply to the heart muscle; usually as a result of occlusion of a coronary artery. See also *myocardial infarction.*

heart failure: after multiple heart attacks, the heart becomes very enlarged and stretched out. It is so weak it cannot supply the body's needs; i.e., it can no longer function to circulate the blood, a result of which is congestion and edema in the tissues. The patient is said to be experiencing heart failure at this time.

hemoglobin: the red respiratory protein of erythrocytes that transports oxygen from the lungs to the tissues

hemorrhage: bleeding through ruptured or unruptured vessel walls

Holter monitor: 24-hour monitoring of the electrocardiogram. Used to detect transient arrhythmias or cardiac ischemia during ordinary activities

homocysteine: a normal breakdown product of an essential amino acid known as methionine, commonly found in red meats and milk products. Recently high levels of homocysteine have been related to the increased risk of developing cardiovascular disease

homocysteinuria: disorder characterized by the excretion of excess homocysteine in the urine

hypercholesterolemia: extremely high levels of cholesterol in the blood

hypertension (high blood pressure): a resting blood pressure above 140/85 or above 150/90 during stress

hypertensive angina: chest pain similar to ordinary angina but lasting longer and due to acute elevations of the blood pressure

hypoglycemia: abnormally low concentration of glucose in the blood

hypotension: abnormally low blood pressure

invasive test: any test that results in the placement of a tube, catheter or device within the blood vessels or heart

ischemia: reduced blood flow to a tissue, organ, or area of the body

isometric grip: exercise involving maximal muscular contractions of the hand, usually accomplished by squeezing a spring-loaded grip device for about one minute. It can cause an acute and significant increase in blood pressure, heart rate and work load upon the heart.

left atrium: upper left chamber of the heart that receives oxygenated blood from the lungs

left ventricle: lower left chamber of the heart that receives blood from the left atrium

lumen: the inside of an artery

magnetic resonance imaging (MRI): a diagnostic radiological imaging modality that provides 3-D images of the body's muscles, bones, blood vessels, nerves, organs and tumor

menopause: cessation of menses

methionine: see *homocysteine*

microcirculation: the vast network of small arteries less than 0.5 mm that supply blood to the heart muscle. Such vessels cannot be seen on an angiogram because of their small size.

microvascular angina: the term used for patients who have chest pain (angina pectoris) but who have normal, unobstructed coronary arteries when they undergo an angiogram. Their chest pain is probably due to reduced blood flow in the microcirculation.

microvascular circulation: the vast network of small arteries less than 0.5 mm that supply blood to the heart muscle. Such vessels cannot be seen on an angiogram because of their small size.

mitral valve: the input valve on the left side of the heart between the left atrium and the left ventricle

morbidity: the frequency of an illness

morphine: a narcotic commonly used for pain relief during a heart attack

mortality: the death rate for an illness

MRI (magnetic resonance imaging): see *magnetic resonance imaging*

myocardial infarction: the medical term for heart attack. It is usually caused by sudden and complete occlusion of a coronary artery causing loss of blood supply to the heart muscle. Whether or not the heart muscle is damaged depends upon whether the heart muscle has a dual blood supply from branches of another coronary artery or from the microcirculation, and on how quickly blood flow is restored.

myocardial ischemia: reduced blood flow to the heart muscle

myocardium: the medical term used to describe the heart muscle

neuropathy: damage to a nerve caused by loss of blood supply or metabolic disorder such as diabetes and pernicious anemia

nitrates: a class of drugs which release a chemical called nitric oxide. Nitric oxide is normally manufactured by the endothelial cells that line the walls of blood vessels. When the vessel wall is damaged because of arteriosclerotic plaque, the production of nitric oxide is greatly reduced.

Nitrates, by supplying the needed nitric oxide, dilate the arteries and increase blood flow to the heart muscle. On the venous side of the circulation, nitrates cause the veins to relax and fill with blood. This reduces the return of blood to the heart, reducing its work load and the energy it expends and, therefore, the amount of blood required by the heart muscle. Thus, nitrates, through their dual actions, can eliminate ischemia.

nitric oxide: the chemical substance produced by endothelial cells that is responsible for maintaining blood flow through the heart muscle

nitroglycerin: a tablet used for the relief of chest pain or shortness of breath that when placed under the tongue releases nitric oxide. This is rapidly absorbed in the circulation within 2 to 3 minutes, relieving the patient's symptoms.

noninvasive: a term used to describe a group of tests that do not require penetration of the skin, invasion of the body or the insertion of any device or material within the body

noninvasive cardiologist: a cardiologist who diagnoses and treats heart disease without the use of diagnostic tests that require the insertion of tubes or catheters inside the body

norepinephrine: a neurohormone that causes constriction of the blood vessels

NSAIDs: nonsteroidal, anti-inflammatory drugs (e.g., ibuprofen) that are commonly used for pain relief. They are capable of causing significant damage to the kidneys and stomach, block the effects of diuretics, cause fluid retention, elevate the blood pressure, and can cause chest pain in people with obstructive coronary artery disease.

oscilloscope: an imaging device like a small television set that is used to monitor the electrocardiogram and other signals generated by the heart

pericardium: a thick membrane that covers the heart, limiting its expansion

PET (positron emission tomography): a radioactive imaging test that allows detection of normal metabolic substances made by heart cells. Radioactive chemicals identical to the chemicals produced by the heart cells must first be injected into the circulation. If these radioactive substances are found within the heart muscle, then that muscle must be alive and functioning. It is used to distinguish live from dead heart muscle cells.

phonocardiogram: a recording of the heart sounds. When a doctor listens to the heart with a stethoscope, there is no permanent record of what he has heard for comparison at a later date. In addition, some of the abnormal sounds generated by the heart have a very low frequency of around 25 Hertz. Therefore, they cannot be heard by the human ear. The phonocardiogram will record these abnormal sounds. The presence of such sounds can be used to monitor the progress of the patient's disease.

placebo: a pill containing inert ingredients that is used in controlled scientific experiments. Both the patient and doctor are unaware of whether the patient is taking an active experimental drug or the placebo. Typically, 30% of patients taking a placebo will get relief from their symptoms or side effects.

platelets: cellular components within the blood that supply fibrinogen, a necessary factor in the clotting of blood

positron emission tomography (PET): see *PET*

pulmonary artery: the main artery exiting from the right ventricle that carries venous blood to the lungs so it can be oxygenated

pulmonary edema: when the left ventricle fails during heart failure, blood will back up into the lungs, filling the tiny air spaces of the lungs so that oxygen cannot enter the blood stream. Unless promptly treated, pulmonary edema is rapidly fatal.

pulmonary hypertension: a rare disorder in which the pressure within the pulmonary artery is markedly elevated

psychogenic amenorrhea: cessation of menses due to psychological reasons

radioactive imaging: a noninvasive test that is used to study the function of heart muscle. When a radioactive substance is injected into the circulation, there should be equal distribution to all areas of the heart. If a coronary artery is obstructed, then there will be a proportional reduction in the amount of radioactive substance that will reach that area of the heart muscle. Radioactive detection devices known as gamma cameras can locate the radioactive areas. If there is a deficiency of the radioactive material in an area of the heart, then that area is said to be either scarred due to a prior heart attack, or merely ischemic due to obstructive coronary artery disease.

radionuclide ventriculography: a radioactive imaging study in which the radioactive material is imaged as it passes through the heart. Changes in the geometry and contour of the radioactive material within the left ventricle allow indirect assessment of the motion of the heart walls. Areas that do not move or move abnormally can usually be identified. The test allows estimation of the ejection fraction.

radiopharmaceutical: a radioactive drug used to study the function of a variety of organs within the body

renal artery: the artery going to the kidney

renin: a substance normally produced by the kidney that contributes to the control of blood pressure

restenosis: a term commonly used to describe the re-narrowing of a narrowed artery after it has been opened up with angioplasty or stents

right atrium: the right upper chamber of the heart that receives blood from the head and lower body

right ventricle: the right lower chamber of the heart that receives blood from the right atrium

risk factor: a condition which increases the likelihood of a disease. For example, smoking increases the risk or likelihood of developing heart disease.

spectral Doppler: a special application of echocardiography that allows the determination of the velocity of blood flow within the heart's chambers on a moment-to-moment basis throughout the cardiac cycle. This allows assessment of cardiac function, particularly during diastole, the filling phase of the heart during its relaxation.

statin drug: one of the cholesterol-lowering drugs

stent: a small tube with scaffolding walls that, when inserted into a narrowed artery, will expand, enlarging the artery. Unfortunately, growth of tissue within the stents often causes it to become obstructed.

stethoscope (electronic; standard): a stethoscope that amplifies heart sounds and murmurs

stress test: see *ECG stress test*

stress thallium test: see *radioactive imaging test.* Such a test is carried out both at rest and during exercise to determine if there is a loss of radioactivity and, therefore, ischemia, only during exercise.

systolic pressure: the blood pressure within the blood vessels and left ventricle during the contraction phase of the heart's cycle. It is the top number of a blood pressure reading. A systolic pressure above 140 is considered abnormal.

thromboxane A_2: a substance involved in blood clotting

thrombogenic: capable of accelerating the formation of a blood clot

thrombus: the medical term for a blood clot

tricuspid valve: the input valve between the right atrium and right ventricle

unstable angina: medical term used to describe the recent onset of angina, or a change in the behavior of previously present angina such as occurrence with less effort, or at rest, lasting longer, or being more severe

vascular disease: damage to blood vessel walls due to the formation of arteriosclerotic plaque within the walls of the arteries

ventricle: the right or left chambers of the heart

ventricular fibrillation: ineffective contractions of the heart muscle at a rapid rate resulting in the inability of blood to be ejected from the heart. If not reversed with an electric shock, it will result in immediate death.

ventricular septum: the muscular wall that divides the heart's chambers into the right and left ventricles

venules: the small veins on the venous side of the circulation that begin immediately after the capillaries

Part I:
Silent Heart Disease

1

THE SILENT DISEASE

If No One Knows It's There,
How Can It Be Treated?

There are many diseases that exist for years before symptoms appear. One only has to think of diabetes, cirrhosis, kidney disease, cancer, hypertension, and AIDS to name a few. Coronary artery disease, which eventually leads to coronary heart disease, is yet another. Its earliest manifestations may be found in young adults as yellow streaks in the wall of the aorta, the main artery exiting from the heart and traversing the chest and abdomen. Arteriosclerotic plaques, as they are called, gradually build up along the wall of the aorta and its branches in individuals who are well under 40 years old. The exact reason why such plaques develop is not known, but it is thought to be due to an interaction involving a change in blood flow, injury to the vessel wall, and various cells within the blood.

In the same way that a rushing torrent of water can sweep away houses, cars and anything in its path, so can blood that is flowing with greater force and speed than normal injure the lining of arteries. This is most likely to occur where blood vessels branch or change course. Once the lining of the artery is injured, an inflammation is likely to occur. Just as a skin perforation may become infected and is infiltrated with pus cells (leukocytes), so does an injured vessel wall become infiltrated with inflammatory cells. In time, the inflamed area is transformed into an arteriosclerotic plaque.

WHERE PLAQUES DEVELOP

While plaques may appear in any artery, they are the most dangerous when they appear on the coronary arteries on the surface of the heart, on the arteries to the brain and kidney, and on the aorta itself. The blockage of blood flow to any of these important organs can have devastating consequences.

Interestingly, plaques never develop in veins. Plaques are limited to arteries in which the pressure is relatively high, and veins are part of a low pressure system. An exception to this is when a vein is used in a coronary artery bypass operation. Here the vein is used as a detour for an obstructed coronary artery. In such instances, one end of the removed vein is connected to the side of the aorta immediately after it exits from the heart. The other end is connected to the obstructed coronary artery downstream from the blockage. In this way, blood can flow around the obstruction, but the vein is now carrying blood at pressures seen only on the arterial side of the circulation. Accordingly, it can and does become blocked, just like the obstructed artery which it replaced. This is one of the reasons why 50% of the patients undergoing bypass surgery have a return of their symptoms within just a few years.

Just as arteriosclerotic plaques are not found in veins in which the blood pressure is low, they also are not present in the pulmonary arteries (the arteries going through the lungs), which similarly are a part of a low pressure system. Plaques are almost never found in the walls of the pulmonary arteries, unless the patient develops a rare disease called pulmonary hypertension. This disease develops when the blood pressure within the pulmonary arteries becomes extremely elevated for reasons that we don't understand. Not surprisingly, we are unable to treat pulmonary hypertension effectively. As a result, the only treatment available for this disorder is a lung transplant.

If high pressure is an important reason why arteriosclerotic plaques develop, is a person more likely to develop such plaques if he or she has hypertension? Absolutely! This subject will be discussed in greater depth later.

CONTENTS OF A PLAQUE AND HOW IT GROWS

Once plaques appear, they gradually increase in size, partially replacing the wall of the artery where they are located. In addition, the plaques encroach upon the lumen of the blood vessel. This is the space inside of the artery where the blood travels. Most of the plaque is made up of inflammatory cells, muscle cells, cellular debris, calcium and fibrin. Contrary to what the public has been led to believe by the media and the pharmaceutical companies that sell cholesterol lowering drugs, arteries do not become "clogged by cholesterol deposits," because in fact less than 5% of the plaque is made up of cholesterol. Cholesterol-lowering drugs and low cholesterol diets have almost no effect on established arteriosclerotic plaque, despite all the hype orchestrated by the pharmaceutical industry.

In a sense, the plaque behaves like bump in the road, and if it becomes ulcerated, it can be likened to a pothole. Just as a passenger in car that hits a bump or a ditch is traumatized, blood also becomes traumatized when it goes over the arteriosclerotic plaque. When this happens, cellular constituents in the blood known as platelets are stimulated to initiate the coagulation cascade that produces a substance called fibrinogen, which is deposited on top of the arteriosclerotic plaque. Under the influence of enzymes secreted by the endothelium (the lining of the artery), fibrinogen is converted into fibrin; and fibrin causes the blood to clot.

It is fortunate that this mechanism exists. Were it not for the ability of the blood to clot, we could bleed to death from a simple injury. Unfortunately, this same protective clotting tendency is responsible for layering fibrin on the surface of the plaque, making it larger. It is worth noting here that the reason aspirin is an effective form of treatment for preventing heart attacks is because it interferes with the conversion of fibrinogen to fibrin, and helps to prevent the formation of a clot on the plaque's surface.

EFFECT OF PLAQUE ON BLOOD FLOW IN ARTERY

If the arteriosclerotic plaque grows large enough, it can interfere with the flow of blood within the artery in several ways. First, enough fibrin may accumulate on the plaque's surface so that it mounds up, partially obstructs

5

the artery, and causes the blood to slow down. Since blood has a tendency to clot when it slows, at some point a clot may form on the surface of the arteriosclerotic plaque. If the clot is big enough, it will completely obstruct the flow of blood in the vessel, and shut off the blood supply to the body tissues nourished by that artery. If this happens to occur in an artery that supplies the brain, it will cause a stroke. If it occurs in a coronary artery, it causes a heart attack (myocardial infarction), provided there is no alternate supply of blood vessels to that area of the heart.

There is a second way arteriosclerotic plaque may affect the flow of blood. Because the plaque is, for the most part, living tissue, it therefore needs a blood supply. Large numbers of tiny vessels traverse the plaque because it is an inflammatory reaction. These vessels are fragile, are exposed to white blood cells and are susceptible to rupture. When this occurs, the bleeding that follows exposes the plaque's contents to the blood flowing over it. This material is highly thrombogenic. In other words, it has a tendency to make the blood clot or form a thrombus (i.e., a clot) that will obstruct the blood flow. Once again, aspirin, because it is also an anti-inflammatory agent, helps to prevent some of this inflammatory reaction and reduces the risk of hemorrhage.

A third type of complication that may affect the flow of blood is when cellular debris and clot-like material break loose from the plaque and travel downstream. When the debris can go no further, it lodges itself in a branch of the artery, blocking off the blood flow to the tissues beyond. This is particularly likely to take place in large arteries such as the aorta, or the carotid arteries in the neck that supply the brain with blood. In either case, such occurrences may result in small strokes and, if they occur repeatedly, there will be a change in the victim's behavior. If it occurs in the victim's heart, it can gradually destroy small areas of heart muscle without chest pain or a heart attack. If this happens often enough, the final result may be heart failure, a condition in which the heart has been damaged so much that it can no longer function.

HEALING OF AN ARTERIOSCLEROTIC PLAQUE

Although many arteriosclerotic plaques result in the formation of a clot and blockage of an artery, many do not. Instead they may heal by becoming calcified. This is the body's way of repairing itself. The result may be an artery with a fixed degree of narrowing. While such an artery may appear to be severely narrowed on an angiogram, it is in no danger of closing off and will remain unchanged over many years. This is a very important to understand, because cardiologists are in the habit of rushing patients in for urgent angioplasty or coronary artery bypass surgery whenever they see artery in this condition. In the process, the patient is frightened into believing that unless one of these procedures is carried out immediately, a massive heart attack or sudden death may occur. It can't be emphasized enough that such tactics are unethical and are certainly not supported by the scientific evidence [1-5] as shown from the following research reports.

RESEARCH STUDIES

A number of studies have been done in an attempt to track the progression of arteriosclerotic plaques over a period of years. In a study of 29 patients who had angiograms before and after their heart attack[1], Dr. William Little of Bowman Gray School of Medicine, found that only 10 (34%) had occluded (i.e., closed off) the most severely narrowed artery up to six years after the initial angiogram. Ninety-seven per cent of the heart attacks took place in vessels that were only mildly to moderately narrowed. Most arteries with severe narrowing remained unchanged. Similar findings were noted by Dr. Giroud and his co-workers at the University Hospital in Geneva, Switzerland.[2] He found that only 32% of his patients who had heart attacks showed a severely narrowed coronary artery. The other patients who had heart attacks did not show significantly narrowed arteries at the time of the initial angiogram before the heart attack. An even fewer percentage of heart attacks resulted from the occlusion of markedly narrowed coronary arteries, according to a study by Dr. John Ambrose of Mount Sinai Medical Center in New York.[3] In this study, only 22% of heart attacks resulted from severely narrowed coronary arteries, the remainder occured in individuals whose coronary arteries were only mildly to moderately narrowed.

It is evident that further narrowing of extremely narrowed coronary arteries takes place either at a very slow rate or not at all. For example, in the Coronary Artery Surgery Study,[4] 298 patients were followed over a five year period. Of these patients, 89 had coronary arteries that were between 81% and 95% narrowed. Yet, only 23.6% of these became occluded during the 5-year study period. Based upon these studies, Professor Nicolas Danchin in France has pointed out that even if a severely narrowed coronary artery does become completely occluded, it is usually well tolerated, and does not cause a heart attack, nor does it significantly impair the function of the heart.[5] He states that although a heart attack is almost always caused by a blocked coronary artery, a blocked artery often does not cause a heart attack. To understand why, read on.

WHEN IS RESTRICTION OF BLOOD FLOW IN A CORONARY ARTERY GREAT ENOUGH TO PRODUCE SYMPTOMS?

The point at which the restriction to blood flow is great enough to produce symptoms depends upon the important factors listed below, each of which is examined more closely in the pages that follow.

TABLE I: FACTORS THAT DETERMINE WHETHER PLAQUES WILL CAUSE SYMPTOMS
1. The degree of narrowing of the coronary artery
2. The rate of narrowing of the coronary artery
3. The number of collateral vessels
4. The heart rate
5. The level of the blood pressure
6. Adaptive response of the heart muscle
7. Amount of blood flow to the remainder of the heart
8. Degree of enlargement of the heart
9. Compensatory enlargement of the artery
10. Triggering mechanisms

1. The Degree of Narrowing of the Coronary Artery

Plaques do not begin to interfere with the flow of blood until an artery is narrowed by at least 75%, for reasons that have to do with simple hydraulic principles. Picture measuring the amount of water coming out of a garden hose at average pressure. Let us say that five gallons of water come out of the hose every minute. If we put a clamp on the hose that reduces its diameter by 50% and measure the flow of water again, we will find that it still empties at a rate of five gallons per minute. This is because the pressure builds up behind the clamp and helps maintain the output of water. Not until the diameter of the hose has been reduced to 75% or more will the flow of water be reduced. The arteriosclerotic plaque behaves the same way. Plaques that cause narrowing of a coronary artery by less than 75% will not interfere with the flow of blood at normal heart rates. Thus, the coronary arteries may have many plaques, and yet there may be no interference with the rate of blood flow. This is not true at higher heart rates, as will be discussed shortly.

2. The Rate of Narrowing of the Coronary Artery

If a clot suddenly forms in a narrowed artery, the subject will probably begin to notice chest pain (i.e., angina) with exertion and perhaps even at rest. If symptoms were present before, then angina will occur with even less exertion. If the amount of heart muscle supplied by the obstructed artery is large enough, a heart attack or even sudden death may occur. In 10% to 20% of cases, sudden death is the first symptom; in 40% of cases, a heart attack is the first symptom. On the other hand, if the degree of narrowing of the coronary artery is gradual, there may be no symptoms, particularly if the heart has adapted by developing new blood vessels to compensate for the reduced flow of blood.

3. The Number of Collateral Vessels

Under a process known as angiogenesis (*angio* = blood vessels, *genesis* = birth of), new blood vessels will bud out upstream from an obstructed artery like branches from a tree. They will connect up to either a nearby healthy artery or they will reinsert into the mother artery downstream from the obstruction. In other words, the heart puts in its own bypasses. These new vessels are called collateral vessels. They are more durable than the kind the surgeon puts in, the procedure does not cause any complications, they last longer, they do not become obstructed, and the patient does not need to have medical insurance to get them. In fact, even if a coronary artery becomes completely obstructed, if there are enough collateral vessels the victim will not have a heart attack and there will be no symptoms during ordinary activities.

The reason collateral vessels do not become obstructed is the same reason veins and pulmonary arteries never become obstructed: they are all part of the low pressure system. A major coronary artery may be anywhere from 4 to 7 millimeters in diameter. A collateral vessel is one-tenth that diameter. As the diameter of a blood vessel gets smaller, so does the pressure within it. Accordingly, the speed with which the blood flows through the artery is greatly reduced. If one has an accident in a car going only 15 to 20 miles per hour, there is not likely to be any serious injury, compared to an accident at 50 to 60 miles per hour. Recall that injury to the vessel wall that is the beginning of the formation of arteriosclerotic plaque is directly related to the velocity of the blood flowing within that artery. The velocity of blood flow within collateral vessels is so slow that no injury will occur to the vessel wall, arteriosclerotic plaques will not form, and no clot will develop to block the artery.

4. The Heart Rate

Symptoms also may occur when a coronary artery is narrowed if the heart is made to speed up sufficiently during exertion. What does heart rate have to do with the development of symptoms? When the heart speeds up, it contracts more forcefully and has to work harder. To accomplish this, the heart muscle requires more energy and oxygen. Therefore, more blood must travel through the coronary arteries to supply these nutrients. If a main coronary artery is sufficiently narrowed, then the flow of blood is affected. Think of a four lane freeway: during the middle of the day, if two lanes are being repaired there may be no back up of traffic. The number of cars on the freeway during those hours is not very great and two lanes are adequate to allow traffic to move at normal speeds. During rush hour, however, it's a different story. Now there are too many automobiles for two lanes, traffic slows down and may even be completely stopped.

The same thing happens in the heart. At normal heart rates, and even at slightly elevated rates, blood flow through a narrowed coronary artery may be adequate to supply the heart muscle, but it is not adequate at very high heart rates when more blood is required. Now the collateral vessels become an important alternate source of blood supply to the heart muscle. Unfortunately, most collateral vessels in humans are quite narrow. Like a narrow coronary artery, they deliver an adequate amount of blood at normal heart rates, but are unable to do so at higher heart rates.

As a result, at very rapid heart rates the heart muscle will not receive enough blood supply and it will become ischemic; *ischemia* is the generic term used to describe this situation. If a brain becomes ischemic for more than five seconds, the victim will faint. If it lasts more than four minutes, he or she will die. If the heart muscle becomes ischemic, the subject will have chest pain. Doctors call such chest pain *angina pectoris*. If the ischemia lasts for 15 to 20 minutes, the heart muscle (myocardium) will be injured but will recover if the blood flow is restored. If the ischemia lasts 30-60 minutes, the victim will have a heart attack, or myocardial infarction.

5.   The Level of the Blood Pressure

By far the most important factor in determining whether arteriosclerotic plaques eventually produce symptoms is the level of the blood pressure. It is a long-known but not a well-known fact that many patients with hypertension develop chest pain whenever their blood pressure rises. Such increases occur during physical exertion, emotional stress, after eating, smoking a cigarette, and many other activities. Why this pain occurs will be discussed later in this book. For the moment, it is enough to understand that individuals with hypertension are highly susceptible to precipitous increases in blood pressure whenever they are under stress. When coronary artery disease is present, angina pectoris often appears. Yet, if the blood pressure is controlled with medication, similar degrees of stress will not produce any chest discomfort. Clearly, whether or not symptoms appear depends primarily on the degree of elevation of the blood pressure.

6. Adaptive Response of the Heart Muscle

Still another determinant of whether symptoms appear is how well the heart muscle adapts to ischemia. Think of the left ventricle (the chamber that pumps blood to the entire body) as an inflated balloon. When air is expelled from the balloon, it deflates. If both of your hands are holding the balloon, then both hands will come together at equal rates. Conversely, with inflation of the balloon, both hands move outward to the same degree. In the case of the heart, during the relaxation phase of the cardiac cycle, blood enters the ventricle from the left atrium. As it does so, the muscular walls of the left ventricle, like your hands on an expanding balloon, move outward in equal amounts.

When the ventricle starts to contract, these muscular walls come together at equal rates and degrees, and eject blood into the aorta. However, if the blood flow to one of those muscular walls is limited due to severe narrowing of a coronary artery, that wall may be able to move only 50% of its normal excursion, i.e., the distance the heart usually moves from its position at the end of the relaxation phase (when it is completely filled with blood) to its position at the end of its contraction phase (when about 75% of the blood in the left ventricle has been ejected). In this situation, the heart moves the opposite muscular wall 150% to compensate. This is a clever way for the heart to adapt, because the amount of compression of the blood within the left ventricular chamber remains the same. Thus, the amount of blood ejected by the heart remains unchanged at normal heart rates, and the patient has no symptoms even though a coronary artery is greatly narrowed.

7. Amount of Blood Flow to the Remainder of the Heart

Still another determinant of whether or not symptoms will occur depends upon the health of the heart muscle opposite the area that can move only 50%. Is it able to compensate by moving 150%? To accomplish this, it must receive a normal blood supply. If it, too, has a reduced blood flow due to a narrowed coronary artery, then it will be unable make up the difference and the patient will develop symptoms. This explains why, when symptoms do finally appear, it is unlikely that the patient's disease is confined to just one of the three coronary arteries. Most patients with symptoms already have advanced disease of all three of their coronary arteries.

8. Degree of Enlargement of the Heart

Unfortunately, there is a price to be paid when one area of the heart has work extra to avoid the development of symptoms. It triggers other adaptive responses in the heart to make it become larger. If the volume of a normal heart is 100 milliliters (about three and a half ounces) and the various organs and tissues of the body need 75 milliliters with every heart beat, then that heart has to contract three-quarters of its volume to expel the required amount of blood. By enlarging to 300 milliliters, the heart no longer needs to contract three-quarters of its volume. One-quarter will still supply the 75 milliliters that the body needs with each beat. For a weakened heart muscle, contracting only one-quarter is far less work than contracting three-quarters. Accordingly, by enlarging, the heart is able to expel its quota of 75 milliliters per heart beat without the non-affected section of heart muscle having to increase its work output 150%.

After many years, the heart may become so enlarged and stretched out that it loses its elasticity and fails completely. Symptoms will now appear. The prognosis for patients with heart failure is very grim— indeed, it is often worse than the prognosis for patients with cancer.

9. Compensatory Enlargement of the Artery

Another factor in determining whether or not symptoms appear with the build up of plaque is the compensatory response on the part of the artery in the region of the arteriosclerotic plaque. You may have read stories in the newspaper about how certain cholesterol-lowering medications actually cause "regression" of the arteriosclerotic plaque. Indeed, the pharmaceutical companies have staged a media blitz in their attempt to convince the public that plaques will decrease in size if you take their cholesterol-lowering medication. In reality, the artery will actually enlarge in the vicinity of the plaque, for reasons that we do not entirely understand. It may be considered an adaptive response on the part of the artery. For instance, if a 2 mm artery is 50% occluded by plaque, the plaque has a diameter of

1 mm. If the artery enlarges to 4 mm but the plaque remains at 1 mm, the artery will be only 25% obstructed. Thus, the plaque will appear "smaller." In truth, the plaque hasn't changed at all. It's a form of illusion. Such adaptive changes naturally occur in obstructed arteries. If you give a cholesterol-lowering drug and then re-study the patient with angiograms after a few years, you will see that the plaque has become smaller. A medical scientist receiving a large grant from a pharmaceutical company to carry out this study might conveniently conclude that it was the cholesterol-lowering drug that was responsible. In fact, it was merely coincidental.

10. Triggering Mechanisms

The last factor that determines whether symptoms of plaque build-up will appear is the presence of certain triggering mechanisms that will cause the sudden disruption of an arteriosclerotic plaque. This may be followed by partial or complete occlusion of a coronary artery. Activation of the sympathetic nervous system through stress, extremes of exercise, and smoking may result in a rapid increase in heart rate and blood pressure. The sympathetic nervous system is the part of the central nervous system that is not under our conscious control. It is responsible for such bodily responses as a change in heart rate, constriction or dilatation of the skin vessels, and enlargement of the pupils. A rapid rise in heart rate and blood pressure increase the force with which blood travels through the circulatory system, as well as the pressure within the arteriosclerotic plaque. The resulting stresses may cause the plaque to rupture or hemorrhage, or both. Since activation of the sympathetic nervous system also increases the tendency of the blood to clot, circumstances are ripe for partial or sudden occlusion of a coronary artery.

We have seen how and where arteriosclerotic plaques form, how they grow and interfere with the flow of blood, how they may trigger the formation of a blood clot that completely blocks the flow of blood, and the various factors that determine whether or not symptoms occur. Yet, in spite of the presence of extensive arteriosclerosis in many arteries of the body, and the heart in particular, most patients do not have symptoms of their disease. In part, this is because their disease has taken decades to develop and the body has time to grow new blood vessels to replace the obstructed ones. Another contributing factor is the fact that most people fail to exercise enough to increase their heart rate to a level that will provoke symptoms. It is also because the coronary arteries adapt to the presence of arteriosclerotic plaques and the plaques become calcified and healed. Finally, it is because of the adaptive response of the heart muscle which allow it to compensate for any muscle that has been damaged, or whose function is impaired. Yet, these adaptive responses may become maladaptive responses that ultimately are harmful to the heart.

On the surface, it would seem to be desirable for patients not to have symptoms from their disease. Nobody likes to have symptoms. But, it is this very absence of symptoms that make coronary artery disease so dangerous. If no one knows it's there, it can't be treated.

Thankfully, there is a great deal we can do about predicting and preventing future heart attacks, as well as the other long-range complications of obstructive coronary artery disease. That's what this book is about.

REFERENCES

1. Little, WC, Constantinescu M, Applegate RJ, *et al.* Can coronary angiography predict the site of a subsequent myocardial infarction in patients with mild-to-moderate coronary artery disease? Circulation 1988; 78:1157-1166.
2. Giroud D, Li JM, Urban P, *et al.* Relation of the site of acute myocardial infarction to the most severe arterial stenosis at prior angiography. Am J Cardiol 1992; 69:729-732.
3. Ambrose JA, Tannenbaum, MA, Alexopoulos D, *et al.* Angiographic progression of coronary artery disease and the development of myocardial infarction. J Am Coll Cardiol 1988; 12:56-62.
4. Alderman EL, Corley SD, Fisher LD, *et al.* Five year angiographic follow-up of factors associated with progression of coronary artery disease in the Coronary Artery Surgery Study (CASS). J Am Coll Cardiol 1993; 22:1141-1154.

5. Danchin N. Is myocardial revascularization for tight coronary artery stenoses always necessary? Viewpoint. Lancet 1993; 342:224-225.

2

ROUTINE MEDICAL EXAMS ARE NOT ENOUGII

If you went to your family doctor and asked for a cardiac examination although you were not having any symptoms such as chest pain, most likely your doctor will take your resting blood pressure, listen to your heart with an ordinary stethoscope (the basic design of which hasn't changed in over 100 years), and give you an electrocardiogram (a test that doctors have used since the early part of this century). Only one out of four individuals with moderate to severe coronary heart disease will have their disease detected by such an examination. Heart disease will not be identified in the remaining three, until two have a heart attack and one dies.

Even if symptoms are present, the ability to detect an abnormal heart with an examination of this type leaves much to be desired. Of the millions of patients who are seen in an emergency room each year for chest pain, 35,000 are reassured their hearts are fine and they are sent home— only to die within the next few days.

Unfortunately, too many doctors are unaware of how insensitive their methods of examination are. When Mr. Jones is seen for a routine follow-up examination a year after his heart attack and tells his doctor he continues to have rare angina whenever he walks fast or uphill, but that it is no different than before, it is unlikely that the primitive examination Mr. Jones is subjected to will uncover any new findings. Not surprisingly, Mr. Jones will be told he is doing well. And when the doctor receives a call from the coroner a few days later that Mr. Jones was found dead in bed, the doctor will blame his death on the unpredictability of coronary heart disease. It will never occur to him that, had Mr. Jones undergone a more careful examination and been given appropriate diagnostic tests, the impending catastrophe could have been recognized, treated and prevented. That doctor will never learn from his errors and will continue to "practice" medicine and bury his mistakes.

How big is this problem? Far bigger than you might imagine. Although it was mentioned earlier in this book, the following is worth repeating: approximately 10,000 Americans die and 20,000 have heart attacks every week. Two-thirds of these victims actually see a physician shortly before their attack and each is told he or she is doing well.

What is the reason for this extraordinary gap in the diagnosis and treatment of heart disease? If you have read the preceding chapter, you will understand why so many patients with coronary heart disease do not have symptoms to warn them that something is about to happen. Unfortunately, in the absence of new symptoms that would dictate the use of more sensitive tests, both patient and doctor are lulled into a false sense of security. But the absence of symptoms is only one part of the problem. Even more significant is the inability of routine methods of examination to detect heart disease.

LIMITATIONS OF THE ROUTINE METHODS OF EXAMINATION TO DETECT HEART DISEASE

1. The Blood Pressure

Let's start with the blood pressure measurement, the usual beginning of all examinations. Is it an accurate exam? Yes, but a mere glance at the statistics suggests something is wrong. Approximately 64 million people in this country have hypertension, the medical term for high blood pressure. It has been estimated that half of these individuals are completely unaware that their pressure is high. Of the half who are aware and who are being treated, half of *them* are unaware that their blood pressure is not under control. This is difficult to understand when you consider that every doctor's office and nearly every drug store has a blood pressure cuff. The explanation, however, is simple. Resting blood pressure is not an accurate guide to what the blood pressure is when the subject is active.

Think about this for a moment: almost everything we do is based upon performance. If we want to buy an appliance, we won't choose one based upon looks alone, but we will try to find out how it performs. If you decide to shop for a car, you are not likely to buy one unless you take it for a road test first. In the same way, an evaluation of the heart is based upon performance. A stress test is a standard method of evaluating the heart. It has long been recognized that although a patient's heart may function normally when he or she is at rest, it may not be true if the patient is experiencing stress of some kind. Yet, paradoxically, a different set of standards are used for blood pressure evaluation. Indeed, even the definition of hypertension is inaccurate. It is assumed that if a patient's blood pressure is normal at rest, then hypertension is absent. Conversely, if the patient's blood pressure is elevated when he or she is at rest, then the patient has hypertension. Unfortunately, it is not that simple.

Each of us have certain feedback mechanisms in our body. If we go without water, our throats get dry. If we do not eat and our blood sugar gets low, we feel hungry. If it is cold, we shiver, and if it is hot, we sweat, but our internal body temperature remains always at 98.6 degrees. There is also a feedback regulatory mechanism to control blood pressure. If we are subjected to a stress, our blood pressure will start to rise, but as soon as it does, feedback mechanisms in the body cause the arteries to dilate, and this lowers the blood pressure. The opposite happens if our pressure becomes too low.

This feedback mechanism gradually begins to malfunction over a period of years for individuals destined to develop hypertension. When an individual with impaired blood pressure regulation is subjected to stress, the blood pressure will rise precipitously in less than a minute. I often see patients who have all of the classic symptoms of hypertension, but whose resting blood pressure is normal. Such patients are usually told that their symptoms are psychosomatic and they are given a tranquilizer. Yet, when these patients are subjected to an office stress test, such as the isometric hand grip test, their blood pressure will usually rise to dangerous levels. For instance, it is not unusual to watch a patient's blood pressure change from 130/80 to 225/120 in only 60 seconds! When the blood pressure remains elevated for any length of time, it can easily trigger a heart attack. Thus, failure to diagnose and treat hypertension may be the equivalent of a death warrant. As discussed in the previous chapter, high blood pressure not only encourages the development of arteriosclerotic plaques in the coronary arteries, but it may cause them to rupture.

2. The Stethoscope

The second reason why the routine examination fails to detect heart disease is the continued use of the stethoscope. Hearts are like motors. When a motor isn't working properly it makes extra noises, and you don't have to be a mechanic to know something is wrong. When the heart is not working right, it makes noises, too. Doctors call these noises heart sounds. Normally the heart makes only two sounds. The first sound occurs while the heart is contracting, and it is caused by the closure of the mitral and tricuspid valves, which are the intake valves of the heart between the atria and the ventricles. They allow blood to flow into the heart, but then close up when the heart contracts to prevent the blood from flowing backwards.

The second heart sound occurs at the end of contraction. As the heart begins to relax, the high pressure within the ventricles begins to fall. When the pressure falls below the pressures in the aorta and the pulmonary arteries, the aortic and pulmonary valves close to prevent blood from falling back into the ventricles. Only the first and second heart sounds are normal. All other sounds are abnormal in adults, and indicate that something is wrong with the structure or function of the heart. Athletes and runners are an exception to this rule.

Abnormal heart sounds occur when the left ventricle does not empty completely. When this happens, some blood is left behind within the cavity of the left ventricle. Consequently, at the next cardiac cycle, only a portion of the next load of blood can enter the ventricle (think of how not every member of a group of people will be able to get onto a elevator that is already crowded). It results in a backup of blood into the left atrium, causing it to stretch. Fortunately for humans, when their atrium is stretched, it behaves like a rubber band— the greater the stretch, the greater the recoil. The result is that the atrium contracts so forcefully that it makes a sound.

We call this sound the "fourth heart sound," probably because it was not noticed until after the first three sounds made by the heart were deciphered. The fourth heart sound occurs just before the first heart sound.

The third sound made by the heart also occurs as a result of the backup of blood and the increase of pressure within the heart's chambers. It occurs after the second heart sound. Normally when the heart begins to fill with blood at the beginning of every relaxation cycle, no sound is created. However, if the pressure within the left atrium is elevated due to a backup of blood from incomplete emptying of the left ventricle, then blood will rush in with such force that it makes a noise (the "third heart sound").

Thus, the presence of third or fourth heart sounds is a red flag indicating incomplete emptying of the heart, usually due to ischemia of the heart muscle, or to an elevated blood pressure that interferes with the emptying of the heart. In both instances, such patients are likely to be without symptoms and have a normal resting blood pressure and electrocardiogram.

Unfortunately, both the third and fourth heart sounds usually have a frequency of about 25 Hertz, a frequency that is too low to be heard by the human ear. Electronic stethoscopes with low frequency amplification will detect such sounds, as well as recording microphones. Unfortunately, neither of these two devices are used for routine examination; consequently, the abnormal sounds go undetected.

There are other kinds of sounds and heart murmurs that cannot be heard with the ordinary stethoscope but which are readily audible with an electronic stethoscope. Thus, both abnormal sounds and murmurs may be present in the diseased heart that are readily detectable with relatively simple listening devices, but not with the ordinary stethoscope.

3. The Electrocardiogram

The electrocardiogram (EKG) is another test that has almost outlived its usefulness. It can be helpful in special instances, bit it is rarely of use for ordinary examinations.

For most of this century, the EKG was a useful diagnostic tool. So entrenched has it become in diagnosing heart disease that countless patients have been led to believe their hearts were normal because their EKG was normal. This assumption is still prevalent today. It was not until the development of alternative ways to diagnose heart disease that doctors began to recognize how insensitive the electrocardiogram really is. We now know that most patients with early to moderately advanced heart disease will have a normal EKG, and that not until a heart attack occurs will an EKG appear abnormal. Indeed, some studies have shown that as many as 50% of patients who are having a heart attack will have a normal tracing for the first few days afterward, but this will then change 3 to 4 days later— that is, if the patient is still alive.

Many victims of a heart attack recover sufficiently enough so that their EKG appears normal. A comparison with a pre-heart attack tracing will usually show some evidence that the heart has changed. However, the patient's previous EKGs are not always available for comparison, particularly if the patient is seeing a new doctor or is seen in an emergency room.

The reason for the insensitivity of the EKG is that not until heart muscle is actually damaged will there be a change in the electrical conductivity of the heart. Damaged tissue conducts electrical impulses differently than normal tissue. This change in conductivity is what alters the EKG wave forms in an unhealthy subject so that the test result is different than it would appear when done on a healthy heart with normal conduction. Thus, a potential victim may have almost complete blockage of a major coronary artery, but as long as the heart muscle receives enough blood to prevent damage, there will be no change in the way an electrical current flows through the heart, and the patient's electrocardiogram will appear normal.

Another limitation of the electrocardiogram is that it correlates poorly with the function of the heart. Not uncommonly, cardiologists will see someone with a terrible looking EKG, but it turns out the patient is an athlete. Basketball players have the worst EKGs.

The reason athletes have abnormal electrocardiograms is because the extreme physical work they perform causes their hearts to enlarge. Basketball players apparently exercise more than any other athlete. Since the heart is a muscle, it will behave like any other muscle. In the same way as the muscles of a weight lifter increase dramatically, so does the heart muscle increase in thickness in athletes. Such changes alter the way electrical current passes through the heart muscle, causing the electrocardiogram to become abnormal. When such changes are due to damage to the heart muscle, they are usually irreversible. In contrast, if the athlete ceases to exercise, his or her heart will return to normal size and usually his or her electrocardiogram also will return to normal.

Conversely, a patient with a completely normal tracing will confess he can't walk one block without chest pain. The reason for this discrepancy is that the EKG measures the electrical output of the heart and not its mechanical function. Using the electrocardiogram to study cardiac function would be like checking the voltage of your car battery and expecting it to relate it to the performance of your automobile.

4. The EKG Stress Test

What about an EKG stress test? Isn't it always used by doctors to check for heart disease? Unfortunately, it is vastly overrated, and more often than not misses heart disease. When the treadmill stress test first began to be used in the 1950s, it was tested on patients with advanced heart disease. Naturally, the test result was abnormal in most of them. After all, if you're going to develop a new test, it has to tested out on people with known disease. Back then, if you had known coronary heart disease and were still alive, your disease had to be very advanced. Not until many years later when we had more sensitive and sophisticated ways of testing for heart disease, did we recognize that patients with lesser degrees of coronary heart disease often had a normal stress test result. Thus, if you performed the test on such people, who were unaware they had heart disease, only a minority of the results would be positive.

There are other problems with the stress test. In order to make the heart muscle ischemic (deficient in receiving blood), it has to work harder and go faster. For example, in the case of a 50-year-old man, the stress test protocol requires that the heart rate reach 144. Most individuals of that age have become deconditioned over time, and are simply unable to reach a heart rate of that magnitude. Even if an individual could, such a rate would not be relevant for a patient of this age. Consequently, it may be difficult for someone with mild to moderate heart disease to reach this level of stress, and impossible for someone with advanced heart disease. As a result, the stress test will not reveal ischemia.

Where does this leave us? An individual may have advanced coronary artery disease (that is, may be on the verge of having one of his or her major coronary artery completely obstructed), and yet may not have any symptoms unless he or she is subjected to extremes of physical or emotional stress. In this case an examination will not show any abnormalities unless very special methods of examination are utilized— methods employed by only a small minority of physicians in this country. Therefore, these patients are a catastrophe waiting to happen: all that is required are the right set of circumstances. This leads us to a discussion of how to identify those of us who are about to become victims.

3

WHO IS AT RISK?

If heart disease can exist for years without symptoms, and if a routine medical examination is unlikely to discover its presence, how do we increase the odds of detecting it? Many new tests are capable of uncovering heart disease at a very early stage, and they will be the subject of a later chapter. Some of these tests are relatively expensive to perform, especially when compared to a test as simple as an electrocardiogram. Some require rather sophisticated equipment and highly skilled personnel.

Logistically, as well as economically, it would be impossible for everyone to undergo all of these tests for a routine examination. However, most individuals who are to become victims of heart disease at a relatively early age have what is known as risk factors. A risk factor is something in your history, in the environment to which you are exposed, in your life-style, or in your body makeup that makes it more likely you will develop heart disease at an earlier age than if the risk factor were not present. Cigarette smoking is the one risk factor with which most people are familiar. If we compare those who smoke with those who do not, the average age of death due to heart disease for smokers may be 5 to 10 years sooner than for non-smokers.

If you know that you are at increased risk for heart disease and then, if you are, inform your doctor, it may make the difference in whether or not you undergo more specialized procedures for the detection of heart disease.

The following table lists the various risk factors that increase the likelihood that heart disease will appear prematurely. Some are of major importance, others are minor and contribute only slightly to the risk of heart disease. Some we cannot control, such as family history. Still others we can eliminate entirely with a change in life-style or with treatment. Obviously, the more risk factors that are present, the greater the chances are for the early appearance of heart disease.

TABLE II: RISK FACTORS FOR HEART DISEASE
1. Family history
2. Male sex
3. Increasing age
4. Hypertension
5. Tobacco/cigarette smoking
6. Exposure to stress
7. Diabetes
8. Obesity
9. Lack of exercise
10. Depression
11. Hostility and anger
12. Early menopause
13. Oral contraceptives
14. Alcohol consumption
15. Extremely high cholesterol levels
16. Homocysteine
17. Antioxidant vitamins
18. Abnormal EKG

1. FAMILY HISTORY

There are several kinds of heart disease that tend to run in families and may cause premature death in adults. Most of these are beyond the scope of this book. They include congenital heart defects, disorders of the heart muscle known as cardiomyopathies, and metabolic defects such as familial hypercholesterolemia or homocysteineuria, in which advanced arteriosclerosis occurs in the teens or even earlier. Fortunately, most of these diseases are extremely rare and are not the subject matter of this book. However, there are families in which various members have had some form of cardiovascular disease at a much earlier age than usual. Often a patient

26

will recall that Dad had a heart attack in his early fifties, Uncle Joe died suddenly at 46, Aunt Mary had a stroke at 59 and older brother Tom underwent a triple bypass at 48. Since coronary artery disease is a multifactorial disease, there is usually not a single factor that is responsible for heart disease in a given family, but it is a combination of factors. For example, this may have been a family in which everyone smoked. Hypertension is often present as well, particularly in those who experience a heart attack or a stroke at an early age. Some members of the family also may have diabetes and are obese.

To express this another way, typical obstructive coronary artery disease that affects most older people is not likely to surface prematurely if it is the sole risk factor. This is fortunate, because if it were not true, there would be little anyone could do about it. Yet if a patient with a positive family history is told to stop smoking and to start an exercise program to lose weight, and if his hypertension and diabetes are treated, then there is a strong probability that premature heart disease either will be greatly delayed or will not occur at all.

2. MALE SEX

At every age men are much more likely to develop heart disease than women. Until relatively recently, it was exceedingly rare for a woman to be diagnosed with heart disease before she experienced menopause. In addition, even when women reach menopause and develop heart disease at an accelerated rate, it is still not as frequently seen in women as it is in men. This is the basis for the treatment of older women with heart disease with estrogens.

3. INCREASING AGE

Increasing age is a major reason why older people are more likely to die as a result of a heart attack. Four out of every five victims who die of a heart attack are over the age of 65. Interestingly, if death is to occur within a few weeks of a heart attack, twice as many older women will die as compared to men. While chronological age is beyond our control, maintaining a healthy life-style with regular exercise, maintenance of normal body weight, avoidance of stress and cigarette smoking can reduce your physiological age by many years.

4. HYPERTENSION

More than any other risk factors except for age, stress and tobacco, hypertension is responsible for the early appearance and the increased frequency of coronary heart disease. Hypertension is to the early development of heart disease what high speed and alcohol combined are to the increased frequency of automobile accidents. Even after the appearance of coronary artery disease, unless elevated blood pressure is properly treated, the added work load will hasten the onset of one of the dreaded complications of coronary heart disease: congestive heart failure. In addition, elevated blood pressure increases the likelihood of stroke, kidney failure, and other vascular complications. Altogether these various diseases can have a devastating effect on the heart, turning less severe forms of heart disease into advanced heart disease, heart failure and premature death. If the victim of combined heart disease and hypertension is also overweight, smokes and doesn't exercise, it doesn't take a doctor to predict what is going to happen.

5. TOBACCO/CIGARETTE SMOKING

There is now overwhelming scientific evidence that tobacco smoking accelerates the appearance of circulatory disease in general— and coronary artery disease in particular— by decades. Smokers have two to four times the risk of sudden death as compared to nonsmokers. Among those who are going to die suddenly and prematurely of a heart attack, the average age of death for nonsmokers is 64 years, but for smokers it is 47 years. Furthermore, smokers are far more likely to die suddenly than are nonsmokers. The greater the amount of tobacco used, the greater the risk of developing early heart disease. Conversely, cessation of smoking reduces the risk of early heart disease, although it takes a while for this risk to decrease.

An immediate benefit of discontinuing smoking is the disappearance of a byproduct of smoking, carbon monoxide. This gas occupies a significant portion of the hemoglobin molecule, the molecule that carries oxygen. In smokers, both oxygen and carbon monoxide compete for space on the hemoglobin molecule; consequently, there is less oxygen available to supply the heart muscle, which already may have a reduced blood supply if its coronary arteries are narrowed.

Cessation of smoking can have other immediate benefits. Smoking causes a rapid increase in heart rate, blood pressure and the velocity of blood flowing through the blood vessels. As discussed in an earlier chapter, increased velocity of blood accelerates the deposition of the clot-like material onto the arteriosclerotic plaque, hastening the obstruction of the artery. Not smoking, therefore, reduces the accelerated rate of progression of the arteriosclerotic plaque.

With cessation of cigarette smoking, risk decreases about 50% the first year, and even more so for heavy smokers. It takes from two to ten years before the risk for former-smokers approaches that of nonsmokers. For those who stop smoking after a heart attack, the risk of a second heart attack is reduced by 20-50%.

Female smokers taking oral contraceptive pills are particularly at risk of developing early heart disease. Also, chronic second-hand exposure to tobacco smoke also increases the risk. It is estimated that approximately 40,000 people die each year from circulatory diseases as a result of chronic exposure to cigarette smoke. So lethal are the effects of smoking that many cardiac surgeons will not do bypass surgery on a patient unless he or she agrees to discontinue the habit. They have learned that those who continue to smoke after coronary artery bypass surgery will rapidly develop occluded bypass grafts within just a few years.

6. EXPOSURE TO STRESS

Exposure to stress may be acute or chronic. It is now well documented that heart attacks may be precipitated by anger, sexual activity, earthquakes, and other acutely stressful incidents.[1-4] During the Gulf War there was an increase in mortality due to heart attacks following the Iraqi missile attacks on Israel. Indeed, more Israelites died from heart attacks than from the missile attacks. Interestingly, heart attacks that occur during sexual activity are much more common when the partner is not the victim's spouse.

Studies of the effect of mental stress using mental arithmetic have been carried out on patients who have had catheters placed directly inside of the heart's chambers after recovery from a heart attack. Heart rate, blood pressure and pressures within the heart increased significantly within a few minutes with a decrease in output of the heart. When patients were asked to perform mental arithmatic exercises during one study, two patients went into pulmonary edema. Pulmonary edema is the medical term used when the lungs become flooded with fluid as a result of the backup of blood from an acute decrease in the output of the heart. In another study using a radioactive imaging procedure called radionuclide ventriculography, 75% of patients demonstrated impaired contraction of the heart muscle during mental stress due to ischemia. Clearly, stress can cause a deterioration of cardiac function. In addition, the rapid increase in blood pressure and heart rate during emotional stress may cause an arteriosclerotic plaque to rupture, followed by the development of an occlusive clot within a coronary artery, and either a heart attack or sudden death.

Chronic stress is of much greater concern than acute stress merely because it is so prevalent. If one interviews patients shortly after having had a heart attack, the majority will confess to having been under much greater stress in the six month period preceding the attack. Numerous studies in humans have documented the occurrence of myocardial ischemia (reduced blood flow to the heart muscle) during mental or emotional stress. In the past 10 to 12 years, the use of 24-hour Holter monitoring has become more widespread. In this procedure, ECG electrodes are strapped to the patient's chest and connected to a tape recorder so that every heart beat for 24 hours is recorded. Unlike a standard electrocardiogram which may record only 10 to 15 beats, a Holter monitor will record 100,000 or more heart beats. If the subject develops cardiac ischemia or an arrhythmia any time while he or she is wearing the monitor, it will be recorded on the tape, even if the ischemia lasts only for a minute or two, or the arrhythmia lasts only for a few seconds. When the tape is reviewed, these abnormalities are detected by a computer program that can read electrocardiograms.

Because arrhythmia and cardiac ischemia may only occur briefly during a 24-hour period, the Holter monitor technique may be the only way such abnormalities are detected. Because of this procedure, we have learned that the vast majority of ischemic episodes are unrecognized by the subject, i.e., they are "silent." Some studies report that nearly 98% of ischemic episodes are silent. This has completely changed the way heart patients are treated. Prior to this knowledge, patients with obstructive coronary artery disease were not given regular medications unless they were having symptoms. Now that we know that ischemia occurs in most patients without chest pain, such patients regularly receive their needed medications prophylactically.

7. DIABETES

Like hypertension, cigarette smoking and stress, diabetes is a major cause of heart disease. Approximately 16 million people in this country have diabetes, and heart disease is the leading cause of their death. The reason why heart disease is so common in diabetics is complex, and has to do with the interactions between the elevated blood sugar and substances in the blood known as lipoproteins. These interactions result in an excess uptake of fatty substances in the coronary artery plaque. The details are controversial and beyond the scope of this book. Paradoxically, however, strict control of the blood sugar level in patients with diabetes has not been shown to reduce the risk of developing coronary artery disease.

Having diabetes increases the risk of developing coronary heart disease by a factor of three or four times. In part this is because the individual with diabetes also is often overweight and has an elevated blood pressure. Women ordinarily do not develop coronary artery disease until 10 years after men, but if diabetes is present, there is no longer a difference in the rate of development of the disease.

Just as patients who have undergone coronary artery bypass surgery are more likely to progress towards coronary disease of greater severity and consequence, diabetes, too, causes it to appear prematurely. As a result, the mortality following a heart attack in diabetics is disproportionately high.

Typically, heart disease may exist and progress in silent form for years before it is detected, often even before the victim is aware that diabetes is present. In part this is because of the diabetic's predilection for neuropathy, a nerve disorder that impairs nerve conduction. Accordingly, they may not be able to detect chest pain. Instead they may have atypical symptoms such as exertional fatigue and shortness of breath. As a result, their disease may be far advanced before it can be treated with sub-optimal results. In such instances, if the victim already has had a heart attack, the damage that was done cannot be reversed. This is compounded by the fact that silent heart attacks are more common in diabetics.

8. OBESITY

Approximately one-third of the adult population is overweight. It is common knowledge that obese people are at much greater risk for having a heart attack or dying suddenly. In part this is because obesity predisposes one to high blood pressure, diabetes, elevated cholesterol and uric acid levels. Obesity also encourages physical inactivity. All of these increase the risk of premature heart disease. In addition, the increased weight greatly adds to the burden of work of the heart. Patients with advanced heart disease who lose a significant amount of weight will show a remarkable improvement in cardiac function.

One of the physical signs of heart failure is profound weight loss. Much like cachexia which is seen in cancer patients, cardiac cachexia is an adaptive response by the body to minimize the work the heart has to do. The victim doesn't look too good, but this does prolong his or her life. Prior to the widespread use of diuretics, such weight loss was concealed by the simultaneous massive edema that resulted from the severe heart disease.

The reason why low-cholesterol diets such as the Pritikin and Ornish programs are effective is not because their subjects are on a low cholesterol diet at all, but because such diets are very low in calories, too. The loss of weight results in a rapid loss of retained fluid, and a marked reduction in load upon the heart. This reduces the heart's need for oxygen and allows it to function better. As a result, there is a decrease in symptoms including chest pain, shortness of breath and exercise fatigue.

9. LACK OF EXERCISE

It is generally believed that lack of exercise and a sedentary life-style will increase the risk of having a heart attack or even sudden death. Conversely, regular physical exercise is thought to protect us from heart attacks, and will aid in recovery after a heart attack. Is there any truth to these beliefs? Perhaps only those individuals with stronger hearts are able to embark on an exercise program, and this is why they do better. If so, then the results of studies claiming exercise provides benefits would be flawed from the start.

Over 50 scientific investigations have studied the relationship between physical activity and heart attacks during the past 50 years. Overall, most of these studies have found that those who regularly exercise, or whose jobs require them to be very physically active, have fewer heart attacks. When such attacks occur, they do so at a later time in life, are less severe, and are accompanied by more complete recovery. A particularly consistent feature of these many studies has been the wide difference between those who do not exercise at all, and those who are regularly active to a moderate degree.

It is not always clear from these investigations whether the beneficial effects of exercise are due solely to the increased physical activity, or because of the other beneficial effects of exercise. For example, exercise is known to cause a reduction in blood pressure, weight loss (or failure to gain weight with increasing age), and to reduce the tendency of the blood to clot. In addition, the socioeconomic status of those who exercise regularly seems to have an important bearing on outcome. Individuals at higher socioeconomic levels exercise more, and have fewer and less severe heart attacks. Also, as mentioned earlier, there may be a natural selection process in which those individuals with weaker hearts cannot engage in work or activities that are strenuous.

The presence or absence of stress also may have an important bearing on the interpretation of the effects of physical activities. One of the earliest studies attempting to relate the amount of physical activity to the frequency of heart attacks was done on London bus employees. The study compared the conductors, who ran up and down the stairs of the double-decker buses, with the drivers, who just sat. It was found that the conductors had significantly fewer heart attacks then the drivers. Not surprisingly, the conclusion was that exercise protects the heart. The problem was that they failed to take into consideration the amount of stress the drivers encountered in having to deal with London traffic all day long.

Nevertheless, the level of physical fitness does have a bearing on the death rate. A study of 10,224 men and 3,120 women by the Cooper Clinic found that the most physically fit individuals had one-third the death rate from heart disease or cancer than the less fit over the eight years of follow-up.[5] This raises the issue of what proportion of the U.S. population are physically inactive? One out of four Americans are physically inactive and an additional one-third do not get any benefit from what little exercise they do. Furthermore, decreased physical activity is also associated with an increased incidence of diabetes, osteoporosis and certain cancers. It has been estimated that approximately 250,000 deaths a year are related to physical inactivity.

10. HOSTILITY AND ANGER

We have already seen how exposure to stress can increase the risk of sudden death or having a heart attack. Related to stress are the emotions of hostility and anger. A number of research studies have now established that individuals who are easily angered or who demonstrate frequent hostility are at increased risk of having a heart attack or dying. They also are at increased risk of developing hypertension, which will accelerate the occurrence of heart disease. The risk may be three to four times higher than that of subjects who do not exhibit such feelings. Events are more likely to occur in victims of a previous heart attack. These psychological stresses, particularly anger, have now been found to trigger even acute heart attacks. Several recent studies have used 24-hour Holter monitoring on patients with known coronary artery disease. Evidence of heart muscle ischemia was readily detected in subjects under emotional stress. Interestingly, the majority of such episodes were unaccompanied by chest pain and, therefore, fell into the category of silent ischemia. Of profound importance was the observation that ischemia could be prevented by treating a subject with beta blockers (this topic will be addressed in a subsequent chapter). Hostility was also found to affect the degree of narrowing of a coronary artery after angioplasty. One of the limitations of angioplasty is the high incidence of what is called restenosis, in which a coronary artery will become narrow again after it has been dilated. Restenosis may occur in 30% to 50% of patients after angioplasty. Patients with high hostility ratings were 2.5 times more likely to develop restenosis.[1,2]

11. DEPRESSION

Approximately 16-22% of patients who have recently had a heart attack are found to suffer from major depression, in contrast to the normal 5% prevalence of this disorder. While mild depression is extremely common following a heart attack (65%), it may be considered a normal response that might follow any major illness.[6] In such cases, the depression usually disappears within just a few days. Major depression, however, is another matter. It may be recognized by the feeling of sadness exhibited by its victim, inability to sleep, absence of signs of happiness such as expressions of humor or smiling, excessive fatigue unrelated to physical activity, particularly in the morning or even all the time, loss of interest in surroundings and activities, and thoughts of death.

Its persistence heralds the development of complications such as recurrent chest pains, arrhythmias, a repeat heart attack, rehospitalization, and increased mortality. Some studies have found that there is more than a four-fold increase in mortality in the six months following a heart attack in those patients with a major depression.[6] In fact, the accuracy of a state of depression to predict future cardiac events was as great as impaired cardiac function. Even before a heart attack, patients with depression may be 2 to 4.5 times likely to have a future heart attack than those without such depression.[7] A study done in the early 1980s by Dr. William F. Eaton of John Hopkins School of Hygiene and Public Health determined that of 1,551 subjects, 444 were diagnosed with depression. After 13 years of follow-up, 6% of those with depression had suffered a heart attack, versus 3% of those without depression. After statistical adjustments of the data, depression was shown to have increased the chances of a heart attack by fourfold.

Why this psychiatric disorder is associated with more heart disease is not understood at present. Perhaps being tired all the time prevents the depressed persons from being on a regular exercise program, while loss of interest in activities prohibits them from taking an active part in their recovery.

12. EARLY MENOPAUSE

Before the age of 50, most women seem to be protected from heart disease. It is unusual for a woman to have a heart attack before this age. The reason is because of the estrogens women produce. The high doses of estrogen given to transsexual men also have a protective effect upon their circulatory system.

While women may have heart attacks in their thirties or forties, it is extremely rare. When it happens, there are usually several other factors that significantly increase the victim's likelihood of developing heart disease. For example, a highly stressful job, a strong family history, cigarette smoking and taking birth control pills. Additionally, if a woman has had to undergo a hysterectomy, and particularly if her ovaries have been removed, then early heart disease is likely. Once past menopause, a woman's risk of developing heart disease increases rapidly, and after about 10 years it is the same as the risk for men. Moreover, when a heart attack does occur to a woman, the mortality rate is nearly double that of men's. This is because they are usually 10 years older than men at the time of their attack and are more likely to have hypertension, diabetes and to be overweight.

Interestingly, a condition known as psychogenic amenorrhea, or interruption of the menstrual cycle due to stress, is characterized by low estrogen levels and a build-up of a hormone known as cortisol. Cortisol is also known to increase in the blood during periods of stress. Among other things, cortisol increases the blood pressure and heart rate and, therefore, the risk of heart disease. These findings also are seen during depression, which is also associated with a higher incidence of heart disease.

13. ORAL CONTRACEPTIVES

It is relatively safe for females under the age of 35 to take oral contraceptives. However, after age 35, the use of oral contraceptives is associated with an increased risk of coronary artery disease under special circumstances. The most significant of these circumstances are cigarette smoking and hypertension. For example, a woman below the age of 40 has twice the risk of having a heart attack if she takes oral contraceptive pills and is 2.5 times more likely to develop an elevated blood pressure. If she smokes, her risk is increased to 13 times that of a woman who does not smoke. If she both smokes and takes oral contraceptives, her risk of a heart attack is over 40 times that of a woman of the same age who neither smokes nor takes the pill.

When a heart attack does occur under the above circumstances, it is not the typical kind that is seen in older patients. Whereas most heart attacks are due to obstruction of a coronary artery associated with the development of an arteriosclerotic plaque, the majority of women who have a heart attack while on oral contraceptives are found to have normal coronary arteries. It is thought that the normal artery in these cases narrows because of a spasm that restricts the flow of blood. Since oral contraceptive medication increases the tendency of blood to clot, a clot or thrombosis occurs at the site of the spasm. This shuts off the blood supply to the muscle, thereby causing a heart attack.

14. ALCOHOL CONSUMPTION

Actually, alcohol is a paradox, in that more than a few drinks a day can have a detrimental effect upon the heart. Alcohol elevates blood pressure, increases the heart rate, causes irregularities of the heart beat known as arrhythmias, and has a toxic effect upon the heart muscle. When taken in substantial amounts, it causes a condition known as alcoholic cardio-myopathy which eventually leads to heart failure and death.

Interestingly, several recent studies have found that moderate consumption of alcohol, i.e., one to two drinks a day, has a protective effect in that it appears to reduce the risk of having a heart attack by 40-50%, as well as sudden death, when compared to people who do not drink. Yet it does not reduce the frequency of chest pain (angina pectoris) due to coronary artery disease. It does not matter whether the alcohol is in the form of hard liquor, beer, or wine, although the effects of red wine have been studied most frequently. The protective effect of red wine seems to lie in its flavonoids, which are not present in white wine (except for champagne). Paradoxically, the French, who eat a diet high in saturated fats, but drink lots of red wine, have a reduced risk of coronary artery disease.

The mechanism of how alcohol works to reduce heart disease is not entirely understood. It is known that the ingredients in red wine and grape juice interfere with certain cellular components in the blood known as platelets. You will recall that platelets play a major role in the clotting cascade that converts fibrinogen to fibrin. Thus, interference with the formation of fibrin reduces the chances of a clot forming and blocking a coronary artery.

It is possible that the perceived beneficial effects of alcohol may not be due to the alcohol alone but the life-style of the people who drink one or two glasses a day. Maybe these individuals take more time out to relax and thus lead less stressful lives. Nevertheless, excessive alcohol is harmful. It is readily recognized as a risk for patients whose heart rate is up to 80-90 beats per minute without obvious reason, and who also have an elevated blood pressure. These individuals clearly are at increased risk of developing heart disease.

15. EXTREMELY HIGH CHOLESTEROL LEVELS

Hardly anyone who can read has not heard that an elevated cholesterol level in the blood increases the risk of heart disease. Because of all the publicity cholesterol receives, one may believe that it must be a very important risk factor. However, the truth is more complicated than this, and it has been placed near the end of the list of risk factors for good reason. To explain the "cholesterol story" completely would require an entire book, but the next chapter provides a good start in understanding how cholesterol relates (or doesn't relate) with heart disease.

It's true that there is an increased risk of having a heart attack if your cholesterol is elevated to *extreme* degrees, but if your cholesterol is only mildly elevated, then the increased risk is minimal. This becomes further complicated by trying to determine what level of cholesterol is normal, for it turns out this depends upon which country you live in and a host of other factors. To confuse things yet more, most patients who have a heart attack have normal or low cholesterol levels. Furthermore, recent studies have established that the lower one's cholesterol, the greater one's chances are of dying from cancer, accidents, suicide and depression. For the moment, then, we will leave the saga of cholesterol to the next chapter.

16. HOMOCYSTEINE

Homocysteine is a sulfur-containing amino acid that is a metabolic breakdown product of the protein we eat. Specifically it has been metabolically converted from another essential amino acid known as methionine. A number of studies have now shown that subjects with elevated levels of homocysteine are twice as likely to develop coronary artery disease as those with the lowest homocysteine levels. It appears to be an independent risk factor for coronary artery disease, meaning it is unrelated to other risk factors. Furthermore, significant coronary artery narrowing may be seen with levels of homocysteine currently considered to be normal.

A rare recessive disease known as homocystinuria, in which there are high blood levels of homocysteine, is accompanied by severe and premature occlusive arterial disease. In part, this is because elevated levels of homocysteine seem to bring about adverse effects on blood platelets, clotting factors and the endothelial cells that line the inside walls of arteries. The result is an increased tendency of the blood to clot. Because blood levels of homocysteine are influenced by both genetic and nutritional factors, it is important to know that both vitamin B6 and folate are necessary for the metabolic breakdown of homocysteine into other essential amino acids. Without these vitamins, homocysteine levels would simply build up in the blood. One interesting study found that the mortality rate for coronary heart disease in men is about three times as great in Northern Ireland as it is in France. These differences were not due an excess of the usual risk factors for coronary heart disease. Blood levels of homocysteine were found to be higher in the Irish than in the French, and higher in men who had heart attacks compared with those who did not. It was felt by the researchers who did the study that the difference in mortality rates was due to the different homocysteine blood levels between the Irish and French.

17. ANTIOXIDANT VITAMINS

Several studies have claimed that consuming large amounts of the antioxidant vitamins A, C, E and beta carotene will reduce the risk of heart disease when compared to people who consume normal amounts. Such studies do not prove that coronary artery disease is a form of vitamin deficiency. It would be inappropriate to assume that failure to take supplemental vitamins would result in an increased risk of coronary artery disease. There will be more about this subject in a later chapter.

18. ABNORMAL ELECTROCARDIOGRAM

The final risk factor that increases the likelihood of heart disease is an abnormal electrocardiogram (EKG). While it may seem that an abnormal EKG already means that heart disease is present, this is not necessarily the case. There are many non-specific and non-cardiac factors that could cause an electrocardiogram to appear abnormal. Medications, metabolic imbalances, too much or too little potassium in the blood stream, and hyperventilation are just of few conditions that can alter an EKG. Also, certain kinds of conduction disorders that block the electrical activation of the heart will make the electrocardiogram appear abnormal in the absence of obstructive coronary artery disease. Nevertheless, an abnormal electrocardiogram in a patient without known cardiac disease is a source of concern. The reason is that heart disease may appear and progress in the complete absence of symptoms. Indeed, as many as one-third of heart attacks may be silent, in that the patient does not recall having chest pain. Symptoms of silent heart attacks may appear in the form of fatigue or flu-like characteristics and they go unrecognized. Accordingly, an abnormal EKG is a source of concern and should be investigated with more specific tests.

FOREWARNED IS FOREARMED

Because of the widespread prevalence of coronary artery disease in the complete absence of symptoms, and the failure of routine methods of examination to detect anything less than advanced coronary artery disease, millions of people are likely to experience a heart attack or die because their disease is not diagnosed or treated in a timely fashion. The presence of one or more of the risk factors described in this chapter should alert the concerned individual that special tests, which will be described in another chapter, are needed to determine if he or she has this disease.

REFERENCES

1. Kawachi I, Sparrow D, Spiro A, *et al.* A prospective study of anger and coronary heart disease. Circulation 1996; 94:2090-2095.
2. Mittleman MA, Maclure M, Nachnani M, *et al.* Educational attainment, anger, and the risk of triggering myocardial infarction onset. Arch Intern Med 1997; 157:769-775
3. Katsouyanni K, Kogevinas M, Trichopoulos D. Earthquake-related stress and cardiac mortality. Int J Epidemiol 1986; 15:326-330.
4. Suzuki S, Sakamoto S, Koide M, *et al.* Hanshin-Awaji earthquake as a trigger for acute myocardial infarction. Am Heart J 1997; 134:974-977.
5. Blair SN, Kampert JB, Kohl HW, *et al.* Influences of cardiorespiratory fitness and other precursors of cardiovascular disease and all-cause mortality in men and women. JAMA 1996;276:205-210.
6. Frasure-Smith N, Lesperance F, Talajic M. Depression following myocardial infarction. Impact on 6-month survival. J Am Med Ass 1993; 270:1819-1825.
7. Pratt LA, Ford DE, Crum RM, *et al.* Depression, psychotropic medication, and risk of myocardial infarction. Prospective data from the Baltimore ECA follow-up. Circulation 1996; 94:3123-3129.

4

HYPERTENSION AND HEART DISEASE

O f the many risk factors discussed in the previous chapter, three warrant additional discussion: hypertension, stress and cholesterol. Two of these factors— hypertension and stress— have not received adequate attention for the role they play in the development of coronary artery disease, while the third— cholesterol— has been given far more attention than it merits.

HYPERTENSION

High blood pressure (i.e., hypertension) is important in the development of vascular disease throughout the body, and not just heart disease. More than any other risk factor, it is responsible for the occurrence of obstructive coronary artery disease, heart attacks and premature death. Chapter 1 explained that arteriosclerotic plaques are rarely seen in blood vessels where the pressure is low. For example, they are not seen in the pulmonary arteries where the pressure is only one-fourth to one-fifth of that in the aorta and other arteries. Neither are plaques found in veins, unless the vein is used as part of a bypass graft where it is then subject to the same pressures as the coronary arteries. All of these observations would suggest that the higher the pressure, the more likely the development of arteriosclerotic plaques.

In general, hypertension is said to exist when blood pressure exceeds 135/85. Some doctors still use levels of 140-150/90-95, and there are a few who will not put a patient on medication even when the blood pressure is up at 150/100.

The presence of high blood pressure increases the risk of coronary heart disease by two to three times. However, because it is so frequently associated with other risk factors such as diabetes, cigarette smoking, an enlarged heart and an elevated cholesterol, it actually may increase the likelihood by six to seven times. In addition, as will be explained later on in this chapter, hypertension may be present even when the blood pressure is normal. A more realistic definition is based less on what the blood pressure is at rest, and more on what it rises too during stress.

WHAT THE NUMBERS MEAN

As a rule, when hypertension occurs, there is an increase in both the systolic pressure (the numerator) and diastolic pressure (the denominator). The systolic pressure is the pressure found in the major arteries of the body when the heart is contracting; the diastolic pressure is the pressure in the arteries during the relaxation, or filling phase, of the heart's cycle. When the heart muscle is electrically activated (as reflected by the spike wave of the electrocardiogram), the muscle begins to contract. At this point, the pressure begins to rise within the heart's chambers. On the left side of the heart, within the cavity of a normal left ventricle, it takes about 70-80 milliseconds for the pressure to reach a level that will force open the heart's exit valve, which is known as the aortic valve. A millisecond is one-thousandth of a second; thus, in less than one-tenth of a second, the pressure buildup within the heart's chamber is enough to force blood out of the heart and into the aorta and all of its branches. In contrast, in a diseased heart, it will take 90-125 milliseconds for the pressure to build up. During the next 300-350 milliseconds, the aortic valve remains open as the heart's muscular walls squeeze blood out into the circulation. Consequently, the pressure within the aorta and its arterial branches is approximately the same as it is within the left ventricle.

When a blood pressure cuff is placed around your arm, and the pressure in the cuff is pumped up to 130 mm Hg, that pressure is transmitted to the tissues of your arm. If the pressure within the brachial artery (the main artery that carries blood from the arm into the forearm and hand), is 120 mm Hg, then the artery will collapse because the pressure outside it is greater than the pressure within it. Listening with a stethoscope reveals only silence, because the artery is collapsed and blood cannot enter. The pressure within the cuff is gradually lowered, and when it falls below 120 mmHg, the artery starts to expand again. It expands slowly because there is still a considerable amount of pressure within the blood pressure cuff and in the tissues that surround the arm. Now, listening with a stethoscope reveals a sound like a heart beat, as a small amount of blood enters the artery with each pump and the turbulence this creates makes it sound like a heart beat. The pressure on the blood pressure cuff manometer at which this sound occurs must equal the approximate pressure within the heart's chamber, and it is called the systolic pressure. This is a measurement of the pressure during systole, when the heart is contracting. It is the numerator of the fraction used to communicate blood pressure.

As the cuff pressure is lowered yet further, the artery continues to expand. When it is fully expanded, the pressure surrounding the artery from the blood pressure cuff will be less than the pressure within the artery; i.e., the artery is fully expanded. Now listening with the stethoscope there is again silence, for the blood flows unobstructed. The pressure at which the sound disappears is called the diastolic pressure, and it represents the pressure within the artery while the heart is relaxing and filling with blood for its next cycle.

WHAT CAUSES HIGH BLOOD PRESSURE?

In most patients with hypertension, there is no obvious cause for the elevated blood pressure. Although we do not know why it occurs, we do know some of the factors that affect it. This type of elevated blood pressure is called essential hypertension and includes about 96% of all hypertension patients. About 1% of the time, hypertension is the result of the growth of a hormone-secreting tumor within the adrenal gland that causes the blood pressure to rise. Removal of the tumor will usually allow the blood pressure to return to normal. In the remaining 2-3% of patients, hypertension is caused by chronic kidney disease, usually secondary to recurring infections or stones.

Since the 1930s, it has been known that placing a clamp around the renal artery, the artery that goes to the kidney, and restricting the blood flow, will result in hypertension. More recently it has been found that if a kidney is transplanted from a hypertensive rat to a rat with normal blood pressure, the recipient rat will develop hypertension. Conversely, if a healthy kidney is transplanted to a rat with hypertension, the blood pressure will return to normal in the recipient rat. The hormone responsible for this is produced by the kidney and is called renin. It enters the circulation and acts upon a substance produced by the liver known as angiotensin I, and it is transformed into angiotensin II by a converting enzyme. Angiotensin II is an extremely powerful constrictor of blood vessels, and this action causes the blood pressure to increase. Thanks to a triumph of modern pharmacology, drugs known as angiotensin converting enzyme inhibitors (ACE inhibitors) block this whole reaction and are therefore highly effective in treating individuals with hypertension.

COMPLICATIONS OF HIGH BLOOD PRESSURE

Most people with an elevated blood pressure experience an increase in both the systolic pressure and the diastolic pressures. About 25% of the time, only the systolic pressure will increase, while the diastolic pressure remains normal or even low. Typically this occurs in older patients. It was believed that this was a normal response to aging, and no attempt was made to treat it. We now know this was wrong; such patients have the same risk of developing complications as those who have elevation of both the systolic and diastolic pressures. Those complications include exertional chest pain (angina pectoris), heart attacks (myocardial infarction), heart failure, premature death, strokes, peripheral vascular disease in the arteries of the lower extremities, and kidney failure.

How frequently do these complications occur? Approximately 50% of hypertensive patients will develop a heart attack, about one-third will have a stroke and 10-15% will develop kidney failure. Most victims suffer multiple complications of their disease, although it may take many years before these complications occur. If a hypertensive patient lives long enough, heart failure is almost inevitable. The Framingham study showed that 75% of all patients with congestive heart failure have hypertension. Also, hypertension is present in two-thirds of patients with diabetes.

The actual mechanism by which hypertension increases the risk of coronary heart disease is not known. In all probability it does so in several ways. One explanation relates to the increased velocity of the blood as it flows through the circulatory system of a hypertensive individual. An analogy would be the dramatic change in the flow of water coming out of a garden hose when one turns the nozzle of the spout from fully open to half open. The water exiting the hose comes out with much greater force and velocity, and travels further merely because it is under greater pressure. In the case of the circulatory system, a combination of factors acting together cause the pressure to become elevated. These include the heart, which contracts with much greater force than normal; a hyperactive sympathetic nervous system, that causes the small arteries throughout the body to constrict; and the endothelial linings of the coronary arteries, which constrict in a paradoxical manner when they are stimulated. The result is an increase in the speed and the force with which blood travels around the body. In the same way that an automobile bounces higher when it hits a bump at a greater speed, so is the blood subject to more trauma at increased velocity. More clot-like material is laid down from traumatized platelets, speeding the buildup of arteriosclerotic plaque.

What is particularly insidious about hypertension is that it is not only a lethal disease in its own right, ultimately causing damage to the brain, kidney and heart, but that it usually exists for years in the absence of symptoms. Thus, its victim is completely unaware of its presence. Even if doctors promptly treated patients with an elevated blood pressure as soon as it appeared, it would be present for years before it was detected. Unfortunately, doctors do not treat hypertension as early as they should because they mistakenly believe that their patients can tolerate moderate elevations of blood pressure without creating any harm. Patients with pressures of 170/80 or 155/100 are reassured that their blood pressure is "okay" for their age. Rarely are the patients given the actual numbers.

I suppose that if Mr. Jones came in with a pressure of 165/85 complaining of headaches and shortness of breath, the doctor might actually be compelled to prescribe something. But most patients do not have symptoms of their disease because their bodies have gradually adapted to the increased pressure over a period of years. This adaptation was dramatically illustrated when my technicians and I were putting on scientific exhibits at various medical meetings throughout the country. We were trying to teach doctors about some of the new noninvasive tests that were available for diagnosing heart disease. As part of that scientific exhibit, we used physicians as subjects to demonstrate to other physicians how to do the tests. The blood pressure of these subjects was routinely taken. We were shocked to discover how many doctors often had extreme elevations of their blood pressure in the total absence of symptoms. They were completely unaware that their blood pressure was elevated. Yet, if anyone were to be aware of the subtle appearance of symptoms, and that it was due to hypertension, it should be a doctor!

FACTORS AFFECTING THE DEVELOPMENT OF HYPERTENSION

Whether or not you develop hypertension will largely depend on your genetic make-up, what kind of stressful life you lead, your diet and weight, how much alcohol you drink, your age, the function of your kidneys, whether or not you have diabetes, and whether you smoke. If one of your parents had hypertension, there is a good possibility that you will get it, too. If both parents had it, you will almost certainly develop elevated blood pressure at a relatively early age.

Evidence that hypertension will develop may be seen even in childhood. Increased activity of the sympathetic nervous system since childhood is consistently present in the early stages of hypertension. Excessive sympathetic tone contributes to the early development of coronary heart disease by increasing the number of red cells in the blood stream, and by causing increased platelet adhesiveness. When platelets cling together, they liberate a substance known as thromboxane A_2 which helps blood clot and aids in the formation of an arteriosclerotic plaque. In the Dutch Hypertension and Offspring Study, heart rate and cardiac output declined in the offspring of hypertensive parents during static exercise due to an increased peripheral resistance (increased narrowing of the small arteries throughout the body), no doubt the result of increased sympathetic activity.[1]

Other studies have shown that individuals exposed to psychological stress whose heart rate increases and blood pressure rises more than 30 mmHg systolic and 15 mmHg diastolic had four times the risk of developing hypertension in later life. Related to this phenomena is the increased risk of heart disease in subjects with easily provoked hostility and anger. Emotional stress will cause the heart rate and blood pressure to increase through activation of the sympathetic nervous system. This increases the amount of oxygen needed by the heart. Also, it may provoke arrhythmias, which means the heart may be beating irregularly and less efficiently. Blood vessels, particularly on the surface of the heart, may constrict; which will further reduce the flow of blood to heart muscle. Thus, there are significant reasons for the heart to be more vulnerable. Indeed, studies have shown that subjects with high levels of anxiety are at increased risk of a heart attack or sudden death.

Excessive weight is another factor that increases the likelihood of developing hypertension, but not until that weight is more than 25-30% of one's ideal weight. Such weight gain is less likely to be caused by excessive eating than inadequate exercise, although overeating certainly contributes to the problem. At one time it was thought that excessive salt intake was a contributing factor to the development of hypertension. Indeed, prior to the introduction of drugs, the only way to reduce blood pressure was to have the patient on a strict, low-salt diet. Many patients had to suffer through a rice diet to bring their pressure down. While we no longer force our patients to undergo this, many physicians still advise their patients not to add salt to their food, or to use a salt substitute. With modern diuretic therapy, this practice is rarely necessary.

Another cause of hypertension is increased consumption of alcohol. Alcohol will activate the sympathetic nervous system, and this increases the heart rate and constricts the peripheral vessels, causing the blood pressure to increase. Oddly enough, excessive drinking of hard liquor is an uncommon cause of hypertension, except in known alcoholics. Increased intake of wine is another matter. Evidently, the drinking of a several glasses of wine with dinner each night is not viewed as drinking but as part of a meal. On occasion, I will see patients with hypertension in association with irregular heart beats and a rapid heart rate. At times the heart rate may be as much as 100-120 beats per minute, and the patient seems relatively unaware of it. If the intake of wine is stopped, the blood pressure, heart rate and rhythm will return to normal.

Smoking is another controllable factor that will increase the occurrence of hypertension both acutely and chronically. Acutely, it constricts the blood vessels and speeds up the heart rate, causing a rapid increase in blood pressure. Chronically, it damages the arterial wall and encourages the development of arteriosclerotic plaques. This results in a stiffer and less distensible artery. Since a stiff artery will not expand with the inflow of blood accompanying each cardiac contraction, the blood pressure will increase more than it would if the artery still had its elasticity. A similar thing happens in diabetic patients: premature vascular disease is a well-known complication of this disorder. Finally, aging also produces the same effect. This is why hypertension is so common in the elderly.

CARDIAC CHANGES CAUSED BY HIGH BLOOD PRESSURE

Because hypertension may be present for years before the subject is aware of it, certain changes may occur in the silent hypertensive that have an important bearing on their ultimate survival. One of the earliest of these changes is an increase in the mass of the heart muscle. Like the weight lifter whose muscles become bigger, the heart, which is also a muscle, increases in size too. Recent studies have shown that subjects who are to become hypertensive develop an increase in their cardiac mass before their hypertension becomes clinically evident. These individuals have a risk of dying that is three times greater than those without an increased mass. In addition, these future victims are likely to have depressed cardiac function. In a 10-year follow-up of 100 patients with depressed cardiac function, 29% had morbid events (defined as any complication of the disease, such as heart attack, heart failure and stroke) and 10% died. In contrast, 11% of those with the lowest cardiac mass had morbid events and only 2% died.[2]

The tragedy of hypertension is that it is the most common disease in this country, one that affects more than 64 million people— or one out of every four of us— and it is a disease that ultimately is responsible for the early development of coronary artery disease, heart attacks, heart failure, strokes and kidney failure, yet goes unrecognized for years before treatment is begun. This is compounded by the fact that most patients are being grossly undertreated. A recent survey revealed that leaders in the field of hypertension graded doctor's treatment of hypertension only a C minus. The major problems were ones of under-diagnosis and under-treatment.

WHY HYPERTENSION IS UNDERDIAGNOSED AND UNDERTREATED

A major reason for the failure of doctors to adequately diagnose and treat high blood pressure can be directly attributed to poor methods of diagnosing its presence, and failure to recognize the functional effects of an elevated blood pressure upon the heart. In addition, because hypertension is so common, and often without symptoms, doctors tend to be rather casual about the seriousness of mild elevations of the blood pressure. This attitude is communicated to the patient. Finally, many doctors have accumulated a considerable amount of misinformation about both the diagnosis and treatment of hypertension. Why doctors fail to detect hypertension was addressed earlier. Their casual attitude is a result of their inability to detect the functional changes and complications of the patient's elevated blood pressure upon the heart. For example, in a recent study comparing the sensitivity of the electrocardiogram and the echocardiogram for detecting increased cardiac mass, the electrocardiogram identified 6-17% while the echocardiogram found 85-100%, depending upon whether the population studied had mild or severe disease. Yet the EKG continues to be the most popular tool for the diagnosis and follow-up management of the hypertensive patient.

Another reason for the gross mismanagement of patients with hypertension is the misinformation on the part of the doctor as to when hypertension is present. So-called "white coat hypertension" is a case in point. It is a popular belief that patients will develop an elevated blood pressure only in the doctor's office but not at home or when they are relaxed. To conclude from this that these elevations of blood pressure are harmless is mere speculation, and it is certainly not supported by the facts. A number of studies have shown that such patients are just as likely as patients with fixed elevations of their blood pressure to develop hypertensive complications in both the structure and function of their heart. Thus, such patients are apt to be undertreated for years before they come down with a major complication of their disease. Even then, the complication may not be recognized for what it is. This is illustrated by the following true case history.

THE STORY OF AK

AK was a 60-year-old foreman in a naval ship-building and repair yard. His job was extremely stressful, for all of the work had to be done in the shortest possible time. There was no room for errors that could slow down production. His stress was not confined to the pressure from upper management, but to the workers who were under his supervision as well. If these workers were not careful and made errors in repairing circuits and installing new equipment on the naval vessels, lives could be lost. AK felt responsible to make sure the work was done carefully.

He began to notice that when he had occasion to help out with the physical work— for example, when he helped to lift heavy equipment— he would experience chest pain. Also, whenever he was in a hurry and had to climb more than one flight of stairs, he would experience the same discomfort. AK remembered that his father used to have chest pain before his fatal heart attack. This was enough to motivate him to see a cardiologist.

The doctor talked with him for only a few minutes before conducting a brief examination of his heart. An electrocardiogram was performed followed by a stress test. AK was told that although his blood pressure and heart sounded all right, the stress test was abnormal and angiograms would have to be done that afternoon. He was told that an angiogram was just a routine x-ray of the coronary arteries. Not having any previous experience in this area and remembering what happened to his father, AK agreed and entered the hospital.

The angiogram revealed moderate narrowing of the circumflex artery, one of the three main arteries on the surface of his heart. This particular artery supplies the back and side walls of the heart. The cardiologist suggested that while AK had a catheter placed in his coronary artery, he should go ahead and perform an angioplasty. The catheter would be inserted into the circumflex coronary artery with a deflated balloon at the tip. When the catheter reached the narrowed portion of the artery, it would be inflated and the arteriosclerotic plaque would be compressed against the vessel wall, thereby reducing the amount of narrowing. AK was not exactly in a position to seek a second opinion and he agreed to the procedure.

The angioplasty was completed successfully and AK returned home and back to work within a few days. For the next six weeks he had no further chest discomfort. Then, once again, his chest pain began to return whenever he carried heavy objects. He returned to the cardiologist who casually informed him that about 50% of the time the procedure had to be repeated because of a complication known as restenosis. This came about when new tissue grew in the wall of the artery where it had been expanded. The reasons for this were not understood, but it could often be corrected by repeating the angioplasty. AK reluctantly agreed to undergo the procedure again. Once more he entered the hospital, had a repeat angiogram followed by the angioplasty without complications. Once more he returned to work and remained symptom-free, but this time for only one month.

Again he returned to the cardiologist and now was told that a "rotor rooter" procedure would have to be done. It is called an atherectomy. This was different than the angioplasty, in that a device would be inserted in the artery to where it was narrowed. In much the same way an old corroded water pipe would be cleaned out, so would the artery be cleaned out. AK did not know enough to ask, and the cardiologist did not bother to explain to him what would happen to all the particles that were removed from the arteriosclerotic plaque. Thus AK was unaware that some of the arteriosclerotic debris could plug off smaller vessels downstream.

AK entered the hospital for a third time, had his rotor rooter procedure, returned to work, and this time remained symptom free for two months. When the chest pains returned, AK returned to his cardiologist for a forth time, and he underwent a stress test once again. The results were essentially the same as before— the test was still abnormal. This time he was told that a stent was going to be put in, and this would keep the artery expanded permanently. AK was told that a stent was like a coiled spring from the inside of a ball point pen. It was constructed in such a way that when inserted into the artery, it would expand and serve as a scaffold to keep the walls of the artery apart. The cardiologist did not bother to explain, nor did AK know enough to ask, what would happen if the stent became blocked by a clot.

The scenario was repeated once more: the stent was inserted and fortunately there were no complications. But the stent was no more successful than the other procedures, and AK returned to the cardiologist two months later. Now he was told that there was no other choice but to proceed to coronary artery bypass surgery. Believing that there were no other options, AK underwent bypass surgery. This time, however, he was not so fortunate. A week after surgery he sustained a small stroke, and although he regained the ability to use his arm and leg, and his speech returned almost to normal, he had serious impairment of the cognitive ability of his brain with considerable loss of reasoning and memory skills. It was sufficient to prevent his return to work in his capacity of a foreman, and AK was forced to retire early.

Sadly, the bypass surgery did not stop his chest pain either. By this time it took much less physical work to provoke his pain. With the urging of his family he finally agreed to seek another opinion and that is when AK came under my care. On physical examination, although his resting blood pressure was still normal at 130/80, when his blood pressure was repeated during a procedure called isometric hand grip stress, it rose to 210/115. AK's symptoms were never due to his coincidental coronary artery disease alone, although it contributed to a small degree. His symptoms were due mainly to a precipitous increase in blood pressure whenever he exerted himself. Undoubtedly, the obstruction of the circumflex coronary artery seen on AK's angiogram had been there for years. By itself, the narrowing was not great enough to cause symptoms. But when it was combined with a large increase in blood pressure, it was enough to restrict the flow of blood in the coronary arteries.

HOW HYPERTENSION RESTRICTS BLOOD FLOW IN THE CORONARY ARTERIES AND CAUSES CHEST PAIN

As was described earlier in this chapter, when the pressure rises within the left ventricle and the aortic valves open, that pressure is transmitted throughout the circulatory system. If the arteries are constricted as a result of the hypertension, the flow of blood out of the vessels into the tissues will be restricted. Thus, there is much more blood entering the aorta than there is is leaving it. There will be a rapid increase in blood pressure that is transmitted back to the heart's chambers. In much the same way as you would inflate a balloon by blowing into it, the heart would inflate from the increase in pressure, were it not for two things.

The first is the thickness of the muscle wall itself, which may be a centimeter or more in diameter. Muscle that thick is not easy to distend. The second factor that prevents the heart from being distended is the thick, tough membrane known as the pericardium that surrounds the heart. Since the heart cannot be distended by a rise in blood pressure, that pressure is transmitted to the muscular tissue itself in the same way that the pressure within an inflated blood pressure cuff is transferred to the tissues of the arm causing the brachial artery to collapse. In the case of the heart, however, the vessels that collapse are the thin-walled distant branches of the coronary arteries. These vessels are known as the microcirculation of the heart and are the major source of blood supply to the heart muscle and its tissues.

For a patient like AK, a mild narrowing, or stenosis, of a coronary artery may exist for years without causing a problem until the blood pressure begins to rise. If that happens rapidly, as might when a patient carries a heavy object or if he or she is under stress, an acute rise in blood pressure within the left ventricle will be accompanied by a dramatic reduction in blood flow to the heart muscle, and this will be followed by chest pain. If the patient's cardiologist "shoots from the hip and asks questions later," then the scenario is not dissimilar to that involving AK. And sadly, such scenarios take place hundreds of times a day. The real tragedy is that the treatment may be worse than the disease. Such things inevitably occur in a small percentage of surgical procedures, and we have to live with that. But it's impossible to accept a complication that changes a person's entire life when that surgery was unnecessary.

Considering that the current fashion in treatment by cardiologists is to recommend either angioplasty or coronary artery bypass surgery as the initial treatment, and since over 2000 patients each day undergo these procedures in this country, the number of patients whose symptoms could be relieved by blood pressure medication instead of surgery is staggering. This will continue as long as the public remains uninformed that there are multiple reasons other than coronary artery disease why chest pain may occur, and that other options beside surgery are available for the relief of symptoms. Both of these topics will be discussed in later chapters.

CONCLUSION

Hypertension will continue to be under-diagnosed and undertreated as long as doctors insist upon using antiquated methods of diagnosis to detect and follow patients with an elevated blood pressure, and as long as they do not take action when patients demonstrate an elevated blood pressure, merely because they have no other symptoms. Patients must assume some responsibility as well: blood pressure levels higher than 135 mmHg systolic and 80 mmHg diastolic are not acceptable, and the patient should let his or her doctor know this. The problem is that this is merely a resting blood pressure, and under stress the blood pressure is likely to go much higher unless measures are taken to adequately control it.

Aside from the usual complete absence of symptoms of hypertension, the relatively primitive diagnostic methods used in the routine examination of the average patient are too insensitive to show the changes that result from the patient's elevated blood pressure. Accordingly, if the damage from an elevated blood pressure takes years before it produces symptoms, if the patient's blood pressure is only mildly or moderately increased, if the patient states he or she feels fine, if the doctor can't hear any abnormality with a stethoscope, and if the patient's electrocardiogram is normal, then it is not surprising that both doctor and patient remain unconcerned. Meanwhile, the patient's blood pressure remains elevated for years without being a problem. When a heart attack or stroke finally does occur, then it's not hard to see why hypertension is not blamed. Unfortunately, too often both the medical profession and the public remain complacent about a lethal disease that is literally a time bomb if not treated promptly.

REFERENCES

1. de Visser DC, van Hooft IM, van Doornen LJ, *et al.* Cardiovascular response to mental stress in offspring of hypertensive parents: the Dutch Hypertension and Offspring Study. J Hypertens 1994; 13:901-908.
2. Devereux RB, de Simone G, Koren MJ, *et al.* Left ventricular hypertrophy and hypertension. Clin Exp Hypertens 1993; 15:1025-1032.

5

THE EFFECTS OF STRESS UPON
THE HEART

How does the stress we face in our daily living affect our health and how long we live? In particular, how does it affects the way our heart functions, how fast it beats, what our blood pressure is, how much adrenaline we secrete, how fast our blood clots, and whether or not we are likely to have a heart attack or die? Do certain types of employment make people more or less likely to experience heart attacks than others, and does our level of education and how much money we make determine whether we will develop heart disease? The answers to all these questions and more will be provided in this chapter.

Dr. John Shannon was an internist, a graduate of Yale, conscientious and well-respected by his peers. He was happily married and had three children. He was a member of a physician's group with three other doctors, all of whom were internists. They practiced in Southern California, and their group had been quite successful for the first 10 years they had been together. In the past two years, however, Dr. Shannon had noted that there were more open slots in his appointment book, and he seemed to have fewer patients in the hospital. Also, there were fewer medical assistants working in the practice than before. No one had been discharged, but when someone left, a new assistant was not hired.

One day in the early 1990s, the senior internist who had started the group called a meeting and explained that a large HMO had moved into the area within the past year. "HMO" and "managed care" were still new terms, and neither doctors nor patients had learned how they operated. What was known, however, was that this particular HMO was well-financed and was aggressively advertising for and getting new patients. Medicare patients, in particular, were lured by television commercials which assured they would get loving, personal attention and annual physical examinations; they would only have to make a small copayment for drugs, and they would not even have to pay monthly premiums because the HMO would be directly reimbursed by Medicare. Not surprisingly, people were signing up in droves.

The senior internist explained further that their group was losing a sizable number of patients to the HMO, and that it wouldn't be long before everyone would have to take a pay cut. However, there was an alternate choice. The HMO had contacted the senior internist and had offered to contract with all four physicians in the group. Although they would be paid a discounted rate for seeing patients, it would be more than compensated for by the increased number of patients they would see. At least, that was what the HMO had promised.

Recognizing their predicament, all four doctors agreed to work with the HMO. For the first six months, everything appeared to be going well. They were all certainly busier again. Indeed, they needed additional help because there were now more administrative problems. It seemed that they had to get approval from the HMO to admit a patient to the hospital or to have surgery. On a few occasions, the doctors themselves had to argue with a clerk to get prior approval. Without that approval, they would not be reimbursed. On one occasion, Dr. Shannon had to talk with several administrators in the hierarchy of the HMO when he had a patient that needed a heart transplant and the procedure could not be carried out in the hospital the HMO used. He was told that cardiac transplants were still considered an experimental procedure and the HMO would not cover it. The doctor became furious and told the administrator the HMO could be sued for negligence. He was reminded by the administrator that the HMO did not practice medicine and that only the doctor could be sued for malpractice. He was further warned that he would not be allowed to offer this treatment to the patient since it was not a covered service.

Things got worse. He was called to the HMO administrator's office one day and was told that he was ordering too many tests and not seeing enough patients. The HMO's profit margin was slipping and it needed to be increased. Dr. Shannon had trouble believing this. There were commercials lauding the HMO every day and one could hardly read a newspaper without seeing large ads about the HMO and how happy the patients were. He had even heard that each of the three top administrators were receiving in excess of one million dollars a year, in salary and bonuses. He was already stretched to the limit in seeing patients.

Before joining the HMO Dr. Shannon always spent 20 to 30 minutes with each patient. As his load of patients increased, he had already decreased the time spent to 15 minutes, and now to 10 minutes. He couldn't practice quality medicine anymore. Depression, anger, aggravation, frustration and enormous stress were now an everyday occurrence. Each evening, he went home exhausted and late. He began to hate the profession that he had once loved so much.

Dr. Shannon knew that he was not doing an adequate job with almost every patient. He used to ask each of them numerous questions to discover a cause for their illness, and would carefully give each one instructions about their treatment. He would always say as they departed, "If you aren't better or have a problem or questions, call me." Now he no longer had time to ask questions except when absolutely necessary. And there was certainly no time to answer telephone questions. Often there wasn't even time to examine the patient. He couldn't even write out prescriptions for the drugs the patient needed because they weren't on the HMO's formulary. The better drugs were too expensive, he was told. Tests that would help him in the diagnosis and treatment of the patient were out of the question. He would have to spend an hour getting permission and he just didn't have the time.

As patients began to pile up in the waiting room, the doctor began to feel the stress even more. He began noting chest pain. In the beginning it was just while he was trying to rush through an examination, or when he climbed a flight of stairs. He had always taken a 15 minute walk after lunch just to get some fresh air. Now he began noting chest and arm pain when he started to walk, but if he kept on walking it would disappear. He was pretty sure it was his heart, but he didn't have time to become ill. Besides, who would he go to? An HMO doctor? They would probably have to get permission to do an electrocardiogram.

Gradually the chest pains became worse. One day it lasted for nearly an hour, but Dr. Shannon kept on working. Finally he had to sit down at his desk and rest. He felt completely washed out. When nurse discovered he was not in the examination room seeing patients, she peeked in his office only to find he was resting with his head in his arms. She gently called him to remind him his next patient was waiting, but Dr. Shannon didn't respond. He could no longer hear. He was dead at age 46.

PREHISTORIC MAN

One hundred thousand years ago, mankind's way of life was vastly different than it has been for the past few thousand years. If a man or woman survived until adulthood, his or her life was a constant struggle between the elements, predator animals, and even fellow humans. Whether or not one survived largely depended upon how quickly one's body responded to a life-threatening situation. Trying to kill a large animal for food or defending oneself against an enemy depended not just on strength, but also on endurance, quickness, and even how quickly the blood would clot. These abilities, in turn, depended upon how high one's blood pressure would rise, and how rapidly one's heart could beat to supply active muscles with energy. Clearly, those who had these gifts survived.

Our ancestors provided us with these gifts, but now, not only are they no longer needed, they also actually backfire on us. When hunter-gatherers became agriculturalists, and then lived in cities, we became civilized. No longer do we cannibalize or enslave our fellow human in most parts of the world. We are more civilized about it: we devour them through due process of law. No longer do we fight or flee when we deal with the enemy— because the enemy might be our boss, a landlord who is threatening to evict us, a doctor who wants to operate, or a life-threatening disease in one of our children. We must stand firm and cope with "the enemy." But the more primitive parts of our brains don't always understand. Our blood pressure rises, our heart rate increases, our blood vessels constrict, and the adrenaline pours out. The muscles no longer need all that energy— there is no place to go. What happens when all these forces mobilize? In the past 20 years we have begun to find out. Following are some of the many studies that are beginning to make all this more understandable. However, first some background information is necessary to fully appreciate what follows.

THE EFFECTS OF STRESS UPON THE HEART: HEART RATE AND BLOOD PRESSURE RESPONSES

Traditionally physicians have been taught that whenever cardiac ischemia occurs (reduced blood supply to the heart muscle), it is preceded by an increase in heart rate. For example, in a UCLA study some years ago,[1] the relationship between heart rate and ischemia was studied in 54 patients with known coronary artery disease while they were performing their normal activities. This information was obtained by having subjects wear a Holter monitor, which records an electrocardiogram 24 hours a day while the subject goes on about his or her usual daily activities. Using this technology, information about how the heart behaves during such things as driving, climbing stairs, stressful encounters, etc. can be monitored.

In this particular study, 89% of the ischemic episodes were preceded by an increase in heart rate of 10 beats or more. Other studies have shown similar findings.[2]

However, at Gupta Medical Centre in Jaipur, India,[3] of a group of 50 patients with suspected heart disease, 76% developed ischemia during physical exercise on a treadmill and 68% developed ischemia during mental stress tasks such as reading aloud in front of an audience, mental arithmetic, or giving an emotionally arousing speech. These ischemic changes occurred at lower heart rates when they were secondary to mental stress, compared to physical exercise. The reason this is of interest is that doctors have always felt that when a heart patient developed chest pain (angina) due to ischemia, it was because the heart had to work harder to increase the heart rate and blood flow to active muscles that needed more blood. This study implies that ischemia may develop for another reason.

For example, stress will stimulate the sympathetic nervous system causing constriction of all the peripheral blood vessels and a precipitous increase in blood pressure. When this increased pressure is transmitted back to the cavity of the left ventricle and to the heart muscle tissues, as previously described, the small vessels that make up the microcirculation will be compressed, blood flow to the heart muscle will be reduced, and ischemia and chest pain will follow. Alternatively, the coronary arteries themselves may constrict, reducing the blood flow to the heart muscle.

Other studies also have found that during mental stress, a high proportion of patients with coronary artery disease will develop both ischemia and a fall in the heart's output known as the ejection fraction at heart rates lower than ischemia produced by exercise. Interestingly, such ischemia is usually silent.

Why does ischemia induced by mental stress occur at lower work loads and with lower heart rates and blood pressures than is seen with physical exercise? One possibility is that mental stress affects the body in a different way than does exercise. This will be examined more closely presently. Another explanation is provided by a study from Toronto, which revealed that patients with mental stress-induced ischemia tended to have more severe disease than exercise-induced ischemia; and more exercise-induced angina at lower increases in heart rate and blood pressure.[4]

SIGNIFICANCE OF MENTAL STRESS-INDUCED ISCHEMIA

What is the importance of realizing that ischemia may be induced by mental stress? Does it have any prognostic value? In other words, can the presence of mental stress-induced ischemia predict an increased frequency of heart attacks or premature deaths? A Duke University study attempted to answer these questions.[5]

Researchers studied a group of 132 patients with documented coronary artery disease who developed ischemia during exercise or mental stress or both, and followed them with ambulatory Holter monitoring during their daily activities. It was found that patients who developed ischemia during mental stress in the university laboratory were more likely to develop ischemia during their ordinary activities than patients who exhibited ischemia only during exercise. Over a five year period, those patients who developed ischemia during mental stress were nearly three times more likely to incur a subsequent fatal or nonfatal cardiac event than were those whose ischemia only occurred during exercise. These events were independent of age, heart function and previous heart attacks.[6] Similar findings were reported in a study of 380 patients who suffered a heart attack. Nearly one-third had experienced three or more stressful life events, in comparison to only 13.6% of healthy controls.[7] In another study from Sydney University in Australia, a group of patients who had their first heart attack were followed for a period of three years. Those who suffered from either acute or chronic stress were three to four times more likely to experience a repeat heart attack or to die.[8]

No doubt a partial explanation for the increased mortality in these patients with coronary artery disease is the likelihood of sudden death during or immediately following a very stressful event. There are numerous reports of such happenings, but rarely are the events witnessed and then followed by an autopsy. In a study from the University of Paris, 43 cases of stress-induced sudden death were studied. All cases were witnessed. In 20 cases, sudden death occurred at the time of the stressful event; in the remainder, it took place within two hours after the event. In all cases death occurred without warning symptoms. The stressful events included fear in 15, altercation in 21, sexual activity in 3, and police questioning or arrest in 4 cases. In 38 of the cases, the cause of death was cardiac.[9] Usually the victims already had advanced cardiac disease. Other examples of death occurring during extremes of stress and fear are found in the many reports of increases in death during earthquakes.[10,11] These deaths usually occur in individuals who have severe heart disease.

MECHANISMS OF THE EFFECTS OF STRESS UPON THE HEART

Heart disease, however, is not necessary for sudden death to occur. Dr. Robert Sapolsky, in his book *Why Zebras Don't Get Ulcers*[12] talks about the subject of voodoo death, a subject that is well-documented. As we have just seen, fear may very well cause cardiac arrest in patients with advanced heart disease. Sudden death in young adults with voodoo death is another matter entirely. It would be most unlikely for such an individual to have advanced heart disease. According to Dr. Sapolsky, such events have been called psychophysiological deaths.

In a way, such deaths can be likened to the porcine stress syndrome. In the late 1960s it was noted that when pigs on their way to market were subjected to routine handling, some would develop red and white areas of discoloration of the skin, followed by an increase in body temperature, and heart failure. Then the pigs went into a shock-like state and died. Further studies were carried out by immobilizing the animal for a period of time. Many of these animals developed changes in their electrocardiogram and died. Autopsy revealed microscopic changes in the heart muscle that could be reproduced by the injection of catecholamines. This is one of the many hormones released during episodes of extreme stress, and is mainly responsible for the increase in heart rate and blood pressure when we become frightened.

When they are released in massive amounts, catecholamines may cause extreme constriction of blood vessels throughout the body, a marked elevation in blood pressure and heart rate, and result in an increased tendency for the blood to clot, reduced blood flow to the heart muscle, an increase in cardiac arrhythmias such as ventricular fibrillation (rapid, erratic, ineffective beating of the heart) and death. The combination of extreme constriction of the blood vessels, which slows the flow of blood, with increased likelihood of the blood to clot, causes what is called intravascular thrombosis (i.e., a blood clot forms within an artery). If the blood vessel happens to be a coronary artery, the victim will have a heart attack. If the artery and the territory it supplies are large enough, and if the victim has preexisting damage from a prior heart attack, then the stressful episode and the cascade of events that follow can cause sudden death.

The underlying basis for all these events is tremendous over-stimulation of the sympathetic nervous system with the overproduction of the neurohormones epinephrine and norepinephrine. The increased amount of these neurohormones can be easily detected in the blood stream of these animals. Certain groups of drugs known as beta blockers interfere with the action of these hormones upon the heart. One might anticipate that if these experiments are repeated in animals that are pretreated with beta blockers, the cascade of events that occurs would be reduced or stopped. This is exactly what happens, and the animals no longer die.

Animals do not always respond the same was as people. Do the same kind of changes take place in us? A variety of studies have attempted to find out exactly what might explain the increased morbidity and mortality that occurs during stress. In a study from John Hopkins,[13] 29 subjects with no evidence of coronary artery disease were subjected to mental stress, and a variety of physiological variables were measured. They noted a substantial sympathetic response characterized by increases in blood pressure, heart rate, output of the heart , and rises in the blood levels of epinephrine and norepinephrine. As a result, the heart became larger and the ejection fraction decreased with each heart beat. A number of subjects exhibited impaired contraction of the heart muscle in spite of the fact that they were said to be free of heart disease.

COMPARISON OF MENTAL AND PHYSICAL STRESS

A recent Henry Ford Hospital study[14] attempted to compare the effects of physical and mental stress on heart rate, blood pressure, cardiac output, and peripheral resistance (the amount of constriction or resistance to the flow of blood in the small blood vessels of the body), and to note the connection of these changes with the amount of epinephrine and norepinephrine secreted by the sympathetic nervous system. It turns out that physical exercise and mental stress produce qualitatively different effects on the cardiovascular system. Mental stress produced a small increase in heart rate, blood pressure, and cardiac output. However, there was a significant increase in peripheral vascular resistance. This means that the increase in blood pressure was largely due to the small blood vessels of the body becoming even smaller. Much like reducing the size of the nozzle of a garden hose, which will increase the pressure in the hose, so does the blood pressure increase when the small blood vessels of the body constrict. These changes correlated with increases in the blood epinephrine level, suggesting that this neurohormone was responsible. Furthermore, although the cardiac output increased during mental stress, the ejection fraction decreased indicating impaired contraction of the heart muscle. Thus it was not surprising that 58% of the patients exhibited ischemia.

In contrast, physical exercise produced a decrease in vascular resistance and a greater increase in heart rate and blood pressure. Ischemia occurred in 92% of the patients. Thus, both physical and mental stress produced ischemia of the heart but in different degrees and through different mechanisms. Indeed, one researcher studied the combination of mental and physical stress.[15] When mental stress was added to steady exercise, there was a significant increase in both heart rate and blood pressure.

EFFECT OF BETA BLOCKERS

Since humans show the same kind of effect as animals with an increase in heart rate, blood pressure, cardiac output, and increased tendency of the blood to clot, it can be predicted that beta blockers protect individuals with coronary artery disease from dying in the same way as it protects animals. Numerous studies have documented the protective effects of beta blockers both during an acute heart attack, and in the period after a heart attack, when the victim is most likely to die or to have a repeat event. Unfortunately, for reasons that are not clear, most patients with coronary artery disease either are taking inadequate doses of a beta blockers, or are not taking any at all.

TYPES OF STRESS

There is overwhelming evidence documenting the harmful effects of stress on the cardiovascular system. However, stress effects people in different ways. A given series of events may be perceived as extremely stressful by one individual, and not at all by another. Who is most likely to be affected by stress? Is one type of stress more likely to be harmful than another? Is it the environment in which the subject lives, and not the stress itself, that contributes more to the degree of stress experienced?

Some responses to these questions arise from the experiments of Dr. Jay Kaplan at Bowman Gray School of Medicine.[16] Kaplan has done extensive work using primates, relating social stress to the development of coronary artery disease. It is well known that monkey communities form a social hierarchy with the one dominant monkey on top and subordinate monkeys at the bottom. The dominant monkeys have much higher levels of sympathetic nervous system stimulation and more evidence of arteriosclerotic plaques, as compared to the subordinate monkeys. By repeatedly introducing new groups of animals at regular intervals, the hierarchy is always fluctuating. The dominant monkey's position is now unstable and is constantly challenged. In these cases, they were incessantly fighting and exhibited increased manifestations of stress, as well as more arteriosclerotic plaques, even when the monkeys were placed on a low fat diet. Presumably the mechanism of increased arteriosclerotic plaque formation is an increase in blood pressure and the force with which blood is transported in the arteries. As a result, there is increased injury to the endothelial lining, increased inflammatory response, increased platelet adhesiveness and aggregation, increased deposition of clot-like material along the wall of the vessel, etc. Kaplan found that the monkeys who developed the most atherosclerosis responded to stress with the greatest increase in activity of the sympathetic nervous system, as reflected by the largest increases in heart rate and blood pressure. Interestingly, when such animals were pretreated with beta blockers, they did not form arteriosclerotic plaques.[17]

INFLUENCE OF SOCIAL ENVIRONMENT

That social environment may strongly influence whether or not heart disease occurs is suggested by a study of a group of secluded 144 nuns living in central Italy who were followed for 30 years, and compared to 138 women from the same region.[16] None of the women were smokers, took birth control pills or estrogen supplements. During the period of observation, the blood pressure remained remarkably stable among the nuns. None of the nuns developed a diastolic blood pressure of more than 90 mmHg, while the lay women showed a rise in blood pressure with age of 30/15. Comparing the two groups, there were 10 versus 21 fatal cardiovascular events and 21 versus 48 nonfatal cardiovascular events, in the nuns and lay women, respectively. The authors concluded that it was the difference in the psychosocial stress between the two groups that were responsible for these results.

Another way of determining whether or not socioeconomic events influence the development of coronary artery disease and its complications is to track what happens to different groups of patients after they have a heart attack. One study related income and marital status to survival and it was found that patients with low incomes below $10,000 a year are twice as likely to die as patients with a higher incomes of $40,000 or more. Also, unmarried patients without a partner were three times more likely to die as married patients.[19] Similarly, both social isolation and lack of education have been found to increase the risk of coronary artery disease.[20] Victims of a heart attack who live alone have a high risk of dying.[21] As a rule, social isolation can be directly related to income. A Danish study found that the higher the social class, the less the risk from coronary artery disease. Indeed, the highest social class had only one-quarter of the risk of having a coronary event as the lowest social class.[22]

The relationship between social class, socioeconomic status and coronary heart disease has been noted in other countries as well. A report from the *British Heart Journal*[23] noted that over the past 40 years there has been an increase in mortality from coronary artery disease among working class men, whereas among white collar men, mortality has remained unchanged. When men with the lowest level of employment were compared with men from top management, the mortality rate was 3.6 times greater among the former. These differences could be attributed only in part to a greater number of risk factors among the workers of lower status. In other words, the lower the social status, the greater the risk.

The entire subject of socioeconomic status and cardiovascular disease was recently reviewed.[24] It was pointed out that the principal measures of socioeconomic status are education, occupation and income. During the past 40 years there has been an inverse relationship between coronary heart disease and the indicators of socioeconomic status. Although the overall mortality from coronary heart disease has declined substantially during that time, the decline has not affected all segments of society equally.

DEPRESSION AND HEART DISEASE

If social isolation increases the risk of dying from coronary artery disease, might not certain types of psychological or emotional problems also influence the occurrence of coronary events? Depression is the first emotional state that comes to mind in light of the studies just cited. Is there a relationship between depression and heart disease? The most likely way to find out the answer to this question is to study the depression that is known to occur following the death of a mate. A number of such studies have been carried out, and it has been found there is a marked increase in mortality in those individuals with prolonged depression following the death of a spouse.[25,26]

Similarly, the presence of depression following a heart attack can predict adverse events. In a study from Germany, 560 survivors of a heart attack were followed over a 6 month period. Twelve cardiac deaths and 17 irregular cardiac rhythm events occurred. They were significantly predicted by severe forms of post-heart attack depression.[27]

Two important studies from Duke University add to the evidence linking depression and heart events. The first, operating under the assumption that depressed patients with coronary artery disease have an increased risk of death at the time of their hospitalization, followed 1,250 patients with coronary artery disease for 19 years.[28] Compared with patients who were not depressed after 5-10 years, depressed patients had an 84% greater risk of death, and a 72% greater risk of death after 10 years. Patients with mild depression had an intermediate degree of risk. The researchers felt that chronic or recurring depression was associated with coronary artery disease progression, triggering of acute events, or both.

The second study followed 58 patients who exhibited cardiac ischemia during their daily activities and attempted to correlate the ischemia with the subject's emotional state.[29] Negative emotions, tension and sadness increased the risk of ischemia by 2 to 3 times. A similar study was carried out at Washington University School of Medicine in St. Louis. Fifty-two patients with documented coronary artery disease were followed for a year after an initial diagnosis was made. The presence of major depression was the best predictor of subsequent cardiac events, and it was independent of disease severity.[30]

JOB CONTROL

Socioeconomic status, social environment, chronic mental stress, and chronic depression all predict an increased occurrence of obstructive coronary artery disease and heart attacks. It would seem logical that a relationship would be found between occupation and work environment, and morbidity and mortality from heart disease. A number of studies have attempted to determine answers to this question.

The common thread among these studies is not so much the degree of stress involved, but whether or not the worker has a degree of control of his work situation. Experiments with monkey, rats and other animals have all clearly shown this to be true. Unfortunately, the following description will not be comfortable to animal rights supporters, while it does yield some interesting theory. Studies were done on two monkeys, each of which was placed in a separate cage. At regular intervals they were subjected to electric shocks. The experiment was arranged so that both animals received the same total number of shocks, but only one monkey was trained to push a button that enabled it to control the number of shocks. This monkey is called the "avoidance monkey." Over a period of time, the other monkey — the "nonavoidance monkey" — developed electrocardiographic changes and died of cardiac arrest, while the avoidance monkey showed no changes on an electrocardiogram. Variations of this kind of experiment have been done many times with similar results.

The most complete investigation done on humans in this area is the well-known Whitehall Study from England.[31] Over 10,000 London-based civil servants were followed for an average of about five years. Both the men and women who had low levels of job control had nearly twice the incidence of newly-reported coronary events during the period of observation than did the civil servants who had high levels of job control. These findings could not be explained by employment grade or any of the classic risk factors.

Another way to study this problem is to compare coronary events in factory workers with executives. At first guess, one might think that the factory workers would exhibit less heart disease in general, because they don't have the responsibilities that the executives do. However, the results are just the opposite: the factory workers exhibit more cases of heart disease. This is because factory workers do not have much control over their work environment. They are stuck in a monotonous job and have little to say about what they do. In contrast, executives usually have more job mobility and can delegate responsibility to others to relieve their stress.

Decision-making control is crucial. If you don't believe this, then get in an automobile with your spouse— but *you* sit in the passenger seat. You will probably be extremely nervous, and it will have nothing to do with your spouse's driving skills. It is because you're not behind the wheel and you have no control over the car. It's okay for you to go 70 miles an hour, but not for your spouse!

TRIGGERING FACTORS

So far we have examined factors that increase the possibility of coronary heart disease over a period of years. Are there factors or types of behavior that can trigger a coronary event? This was briefly addressed earlier in this chapter, under the subject of extreme fear. Fortunately, this is not a common emotional state unless you're in the habit of going to horror movies. Yet this subject is important, because it suggests that heart attacks may not always be random events. If there are triggers, then awareness of these triggers might prevent a catastrophic event from happening.

Researchers at Harvard studied 894 patients to determine whether a triggering event was responsible for a recent heart attack.[32] In nearly half of the patients, a possible trigger was identified. For 18%, the trigger was an emotional upset, for 14%, it was physical activity; and for 13%, multiple triggers were identified.

A more direct approach was taken by Stanford researchers when 12 patients with angina due to coronary artery disease were studied while coronary angiograms were being performed.[33] Arteries that were narrowed due to obstructive coronary artery disease were compared to arteries with a normal diameter. The patients were then asked to recall an incident that made them angry. No changes were noted in the normal arteries. However, in the diseased arteries, there was a significant decrease in the diameter and, presumably, a decrease in blood flow to heart muscle.

A recent study from the Harvard School of Public Health supports the claim that anger may be an important trigger of coronary events.[34] In the Veterans Administration Normative Aging Study, 1,305 men who were free of coronary artery disease were examined with the Minnesota Multiphasic Personality Inventory Test and followed for 7 years. Individuals who had the greatest problem controlling their anger were compared with those who had the least amount of anger. During the period of the study, 110 subjects had a coronary events including fatal heart attack (20), non-fatal heart attack (30), and angina pectoris (60). Those with the highest level of anger were more than three times as likely to have a coronary event than were those with the lowest level of anger.

In another Veterans Administration study,[35] researchers were able to compare 15 patients with coronary artery disease who showed an ischemic response with radioactive imaging during mental arithmetic with a different group of 15 patients who also had coronary artery disease, but who showed no ischemia during mental stress. There were no differences between the two groups in terms of heart rate and blood pressure. The group with the ischemic response had higher anger and hostility scores on their psychological profile than the group that did not.

Clearly, anger and coronary events are related. One interesting relationship that has emerged from these studies on anger and heart attacks has been the influence of education on coronary events. In another study from Harvard,[36] 1,623 patients were interviewed an average of four days after their heart attack. Episodes of anger triggering the heart attack were related to levels of education. It was found that the risk of a heart attack declined with increasing levels of education. The relative risk was twice as high among those with less than a high school education.

PERSONALITY TYPES

The fact that both depression and anger in some way encourage the occurrence of coronary heart disease raises the question as to whether certain personality types are more likely to have a heart attack. Back in the 1960s, it was claimed there was such a personality type, and it became known as Type A. Type A behavior was described as impatient, hostile, aggressive, hard-working, competitive and having an urgency about time. A Type B personality was also identified as an absence of these characteristics and was noted to have a reduced risk of developing coronary artery disease. A restudy of the original groups of patients established that it was not the competitive, time-constrained overachiever who was at risk, but the individual who exhibited the most hostility. Such subjects have more coronary artery disease and higher mortality rates.

One of the criticisms that might be directed toward the concept of a specific emotional state or character pattern causing a heart attack is that it places the cart before the horse; that is, perhaps the environmental situation is responsible for the depression, hostility, and anger. A number of different stressors have been linked to coronary heart disease. They include unhappy marriages, dissatisfaction with one's work, too much work responsibility, sudden loss of self-esteem, and death of a spouse. In one study of 35 patients who suffered a heart attack before the age of 40, the following stressors were identified: 51% had to meet deadlines, 46% had extraneously determined interruptions, 43% had multifunctional task demands, 35% had to maintain a second job, and 31% had stressful work hours. Similarly, a number of social factors have been found to correlate with an increased incidence of coronary heart disease. These include the process of urbanization, geographic mobility, lack of social support and family ties.

It is possible to place these various psychosocial risk factors into four groups:

1. Exaggerated, illogical emotions such as chronic anger, depression and hostility that are often out of proportion to their underlying cause.
2. Chronic dissatisfaction with work due to lack of latitude in decision-making, monotony, little job mobility, lack of appreciation of one's work, overwork and stressful demands.
3. Those who live in lower social strata with its associated lack of education, isolation and lack of social support.
4. Those who, through no fault of their own, experience stressful life events and are unable to recover.

Regardless of the underlying cause, stress acts upon the central and autonomic nervous system, producing a cascade of physiological changes in vulnerable individuals that lead to arteriosclerotic plaque formation, cardiac ischemia, plaque rupture, coronary thrombosis and often death.

These are all byproducts of our modern civilization. Their effects on the cardiovascular system can be devastating. Yet these effects can be minimized and even prevented with awareness of their impact, and with the careful use of modern drug therapy.

REFERENCES

1. Rozabnski A, Bairey CN, Krantz DS *et al.* Mental stress and the induction of silent myocardial ischemia in patients with coronary artery disease. N Engl J Med 1988; 321:1005-1012.

2. Panza JA, Diodati JC, Callahan TS, *et al.* Role of increases in heart rate in determining the occurrence and frequency of myocardial ischemia during daily life in patients with stable coronary artery disease. J Am Coll Cardiol 1992; 20:1092-1098

3. Gupta R, Gupta KD, Induction of myocardial ischemia by mental stress in coronary heart disease. J Assoc Physicians India 1993; 41:75-78.

4. Legault SE, Freman MR, Langer A, *et al.* Pathophysiology and time course of silent myocardial ischemia during mental stress: clinical, anatomical, and physiological correlates. Br Heart J 1995; 73:242-249

5. Blumenthal JA, Jiang W, Waugh RA, *et al.* Mental stress-induced ischemia in the laboratory and ambulatory ischemia during daily life. Association and hemodynamic features. Circulation 1995; 92:2102-2108.

6. Jiang W, Babyak M, Krantz DS, *et al.* Mental stress-induced ischemia and cardiac events. JAMA 1996; 275:1651-1656

7. Siegrist J, Dittmann K, Rittner I, *et al.* In: *Myocardial Infarction and Psychosocial Risks.* New York: Springer-Verlag, 1981, page 52.

8. Tennant CC, Palmer KJ, Langeluddecke PM, *et al.* Life event stress and myocardial reinfarction: a prospective study. Eur Heart J 1994; 15: 472-478.

9. Lecompte D, Fornes P, Nicolas G. Stressful events as a trigger of sudden death: a study of 43 medico-legal autopsy cases. Forensic Sci Int 1997; 85:159-160.

10. Katsouyanni K, Kovevinas M, Trichopoulos D. Earthquake-related stress and cardiac mortality. Int J Epidemiol 1986; 15:326-330.

11. Dobson AJ, Alexander HM, Malcolm JA, *et al.* Heart Attacks and the Newcastle earthquake. Med J Aust, 1991; 155:757-761.

12. Sapolsky RM, In: *Why Zebras Don't Get Ulcers.* New York: W. H. Freeman and Co., 1994, page 28.

13. Becker LC, Pepine CJ, Bonsall R, *et al.* Left ventricular, peripheral vascular, and neurohumoral responses to mental stress in normal middle-aged men and women. Circulation 1996, 94.2768-2777.

14. Goldberg AD, Becker LC, Bonsall R, *et al.* Ischemic, hemodynamic, and neurohormonal responses to mental and exercise stress. Circulation 1996; 94:2402-2409.

15. Siconolfi SF, Garber CE, Baptist GD, *et al.* Circulatory effects of mental stress during exercise in coronary artery disease patients. Clin Cardiol 1984; 7:441-444.

16. Kaplan JR, Adams MR, Anthony MS, *et al.* Dominant social status and contraceptive hormone treatment inhibit atherogenesis in premenopausal monkeys. Arterioscler Thromb Vasc Biol 1995; 15:2094-2100.

17. Kaplan JR, Manuck SB, Adams MR, *et al.* The effects of beta-adrenergic blocking agents on atherosclerosis and its complications. Eur Heart J 1987; 8:928-944.

18. Timio M, Lippi G, Venanzi S, *et al.* Blood pressure trends and cardiovascular events in nuns in a secluded order: a 30 year follow-up study. Blood Press 1997; 6:81-87.

19. Williams RB, Barefoot JC, Califf RM, *et al.* Prognostic importance of social and economic resources among medically treated patients with angiographically documented coronary artery disease. JAMA 1992; 267:520-524.

20. Ruberman W, Weinblatt E, Goldberg JD, *et al.* Psychosocial influences on mortality after myocardial infarction. N Engl J Med 1984; 311:552-559.

21. Case RB, Moss AJ, Case N, *et al.* Living alone after myocardial infarction: impact on prognosis. JAMA 1992; 267:515-519.

22. Suadicani P, Hein HO, Gyntelberg F. Are social inequalities as associated with the risk of ischemic heart disease a result of psycho-social working conditions? Atherosclerosis 1993; 101:165-175.

23. Rose G, Marmot MG. Social class and coronary heart disease. Br Heart J 1981; 45:13-19.

24. Kaplan GA, Keil JE. Socioeconomic factors and cardiovascular disease: a review of the literature. Circulation 1993; 88:1973-1998.

25. Prigerson HG, Bierhais AJ, Kasl SV, et al. Traumatic grief as a risk factor for mental and physical morbidity. Am J Psychiatry 1997; 154:616-623.

26. Martikainen P, Valkonen T. Mortality after the death of a spouse: rates and causes of death in a large Finnish cohort. Am J Public Health 1996; 86:1087-1093.

27. Ladwig KH, Kieser M, Konig J, et al. Affective disorders and survival after acute myocardial infarction. Eur Heart J 1991; 12:959-964.

28. Barefoot JC, Helms, MJ, Mark DB, et al. Depression and long term mortality risk in patients with coronary artery disease. Am J Cardiol 1996; 78:613-617.

29. Gullette EC, Blumenthal JA, Babyak M, et al. Effects of mental stress on myocardial ischemia during daily life. JAMA 1997; 277:1521-1526.

30. Carney RM, Rich MW, Freedland KE, et al. Major depressive disorder predicts cardiac events in patients with coronary artery disease. Psychosom Med 1988; 50:627-633.

31. Bosma H, Marmot MG, Hemingway H, et al. Low job control and risk of coronary heart disease in Whitehall II (prospective cohort) study. BMJ 1997; 314:558-565.

32. Tofler GH, Stone PH, Maclure M, et al. Analysis of possible triggers of acute myocardial infarction. Am J Cardiol 1990; 66:22-27.

33. Boltwood, MD, Taylor CB, Burke MB, et al. Anger report predicts coronary artery vasomotor response to mental stress in atherosclerotic segments. Am J Cardiol 1993; 72:1361-1365.

34. Kawachi I, Sparrow D, Spiro A. A prospective study of anger and coronary heart disease. The Normative Aging Study. Circulation 1996; 94:2090- 2095.

35. Burg MM, Jain D, Soufer R, et al. Role of behavioral and psychological factors in mental stress-induced silent left ventricular dyusfunction in coronary artery disease. J Am Coll Cardiol 1993; 22:440-448.

36. Mittleman MA, Maclure M, Nachuani M, *et al*. Educational attainment, anger, and the risk of triggering myocardial infarction onset. The Determinants of Myocardial Infarction Onset Study Investigators. Arch Intern Med 1997; 157:769-775.

6

NONCARDIAC CAUSES OF CARDIAC SYMPTOMS

Tom Brown was a 62-year-old, recently retired airline pilot who had been looking forward to his time off so that he and his wife could spend their later years traveling around the country in their motor home. He was tired of flying, the long hours, and the time away from his family while his children were growing up. Now his three daughters and one son were scattered around the country, and he and his wife were joyfully anticipating visiting them all. The only problem was that in recent months he had been having recurring episodes of chest discomfort. He had told the doctor about it at time of his retirement physical. His heart had been carefully checked, and a stress test had been administered but no abnormalities were found.

Lately, perhaps with the stress of a change in life-style due to his retirement, his chest pain had been increasing. He knew that heart pain typically occurred during exertion. In the past his symptoms had always been at rest; however, now it was occurring while he was walking. One night he awakened with severe chest pain. It felt as if his chest were in a vise. Frightened, he asked his wife to call the paramedics. They quickly arrived and he was rushed off to the emergency room of a nearby hospital accompanied by his wife. Fortunately, he was given prompt attention. An electrocardiogram was taken, along with blood from both an artery and a vein. A chest x-ray was also performed. Finally, the emergency room doctor said that it was not clear why he was having the chest pain, because there seemed to be no evidence of a heart attack. He recommended to Tom that he undergo angiograms to obtain further information.

Tom agreed to have the angiograms and underwent the procedure without complications. Afterwards he was advised by the hospital cardiologist that he had disease in all three vessels. Although none of the vessels were severely narrowed, in view of his symptoms and in view of the recent knowledge that even mildly narrowed vessels could undergo rupture of an arteriosclerotic plaque, he recommended that Tom undergo coronary artery bypass surgery. He was not informed of other tests that might determine whether the blood flow to the heart muscle was reduced. Nor was the subject of medical treatment of his symptoms with drugs discussed. Tom was afraid that on one of the motor home trips he and his wife planned to take, that these symptoms would reoccur in an isolated area, and that he might not survive. Accordingly, he agreed to the surgery.

A few days later, a triple bypass procedure was carried out with no complications. Tom was fortunate in that a skilled surgeon with a low complication rate had operated upon him. Also, the nurses responsible for his post-operative care were outstanding. He was in a great deal of discomfort from the procedure, and continued to have a lot of residual soreness in his chest where his sternum (breastbone) had been split open to get at his heart. He also had considerable soreness in his legs where veins had been removed to supply the bypass grafts. Slowly he recovered and after two months had regained his former strength and activities.

One night the pain returned. It was exactly the same as the pain that had forced him to be taken to the hospital a short time before. Tom again became frightened, called the paramedics, and was taken to the hospital. This time he was told that in all likelihood one of the bypasses had closed off and would have to be reopened. Again he underwent a coronary angiogram only to find out that all three grafts were functioning well. The cardiologist reluctantly admitted he did not know why Tom had a return of his chest pain but said one possibility was that one of his arteries had gone into spasm. He would be allowed to return home, and advised Tom to take a calcium channel blocker that was effective against such spasm.

Tom followed his advice, but he was worried whether there was some other cause for his symptoms that had nothing to do with his heart. He went to the library, to the book stores and even began using the Internet. He began to find other conditions that would cause chest pain, and on several occasions the same term was repeated— a condition called GERD. Tom decided to see what he could find on the Internet. He had heard that the National Library of Medicine, the reference source used by doctors, was now available to the public for free. Eventually he found the address and brought it up on his computer screen. He typed in GERD and in 10 seconds had over 200 references. The more he read, the more convinced he became that he was not having heart pain but GERD, gastroesophageal reflux disease.

Tom promptly made an appointment to see a gastroenterologist, a digestive disease specialist. When he did see the doctor, one of the first questions he was asked was whether he had indigestion, heartburn or other digestive symptoms. Tom had never been asked those questions before. He admitted he often had heartburn but could control it with antacids. It never had occurred to him that the heartburn was related to his chest pain. The gastroenterologist recommended that Tom undergo a simple procedure known as endoscopy. A flexible, optical tube would be gently inserted into the throat under local anesthesia, and passed down to the lower end of the esophagus and stomach. Under direct vision, the lining of both organs could be examined for evidence of disease. The procedure was accomplished without incident. Tom was told that there clearly evidence of inflammation of the lower esophagus, and that the lower esophageal muscle was not able to completely close off the sphincter at the end of the esophagus. Accordingly, at times there was regurgitation of gastric acid into the esophagus, and if enough backed up, Tom could have chest pain.

Tom was started on a class of drug that was called a proton pump inhibitor along with an antibiotic. Within a few days his heartburn was gone. He was assured that it was very unlikely his chest pain would return. Tom was afraid to ask the question, and never did, whether the symptoms that led to his bypass surgery and both angiograms never were due to his heart, but were caused by his GERD.

How often do the Toms of the word undergo unnecessary coronary artery bypass surgery? No one really knows. It has been estimated that somewhere between 25 million and 40 million Americans have GERD. Estimates of the number of patients seen in emergency rooms with chest pain vary between three million and six million. Two million people undergo angiograms each year and 800,000 undergo angioplasty or coronary artery bypass surgery. Whatever the number is that undergo unnecessary cardiac procedures and surgery, when the real problem is GERD, that number must be very large indeed. If it were only 10%, then each year there must be at least 80,000 people like Tom. This number does not include the many other diseases and conditions that also will cause chest pain that are mistaken for the pain of coronary artery disease. Also, there are a variety of disorders that may trigger previously silent coronary artery disease and cause chest pain. These topics will be the subject of the remainder of this chapter.

DISEASES AND CONDITIONS THAT MAY CAUSE CHEST PAIN

Esophageal Causes Of Chest Pain

Disorders of the esophagus such as spasm and inflammation of the lining may produce pain that is very similar to angina pectoris, including the fact that it may be precipitated by exertion and relieved by sublingual nitroglycerin. In fact, esophageal disorders often coexist with coronary artery disease. Pain from esophageal disorders is usually precipitated by eating or by lying down after eating, and it can be relieved by antacids and milk. Often it is accompanied by heartburn and difficulty swallowing (dysphagia).

Unlike angina pectoris, which typically radiates across the upper and mid-chest, esophageal pain tends to be located at the lower end of the sternum (breastbone) and radiates to the epigastrium. Certain kinds of food more characteristically produce esophageal pain. These include alcohol, spicy food and coffee. Unlike angina, which tends to last less than 5 to 10 minutes, esophageal pain may last for hours and fluctuates in intensity.

Hiatal Hernia

A hiatal hernia, also called a diaphragmatic hernia, is an abnormally large opening in the diaphragm where the esophagus connects to the stomach. As a result, the upper end of the stomach may herniate into the chest cavity. This is not likely to occur while someone is sitting or standing. Consequently, symptoms, when they appear, do so only when the subject is either lying down or leaning forward after a heavy meal. The pain that develops is a constricting or burning discomfort that appears in the mid and left chest regions, and may last for 30 minutes or longer. On occasion it may radiate to the left arm. It may be temporarily relieved by belching or assumption of the upright position. Sublingual nitroglycerin does not relieve the pain.

Pain From Other Areas Within The Chest

Lungs

A variety of disorders involving the lung may be associated with chest pain. Pneumonia is one of the most common, particularly when it involves the lining of the surface of the lung known as the pleura. Inflammation of the pleura is called pleurisy, and pleuritic pains tend to be sharp, and of brief duration. Typically the pain comes and goes over a period of hours, and it tends to occur only during inspiration. When associated with pneumonia, pleurisy is usually accompanied by a cough and fever. It also may be a symptom of a pulmonary embolism (see the following section), the site of metastasis of a malignant tumor, or a sign of one of the autoimmune diseases such as lupus erythematosus. Although pleurisy tends to be localized to a relatively small area of the chest, at times, with the more infectious type, the chest pain may be generalized and cause shortness of breath.

Pulmonary Embolism

Another major cause of chest pain is a pulmonary embolism. An embolism is a mobile blood clot that usually occurs after a surgical procedure, particularly if the patient has been lying immobile in bed for several days. Immobility and the stress of surgery are associated with stasis of blood in the lower extremities and pelvis. This encourages the formation of blood clots in these areas. An injury to the lower extremities also may result in the formation of a clot, days or even weeks later. Whatever the origin, portions of the clot may break off and migrate to the lungs. This is most likely to occur when attempts are made to ambulate a patient in the post-operative period. Usually such a clot lodges in the small blood vessels in the lung. If the clot is a large one, it may be associated with coughing up of blood, shortness of breath, pain intensified by deep breathing, and even sudden death. The pain associated with a pulmonary embolism may be indistinguishable from both cardiac ischemia and the pain of an acute heart attack. Chest pain may be the first clue that a clot is present in the legs or thighs. In general, prolonged bed rest for any reason encourages the formation of blood clots in the lower half of the body followed by a pulmonary embolus. Usually the diagnosis of an embolism can be made by chest x-ray, however, special tests and procedures may be required in more obscure cases.

Pneumothorax

A pneumothorax is an important cause of chest pain. It occurs when air perforates the outer surface of the lung, forcing ambient air into the chest cavity. When this happens, the victim suffers chest pain, followed by the collapse of the perforated lung and shortness of breath. Usually the pain is in the lateral chest rather than the center of the chest, and it may be aggravated by breathing. The diagnosis of pneumothorax can readily be made with a chest x-ray. It also may be identified on physical examination, if the doctor takes the trouble to listen to both lungs.

Mediastinal Emphysema

Mediastinal emphysema refers to the presence of air in the central portion of the chest cavity that contains the heart. Because the air may create pressure and stretching of the structures and nerves within the mediastinum, severe pain may result. In addition, because the stretched nerves involve the same nerve roots as the nerves coming from the heart, it may be very similar to cardiac pain. Usually the pain is more superficial and tends to be modified by respiration and body position. This disorder can be diagnosed by a chest x-ray.

Pulmonary Hypertension

Pulmonary hypertension is a rare cause of chest pain. It is an elevation of the pressure in the pulmonary artery, the artery that exits from the right ventricle. Before it enters the lungs and branches into tiny blood vessels, it contains unoxygenated, venous blood.

A number of diseases may cause the pressure in the pulmonary artery to become elevated, including various forms of congenital heart disease, mitral stenosis (obstruction of the mitral valve), chronic lung disease, and primary pulmonary hypertension. Although primary pulmonary hypertension is an extremely rare disease, it has recently been found to be a side effect of certain medications used for weight loss. The chest pain associated with pulmonary hypertension occurs with exertion and is relieved by rest, and may be indistinguishable from the pain associated with cardiac ischemia. Indeed, it is thought that the pain seen in this condition is due to ischemia of the right ventricle. Except for chronic lung disease, the various conditions giving rise to pulmonary hypertension occur in a much younger group of people, and the pain that develops does not respond to the usual cardiac medications. The diagnosis of all these disorders can be made from a careful physical examination, chest x-ray, and even the electrocardiogram.

Aortic Valve Disease

The aortic valve is the exit valve of the heart and all blood must leave the heart through this opening. Immediately after the aorta exits from the heart, the coronary arteries arise and supply the heart muscle with blood. If the aortic valve is diseased and obstructed, the blood flow exiting from the heart eventually will be reduced, even though the pressure within the left ventricular chamber becomes markedly elevated. At the same time, the pressure within the aorta beyond the valve will be reduced. The amount it is reduced depends upon how obstructed the aortic valve becomes. If pre-existing coronary artery disease is present, a previously insignificant degree of narrowing in a coronary artery may now become very significant. The result will be a reduction in blood flow and chest pain. Usually, if significant aortic stenosis is present, the murmur associated with it is readily heard. Unfortunately, the modern cardiologist has become so technology-oriented that frequently he does not even bother to listen to a patient's heart with a low technology instrument such as the stethoscope. Even if he does so conscientiously, the blood flow through the valve may be so reduced that no murmur can be heard.

Mitral Valve Prolapse

When the heart contracts, the mitral valve (the intake valve between the left atrium and left ventricle) closes so that blood does not flow backwards into the lungs. If the leaflets of the mitral valve fail to close then blood will be regurgitated into the left atrium and mitral regurgitation is said to be present. A variety of conditions may be responsible for the presence of mitral regurgitation that are beyond the scope of this book. Some, such as rheumatic valve disease, actually damage the leaflets. Some result from aging with the formation of calcium on the leaflet that interferes with its closing. One common cause is mitral valve prolapse. In this condition, the valves are not damaged but fail to close properly while the heart is contracting. Sometimes it is because one leaflet of the valve is deformed, sometimes it is because there is a loss of support of the tissues surrounding the valve that make up the mitral valve apparatus (mitral valve, chordae tendineae and papillary muscles), and sometimes it is because the ventricle has become enlarged from another disease such as hypertension.

Mitral valve prolapse has been claimed to cause chest pain also. There is no anatomical reason why mitral valve prolapse should cause chest pain. Because both this disorder and recurring chest patient pain are so common, mitral valve prolapse is often discovered coincidentally in the evaluation of a patient with chest pain symptoms. Also, mitral valve prolapse may accompany obstructive coronary artery disease; however it is the coronary artery disease that produces the chest pain and not the mitral valve prolapse.

Pericarditis

Pericarditis is the inflammation of the pericardium (that is, the membrane surrounding the heart), and it is accompanied by unique changes in the electrocardiogram. Viral and bacterial infections may sometimes involve the pericardium and will produce chest pain very similar to that seen with cardiac pain. The pain of pericarditis, however, is aggravated by deep breathing and influenced by changes in body position. It may cease when the breath is held or if the victim leans forward. Pericarditis is not a common disorder. Because of its similarity to cardiac pain, and the unique changes seen on the electrocardiogram, it easily can be mistaken for an impending heart attack. If coincidental coronary artery disease is found on an angiogram, and if the doctor seeing the patient is an aggressive cardiologist, potentially dangerous coronary artery bypass surgery may be performed that not only is unnecessary, but possibly harmful to the patient.

Dissecting Aneurysm of the Aorta

This is an enlargement and separation of the wall of the aorta, the main artery exiting from the heart. When present, dissecting aneurysms of the aorta may cause chest pain and be mistaken for an acute heart attack. When chest pain is present, it usually is severe, may involve the back and even the abdomen, and is a medical emergency. If the artery ruptures through the weakened portion of the aortic wall, death is immediate. Milder forms of dissection may be confused with a heart attack but can usually be diagnosed by a simple chest x-ray. However, if an x-ray is not taken, and the patient is made to undergo angiograms, there will be prolonged delay during which the aneurysm may rupture. The usual treatment for a dissecting aneurysm is immediate surgery.

Premature Beats

Premature beats may be accompanied by a sharp, stabbing pain over the heart area, and occasionally may be associated with a fleeting choking sensation. Usually such symptoms occur at rest and decrease during physical activity, but may reoccur when activity ceases.

Chest Pain Wall

Cervical Disk

A cervical disk may irritate the nerve roots going to the chest wall and produce chronic pain that is aggravated by walking and certain body positions. The pain tends to be more superficial than that seen with obstructive coronary artery disease and it is more likely to be present at rest.

Thoracic Outlet Syndrome

The nerves and blood vessels that enter the arm often have to go through a bottleneck of muscles. If a blood vessel or a nerve is kinked by a muscle or a rib, chest and arm pain may develop that is associated with walking. Since exertional chest pain is a hallmark of coronary artery disease, it is easy to see why confusion may arise. The pain is induced by swinging of the arms, and can be reproduced by elevating the arm and rotating it.

Tietze's Syndrome

Inflammation and swelling of the cartilage between the rib and breastbone (costochondral or chondrosternal joints is known as Tietze's syndrome. Such pain tends to be superficial rather than deep, is aggravated by breathing, and is very tender if the area is pressed.

Tenderness of the Muscles of the Chest Wall

A variety of factors may be responsible for tenderness of chest wall muscles, including injury from direct trauma (usually several days before the onset of pain), coughing, and weight lifting, which may cause a pulled muscle. Usually the pain is localized to a small area, lasts briefly, is aggravated by chest wall movements, turning, twisting and deep breathing, and may last many hours.

Herpes Zoster

Herpes zoster is a severe skin rash that does not spread beyond the midline, and it may cause extreme chest pain in the pre-eruptive stage. Typically the skin is extremely sensitive over the involved area. Herpes may not be suspected until the skin eruption actually occurs.

Hyperventilation Syndrome

Hyperventilation syndrome is an extremely common cause of chest pain. Hyperventilation is simply over-breathing as a result of anxiety or fear. It also has been called a panic attack.

Typically the subject unconsciously starts to breath more rapidly and deeply when under stress. The over-breathing is often interspersed with deep sighs. In its acute form it will quickly produce a variety of symptoms including lightheadedness, dizziness, a far away feeling, numbness, palpitations, blurred visions, flushing, and tingling of the hands and around the mouth. Sometimes the victim will even faint. In its milder form, the subject may be constantly over-breathing throughout the day. In so doing there is increased use of the chest muscles. If there is enough overuse of these muscles, they will become painful, producing chest pain.

Usually the victim is not consciously aware that he is over-breathing, but feels simply short of breath. When this is associated with pounding of one's heart, dizziness, blurred vision and the other symptoms of hyper-ventilation, it is not hard to understand the panic that may accompany this disorder. Because the symptoms are due to over-breathing and blowing off of carbon dioxide from the lungs, the chest pain and shortness of breath do not occur during exertion but rather at rest. Indeed, physical exertion, which will produce carbon dioxide, makes the victim feel better.

Primary Muscle Pain

Primary muscle pain includes some poorly understood disorders that have been called fibrositis, myalgia and neuralgia. The pain of these disorders tends to be chronic and ill-defined by the patient, is usually not related to exertion, and is confined to localized areas of the chest in locations that are different than what is seen with cardiac pain. The patient is usually more concerned about the significance of the symptoms, and whether it is a sign of heart disease, rather than the intensity of the pain.

Cancer

Cancer may originate or spread to any structure in the chest, including the heart, and cause chest pain. Such pain tends to be continuous and is not related to physical exertion. The diagnosis often may be made by a chest x-ray. Cancer also may spread to the spine and vertebrae with irritation of the nerve roots that go to the chest. Such pain may be quite severe and will not respond to the usual cardiac medications.

Abdominal Causes of Chest Pain

Perforation of a Peptic Ulcer

Bleeding from a peptic ulcer may cause lower chest pain, a rapid heart rate, low blood pressure, and even electrocardiographic changes. Thus, it erroneously might be interpreted as a heart attack. Massive bleeding from such an ulcer will be accompanied by black, tarry stools and be readily evident. However, if there has been low grade, chronic bleeding, the presence of blood in the stools will not be obvious. The only symptoms might be a discomfort that is mistakenly thought to be coming from the chest. The fact that the pain is related to food ingestion rather than exertion usually differentiates the two, but that distinction is not always clear.

Pancreatitis

Acute inflammation of the pancreas may cause severe pain that, although predominantly in the epigastrium, also radiates to the chest. Such pain is often accompanied by changes in the electrocardiogram. However, patients with pancreatitis usually have a history of alcoholism and gallbladder disease. In addition, unlike the pain of a heart attack, the pain of pancreatitis radiates to the back and can be partially relieved by leaning forward.

Gallbladder Disease

In the acute stage of a gallbladder attack, pain may be referred to the lower chest. The pain is often severe, steady in character, and may cause changes to appear in the electrocardiogram. Gallbladder colic may also trigger chest pain in someone with silent coronary artery disease. Chronic gallbladder disease may produce recurring lower chest and upper abdominal chest pain. Gallstones are readily identified with an abdominal ultrasound examination.

Splenic Flexure Syndrome

This is the term given to distension with gas of the part of the large intestine in the region of the spleen. Because the colon makes a 90 degree turn here, gas may get trapped, causing the colon to distend. Since this location is just beneath the diaphragm, the pain appears to be coming from the lower left chest. It may be distinguished from cardiac pain by its intermittent, colicky behavior, and fluctuations in intensity of the pain. Also, passage of flatus gives temporary relief.

Miscellaneous Conditions

Abnormal Fluid Retention

A variety of conditions may cause abnormal retention of fluid. It may increase the blood pressure and cause a secondary reduction of blood flow to the heart muscle by compression of the microcirculation within the muscle. This is due either to an increase in pressure within the cavity of the left ventricle that is transmitted to the muscular walls of the heart, or it may result from an increase in fluid within the muscle itself, causing an increase in tissue pressure (similar to the swelling that accompanies a local inflammation). One of the most common causes of fluid retention of this type is the use of NSAIDs (non-steroidal, anti-inflammatory drugs) containing ibuprofen or a similar acting compound. These drugs may cause profound fluid retention and can interfere with the flow of urine. The excess fluid usually lodges in the tissues of the body, and can cause a weight gain of several pounds. Because this fluid must enter the blood stream to reach the kidney, it can result in fluid overload and chest pain.

I recall one patient who came to see me for a second opinion because he had been advised to undergo coronary artery bypass surgery. Although his coronary artery disease had been stable for several years, in recent months his chest pain had become more frequent. The findings of his noninvasive examination suggested fluid overload. When I asked if he was taking any medication for pain or for arthritis, his eyes lit up and he replied, "Yes, I take six Advils a day." I told him to stop taking the Advil and to substitute plain aspirin. This he did, and his symptoms promptly disappeared.

In addition to NSAIDs, fluid retention may occur with a variety of urinary tract problems which interfere with the formation and excretion of urine. These include kidney or bladder infections, prostate infections in men and kidney failure. Many patients undergo unnecessary angiograms for chest pain with subsequent coronary artery bypass surgery or angioplasty for coincidental coronary artery disease, when all they really need are antibiotics for their prostatitis.

Fluid Retention

Intense stress may trigger a cascade of hormonal effects involving the pituitary gland, the adrenal gland and the kidney. The ultimate effect is the retention of water by the kidney followed by weight gain. The mechanism, in part, is similar to premenstrual edema. Interestingly, the fluid retention is not immediate but is delayed for 24 hours. If the stress is low grade and over a period of days, the weight gain is gradual and may go unnoticed unless the victim measures his or her weight on a daily basis. Intense stress may result in a weight gain of 5 to 10 lbs in 24 hours. Much of the fluid enters the circulatory system and can cause chest pain, as previously described. Fluid retention of this type can be eliminated and prevented with diuretics. Indeed, the diuretics may be used prophylactically in the anticipation of stress.

Anemia

Anemia is another unsuspected cause of chest pain. Anemia may have a variety of origins, and a discussion of these is beyond the scope of this book. A few of the more common causes, however, are bleeding from a peptic ulcer, a tumor or polyp in the colon, bleeding hemorrhoids, inadequate nutrition with lack of iron in the diet, pernicious anemia (a form of anemia due to a deficiency of vitamin B_{12}), and chronic kidney disease. If the blood count is low enough, it will produce cardiac symptoms such as palpitations and shortness of breath with exertion, chest pain and fatigue. A simple blood count can readily determine whether anemia is present.

Thyroid Disease

Either an underactive or an overactive thyroid can cause previously silent coronary artery disease to become symptomatic. An overactive thyroid, or hyperthyroidism, may result in chest pain because the heart is simply overworking. Typically the heart rate is in the nineties or low one-hundreds even at rest or while the victim is asleep. Silent coronary artery disease is usually present in such individuals and, by definition, is not symptomatic at normal heart rates. If there is enough narrowing of the coronary arteries, blood will not be able to get through at higher rates and chest pain will result. With hypothyroidism or an underactive thyroid, the heart rate will be very slow, and the function of the heart will be impaired enough so that pain may occur during exertion. In both of these thyroid disorders, the disease is easily corrected with appropriate medication.

Cigarette Smoking

There is hardly anyone who is not aware that smoking has serious side effects. That it can produce heart disease and cancer is now common knowledge. However, many people are not aware that smoking also may produce chest pain. Smoking increases the heart rate, blood pressure and work load upon the heart. If there is pre-existing coronary artery disease, but adequate blood flow at rest, the increased work produced by smoking, as well as the increase in concentration of carbon monoxide carried by the blood in place of oxygen, may be enough to produce chest pain.

Chest Pain Related to Miscellaneous Problems with Medications

Many patients with coronary artery disease can live a normal life on a medical program. They have little or no chest pain, and are not considered as subjects for angioplasty or coronary artery bypass surgery until their chest pain returns, or becomes more frequent or severe. The immediate concern voiced by the cardiologist is that their coronary artery disease is getting worse, and that an obstructed artery is getting ready to close off. Often the patient is literally frightened into having surgery. In fact, in the majority of instances, the recurrence or change in symptoms is rarely due to progression of the patient's underlying disease, but due to a problem with the patient's medication. A common problem is that the pharmacy where the patient purchases his or her medication substitutes a generic preparation for one of the patient's prescriptions, and this form may not be as readily absorbed from the gastrointestinal tract. At other times, the patient may have developed a tolerance to the medication he or she has been taking so that the drug is no longer effective. Also, some patients will arbitrarily reduce the dose of a given drug merely because they think they are taking too much medication.

Use of Diuretics

Another extremely common problem arises with the use of diuretics. When diuretics are initially used, the subject often will have to void a great deal. This is a real problem with many women who have had several children and who no longer have full bladder capacity. Going shopping and running errands are particularly difficult. Accordingly, they will only take their diuretic when they are overloaded with fluid. The result is that they are running to the bathroom all day long.

It is necessary to explain to these patients that the body takes up fluid like a sponge. If a sponge is filled with water, it doesn't take much squeezing to get a lot of water out of it; however, if it is dry, additional squeezing won't have an effect. The body works the same way. If it is overloaded, even one diuretic pill will get rid of a great deal of fluid. If they continue to take the diuretic, its effect will be diminished and the situation will be more tolerable.

Coincidental Illness

Another reason patients often arbitrarily reduce the amount of medication they are taking is when they develop a coincidental flu infection or gastrointestinal problem with diarrhea, and wrongly blame it on their medication. When they get better, they are convinced that it was the reduction in their medication that did it, rather than the coincidental and spontaneous improvement in their illness.

Finally, some patients take their medication too close to meals, and it interferes with the absorption of the drug. Accordingly, it is important that someone examine the patient's medical program to be sure it is correct.

Weight Gain and Deconditioning

Other factors that can produce symptoms and which may be misinterpreted as progression of the underlying coronary artery disease include: weight gain, deconditioning, inappropriate timing of exercise, and even weather changes. For a variety of reasons, at times patients with stable and silent coronary artery disease cease to exercise, and they may gain a significant amount of weight. Perhaps they are too busy, or they may have sustained an injury to their back or leg, or they merely may have been on vacation. Whatever the reason, weight gain invariably is accompanied by some deconditioning. When the patient finally decides to resume exercising, chest pain returns. Only through careful questioning and weighing of the patient at each visit can these explanations be uncovered.

Weather Changes

Another reason for the flare-up of chest pain is a change in the weather. Patients with coronary artery disease are much more apt to have pain in cold weather than in warm weather. In this case, merely dressing warmly or avoiding cold wind may be enough to eliminate the occurrence of chest pain.

Exercise Timing

Another cause of recurring pain is when patients decide to embark upon an exercise program, but do so not long after eating a meal. While few people would be foolish enough to vigorously exercise, many patients think a walk after dinner is acceptable. When they begin to have pain they become frightened. Advising patients to walk before dinner instead of after their meal may effectively stop the pain.

Alcohol

Finally, some patients drink too much. Often it is thought to be harmless, but close questioning may reveal that the patient is drinking as much as a half a bottle of wine with evening meals. Alcohol is toxic to the heart, and causes it to beat faster and harder. The alcohol may even produce irregular and ineffective heart beats. The heart's increased need for oxygen may be sufficient to produce chest pain. Cessation of the alcohol is all that is needed to eliminate chest pain.

CONCLUSION: MAKING THE CORRECT DIAGNOSIS

It is apparent that patients with coronary artery disease may develop symptoms for many reasons. While patient and doctor alike become concerned that the new onset of symptoms or a change in previous symptoms implies an impending catastrophe, numerous observations and studies have established that emergency action is rarely necessary, or even indicated. It has been my personal experience that a recent increase in the degree of coronary artery narrowing is hardly ever responsible for a change in the patient's symptoms. Consequently, a cardiologist's immediate response to rush the patient in for angiograms followed by angioplasty or coronary artery bypass surgery is totally inappropriate. Most of the time the cause of a flare-up in patient's symptoms can be determined by carefully asking the appropriate questions and performing an adequate examination. Too often that is not done, and the patient is scheduled for an array of high tech tests. And even when those tests are abnormal, there are typically no prior tests to compare them with. Accordingly, the cardiologist has no way of knowing whether the abnormality found on an echocardiogram, radioactive imaging study or angiogram is the direct cause of the patient's symptoms, or is coincidental and there is some other reason for the patient's complaints.

In our modern, hurry-up world where both patient and doctor expect immediate relief, the outcome is one in which the doctor urges the patient to undergo immediate surgery. Oftentimes the reason for such recommendations are more for the benefit of the doctor than the patient. While patients actually may have some temporary improvement in their symptoms after a surgical intervention, there are many reasons why a symptomatic patient may obtain relief that has nothing to do with the surgery or procedure performed. Thus, merely the fact that the patient feels better afterwards does not mean their surgery or angioplasty was needed. Later chapters will address why a patient may experience some relief of symptoms following an unnecessary intervention such as angioplasty or bypass surgery.

It may take a great deal of time to sort out all the possible reasons why someone may develop chest pain. It can take months to eliminate other diseases that may result in similar symptoms, or other diseases that cause previously silent coronary artery disease to become symptomatic. Even when obstructive coronary artery disease is the source of the patient's symptoms, it may still be weeks and even months before their chest pain is eliminated. Accordingly, it cannot be over-emphasized that you should never allow yourself to be rushed into the cardiac laboratory for emergency angiograms as a prelude for surgery. Nor should you ever accept the explanation that coronary angiograms are needed to determine the cause of your chest pain, or whether a heart attack is occurring, or how you should be treated. Angiograms cannot provide answers to these questions. However, a variety of noninvasive tests will readily provide such information. This will discussed more fully in later chapters.

Rarely, a patient may require emergency surgery because of a vascular accident. Examples include: rupture of a muscular wall of the heart, massive leakage of one of the valves of the heart, rupture of an artery and shock. Such catastrophic accidents can be readily diagnosed without angiograms. Knowledge of your disease, which tests are indicated, *which tests are not indicated*, and what your various treatment options are, will greatly increase your chances of receiving the best and safest treatment possible.

7

HEART FAILURE

Henry was only fifty years old when he had his heart attack. It had not begun with chest pain. In hindsight, he realized he had been extremely tired for the few weeks preceding the attack. Work had been stressful, and there had been family worries concerning his daughter's impending divorce and a son's continued battle with drugs. Financial problems were present as well, with a second son soon starting college and tuition so much more expensive these days...

The chest pain began at work. It started as a mild tightness across Henry's whole chest that gradually became more intense. Before long, it was present in his neck, jaw, and both arms. He was very sure he was having a heart attack. Trying not to panic, he asked one of his co-workers to take him to the nearest emergency room. Fortunately, a large hospital was close to where he worked. When he arrived at the emergency room, one look by the nurse of his ashen color and he was promptly ushered into a room and oxygen started. He was quickly examined by a doctor and given an injection of morphine. Before long the pain began to ease. Within a few minutes the EKG technician entered the room, took an electrocardiogram and handed it to the doctor. He studied it only briefly before saying, "You're having a heart attack. I'm going to send you to the catheterization laboratory for angiograms. We prefer to treat heart attack patients with angioplasty or coronary artery bypass surgery."

When Henry heard this, he recalled reading about a recent study from the Veterans Administration that compared aggressive interventional treatment with conservative medical treatment. The mortality rate with the aggressive treatment was three to four times higher than that of medical treatment. Henry also personally knew of a few of his friends who had undergone emergency bypass surgery when they had their heart attack. Neither one was doing very well. Indeed, one had nearly become an invalid. Now that his pain was subsiding and he felt less apprehensive, Henry didn't hesitate to say, "Doctor, I don't want to undergo these procedures. I prefer to be treated with medication." Although the doctor was obviously displeased, he had to abide by his patient's wishes.

Henry remained in the hospital for a week and seemed to recover without incident. He underwent an echocardiogram, which established that he had suffered a heart attack in the region of his ventricular septum. At the time of discharge, the cardiologist started him on a cholesterol lowering medication, aspirin and nitroglycerin tablets in case he had any more chest pain. He was also advised to go on an exercise program, but he really didn't have time for that. Was it Henry's imagination that when the cardiologist had learned of his refusal to undergo angioplasty, he no longer seemed interested in his welfare? Why else did he fail to have him come back for follow-up visits?

Henry's recovery over the next few months was uneventful. In the beginning, he did manage to walk at regular intervals, but he was too busy to keep it up. Since he wasn't having any chest pain, Henry soon slipped into the old way of doing things; however, he did see the cardiologist once or twice a year, and continued to take the medication he had been given.

Over the next few years Henry almost forgot that he had suffered a heart attack. He had no symptoms that he was aware of; but then, he rarely did anything physical. On the rare occasions that he did— for example, when he carried luggage at the airport— Henry experienced some shortness of breath, but he blamed that on being overweight and deconditioned.

Gradually, Henry began to note more fatigue with just ordinary physical activities. When he paid attention, it seemed he also was getting short of breath. He decided to check with the cardiologist, but learned that he had given up his practice and had moved to another area. A new cardiologist had taken his place and Henry agreed to make an appointment. The doctor did his examination, had him undergo an echocardiogram and a chest x-ray followed by a treadmill test. "You've gone into heart failure," the cardiologist told Henry. "Your heart has become very enlarged and you've developed some leakage of your mitral valve; that is, the intake valve on the left side between the left atrium and the left ventricle."

"Can it be treated?" asked Henry.

"Not very well", confessed the doctor. "Medicine will help for awhile and you're not too old for a heart transplant. I'm afraid the mortality rate is very high for this disease. As high as 50% in 3 to 5 years."

Henry was stunned. He tried to get more information, but the doctor seemed reluctant to elaborate. He was given some prescriptions and told to make an appointment with the dietician. He was also given an appointment to return in one month. Henry wondered if he would still be alive.

THE STORY OF SALLY

Sally was a 58-year-old widow. Except for her high blood pressure, she had always considered herself to be in good health. She did have a couple of kidney infections shortly after her second child, but hadn't had any symptoms for many years and she assumed her kidneys were healthy. The doctor always said her blood pressure was good for her age. On two occasions, she recalled her pressure was 155 and 160. When she asked if that was too high, the doctor said she was probably excited, and told her not to worry. After all, she was taking a calcium channel blocker and that was keeping it under control.

Typically Sally spent less than five minutes in her doctor's office, every three months. The nurse always took her blood pressure and the doctor listened to her heart for no more than 10-15 seconds. Sometimes, when he was busy and the waiting room was crowded, the doctor didn't even bother to listen to her heart. But this was South Florida, there were a lot of retired people, and this was an HMO. Sally felt it was all she could afford since her husband's death a few years before.

Of late, Sally had noticed some swelling of her ankles, and at times even her legs. She had asked the doctor about it but all he did was look at her legs and tell her she had varicose veins. If she wanted to get rid of the edema, the doctor said, she should elevate her legs. Then, the shortness of breath began.

At first it only occurred while she was asleep. It was so bad she had to get out of bed and sit in a chair. After 10-20 minutes it would subside and she could go back to bed. Some nights this didn't happen, particularly if she had only eaten a light supper. Then she began to notice it with walking and climbing the one flight of stairs to her apartment. Now she began to worry. One night the shortness of breath was so bad that she had to call her neighbor. One look at Sally and her neighbor promptly called the paramedics. Shortly thereafter, Sally was being seen by the emergency room doctor. The next thing she knew she had been admitted to the hospital and was given an injection in her arm along with several other medications intravenously.

The following morning Sally felt considerably better. Before long a doctor came by and asked a lot of questions. Finally he explained that she had gone into heart failure. "Did I have a heart attack?" asked Sally.

"No," said the doctor. "But your blood pressure was very high and your heart is quite enlarged. It must have been elevated for a long time for your heart to have become so enlarged."

Sally remained in the hospital for the next week and was discharged on three medications, none of which were a calcium channel blocker. The doctor had arranged for her to come back to the hypertension clinic at the hospital at regular intervals. He assured her that her blood pressure problem would be taken care of much better than it had been. They would use her as part of a research study on a new drug, and it would not cost her anything. That was good for Sally— the doctor had not told her that her life would be considerably shortened because of her heart failure. She might only live a few more years. Nor did he tell her that the complications of her hypertension all could have been prevented had she been on an adequate medical program from the beginning.

WHAT WENT WRONG?

In spite of the fact that both Henry and Sally had two entirely different diseases, both eventually developed heart failure for the same reason. It was not because their doctors failed to make a correct diagnosis. Henry clearly had obstructive coronary artery disease complicated by a heart attack, while

Sally had hypertension. In both cases, the doctors failed to start and maintain their patients on an adequate medical program because neither one had symptoms until shortly before their hospitalization. If Henry were having recurring chest pain with exertion and Sally severe headaches, they both would have received more medication for relief of their symptoms, and this might have been sufficient to delay or prevent the development of their heart failure.

Patients with obstructive coronary artery disease require four and often five drugs, particularly if there is evidence of impaired blood flow to the heart muscle. Hypertensive patients usually require at least two and often three drugs to adequately control their blood pressure. Failure to prescribe the appropriate amount of medication indicates a lack of understanding by the doctor of the long-range complications of the disease he or she is treating. Even if the patient belongs to an HMO where undertreatment is a way of life, there are certain basic drugs that must be prescribed if heart failure is to be avoided. Obviously such drugs are not being utilized because, aside from heart attack, heart failure is the most common diagnosis listed at discharge from hospitals. Over 400,000 of such cases are listed each year. Approximately half are readmitted within the three to six months following discharge. In part this is because heart failure often is a terminal diagnosis; however, it is also because most heart failure patients are undertreated. Numerous studies have established this fact beyond any doubt. One report from the University of Michigan evaluated the medical program of 65 patients who were referred because they had not responded to medical treatment. The study found that 54 patients (83%) were rendered chest pain free after more aggressive medical therapy.[1]

WHY PATIENTS WITH CONGESTIVE HEART FAILURE ARE UNDERTREATED

When an individual first develops symptoms of heart disease, doctors naturally focus their attention on the immediate relief of those symptoms and the avoidance of any impending catastrophic event. This is as it should be. Sadly, most of these doctors then fail to treat the patient for the long-range complications of their disease. Indeed, this is one of the major weaknesses of modern medicine. Doctors are trained to practice a reactive type of medicine, and they wait until their patients develop symptoms before treatment is started. This is like waiting until the house has nearly burned to the ground before calling the fire department. By the time symptoms do appear, it is usually too late. This is why both Henry and Sally had so much trouble when their heart failure finally occurred. Unfortunately, once heart failure develops and the heart loses its elasticity, it cannot be recovered. Accordingly, it would be wise for every patient with a heart condition to know what the long range complications of his or her disease are, how and why they occur and what can be done to avoid those complications.

Heart failure is the end result of all heart diseases that are either improperly treated, or for which no treatment is available. In order for heart failure to develop, heart function must be severely compromised over an extended period of time. It does not matter whether the original disease is a heart attack with extensive damage to the heart muscle, a damaged valve that reduces the output of the heart, severe hypertension with cardiac enlargement, or inflammation of the heart muscle from a viral infection. Whatever the reason, the result is the same: the heart is unable to pump an adequate amount of blood. Since it is easier for a large heart to pump a small amount of blood than a small heart to pump a large amount of blood, the heart attempts to adapt or compensate by enlarging. This may be successful for a period of years. Eventually, however, the heart over-compensates, converting the adaptive response to a maladaptive one by becoming so enlarged and stretched out that there is a loss of elasticity and a weakening of the muscle. When the heart fails to pump an adequate amount of blood to meet the needs of the body, heart failure is present.

Typically, in the early stages of the various diseases that lead to heart failure, the heart adapts quite well through several mechanisms. One mechanism is an increase in heart rate. Normally the heart rate increases whenever we exert ourselves. Unless the exertion we undertake is quite strenuous, the increase in rate is not likely to be more than 5 to 10 beats per minute, and it returns to a resting rate of 60-75 bpm within a few minutes. A clue that the heart has already begun to make adaptive changes is when the resting heart rate does not return to normal, but continues to beat in the

80-90 bpm range. At this rate, there is less time for the ventricle to fill with fresh blood from the left atrium during the relaxation phase of the cardiac cycle, and some blood will remain in the atrium. At the next cardiac cycle, the situation still exists, and so even more blood remains in the left atrium. Eventually, the pressure within the atrium begins to increase as it becomes engorged, forcing it to stretch and dilate.

Fortunately, when the atrium is stretched, it starts to function like a rubber band: the greater the stretch, the greater the elastic recoil. Now all that blood is forced into the left ventricle under pressure. In the same way that a balloon will expand when the pressure inside is increased by blowing air into it, so will the ventricle expand and become larger. For a while, this enlargement will actually make it easier for the heart to function. Unfortunately, the larger the heart becomes, the more energy it requires. Eventually, unless something is done to correct the problem, the heart will fail completely. It will no longer be able to pump blood, blood will back up into the lungs and the victim will die.

How quickly do these events take place? First, it depends upon the underlying disease and how that disease is usually treated. If it is a valve problem, death might take anywhere from 10 to 50 years. What happens to the patient will largely depend upon how much elasticity has been lost during the adaptive process, and how large the heart becomes. If it is not too enlarged and the elasticity has been preserved, then the valve can be replaced or repaired, and a great deal of recovery is possible. Valves tend not to be a problem. There are well-defined criteria for deciding when a valve should be operated upon, and surgeons do a splendid job here and valve replacements are quite good. Today, valve repair is often carried out at the first onset of symptoms, and sometimes even before.

In contrast, if the causative problem is obstructive coronary artery disease that leads to a heart attack, how long it takes for the heart to fail will depend upon the amount of damage suffered by the patient, and the function of the remainder of the heart. If the area of the heart that is destroyed is not too large and the remainder of the heart is healthy, heart failure may take many years to develop. However, if the rest of the heart has already suffered damage from previous heart attacks, even a small amount of damage may be "the straw that breaks the camel's back." In these cases, heart failure may develop in minutes, hours or days.

Can the doctor determine whether heart failure is about to take place or is already present? Most well-trained doctors who perform a careful cardiac examination can usually tell if there is obvious heart failure. Careful questioning of the patient for the presence of exertional fatigue, shortness of breath with less than ordinary activities, a history of awakening with shortness of breath in the middle of the night, swelling of the ankles or legs, a cough, or abdominal discomfort from engorgement of the liver, will alert the astute doctor that heart failure may be present. The findings on a careful physical examination will confirm that heart failure is present. On the other hand, a doctor who performs a hasty examination and does not question the patient carefully will often fail to come up with the proper diagnosis. While the diagnosis will be easy if the patient provides a litany of symptoms that even a medical student will recognize, all too often patients do not volunteer their symptoms unless they are closely questioned.

While obvious congestive heart failure can be readily diagnosed, the detection of impending heart failure is another matter entirely. Even highly skilled cardiologists may not be able to accomplish this task unless they have the proper diagnostic equipment. Yet, sometimes simple measurements may provide a clue. By carefully and regularly weighing every patient at every visit, the experienced doctor will recognize a weight gain of several pounds that is not from overeating, but from fluid retention (heart failure patients do not have good appetites). There are also ways of detecting impending heart failure, but a description of them is too technical for this context. Nonetheless, it can be done, and the benefits are enormous. An analogy would be as follows: If you wished to fill a 10 foot high, open tank with water, but if there were no way to determine the water level in the tank, then you would not be aware that it was going overflow even moments before it did so. And when it overflowed, there would be quite a mess to clean up. The same thing can happen to patients with severe heart disease and incipient heart failure, literally. The "mess" in this case might be sudden death.

Both with the water tank and the heart failure patient, prevention is the key to successful recovery. I remember a patient who was admitted to the hospital because of chest pain. When I first saw him, he was sitting up in bed and appeared to be in no distress. He was breathing normally and his color was good. As I was asking questions about his symptoms, I noted he was becoming breathless. Literally, within the next few minutes, his lungs began to fill with fluid as his heart failed. He was experiencing pulmonary edema. Fortunately, I was able to inject digitalis, morphine and amino-phylline intravenously from the emergency tray just outside of his room. In the space of a few minutes his breathing returned to normal and his pulmonary edema disappeared.

What can be done to correct the problems of neglecting to diagnose an impending catastrophe, and the chronic undertreatment that forces the patient and his or her disease into this situation? It would be too much to hope that every doctor would have the necessary diagnostic equipment in his or her office, and be skilled at using it. However, there is nothing to prevent the patient or a member of the family from asking for more sensitive diagnostic testing at regular intervals. Examination with a traditional stethoscope and EKG is almost useless in this situation. Merely talking with the patient to determine whether his or her symptoms are better or worse will certainly provide more information than these obsolete methods.

An even better way to determine whether proper treatment is being administered is for every patient to know which drugs are recommended for this condition. At the very least, heart failure patients should be on *adequate* doses of a beta blocker, a diuretic, an ACE inhibitor, aspirin, and nitrates to dilate the coronary arteries. These drugs will be discussed in more detail in a later chapter. Accordingly, if a heart failure patient is receiving only one or two of these medications, then the treating doctor must be told that he or she is not following recommended guidelines. Particularly in HMOs where the available drugs are restricted by a formulary or where doctors must pay for some of the medications themselves if they go over the budget allowance for each patient, a heart failure patient may be grossly undertreated. The doctor might use the excuse that additional medication will cause side effects, but this explanation is unacceptable. All medications have side effects with excessive dosage, but when properly used they may save lives. Besides, the side effects of not using the appropriate medications may be more dangerous— e.g, sudden death— than the temporary discomfort of a drug's side effect. As long as the patient and his or her family are unaware of these facts, the patient will remain undertreated.

WHY PATIENTS WITH SEVERE DISEASE OFTEN DO NOT HAVE SYMPTOMS

One of the more serious consequences of long-standing coronary artery disease is the gradual limitation on the part of the patient of activities that produce symptoms. When elderly Mr. Lewis is asked whether he is short of breath, he will truthfully answer that he is not. But then, he has learned not to do those tasks that make him short of breath. He might add that if he does too much, he will get tired. However, he is old and is "supposed" to get tired. At least, that is what both he and his doctor think. In general, though, Mr. Lewis feels just fine. On examination, there are usually no loud heart murmurs to remind the doctor that the patient's disease is getting worse. The few abnormalities that are present will not be heard by 75-80% of doctors.[1] Accordingly, both doctor and patient are lulled into a false sense of security and do not recognize the impending disaster. Indeed, at least two-thirds of the 4,400 patients who have heart attacks or die every day were recently seen by a doctor and told they were doing well.

This typical scenario is acted out many times over a period of years. If the doctor merely took the patient for a walk up one flight of stairs, he or she would quickly discover how sick the patient was. Or if the doctor spent some time with members of the family, they would be able to provide the doctor with more information than any routine test is able to provide. Unfortunately, when the doctor is seeing 30-40 patients a day, there is little time to ask about such details. Not until the patient is on the verge of dying, and often does, will the doctor finally recognize the situation. Unfortunately, by the time patients like Mr. Lewis are treated, it is often too late.

Another reason why patients with coronary artery disease so often develop heart failure is because of the current fashion of urging all patients with coronary artery disease to undergo coronary artery bypass surgery or angioplasty immediately, even in the absence of symptoms. Doctors who recommend, urge or frighten patients into one of these procedures, usually for economic reasons, seem to have limited familiarity with the success of using drugs to medically treat coronary artery disease. Consequently, these doctors commonly fail to place the patient on a full medical program to prevent the long-range consequences of their disease. The surgical interventions are only quick fixes for treating a complicated disease, and do not solve the basic problem of reduced blood flow. Numerous studies have shown that either blood flow is not restored to ischemic muscle by surgery or, if it is, it is only partially restored. At the same time, bypass surgery and angioplasty accelerate the progression of the very disease that they are supposed to treat.

A remarkably large number of cardiologists and surgeons think that coronary artery bypass surgery and angioplasty are definitive treatments, and that nothing further needs to be done. Typically, a patient who has been advised to undergo one of these procedures will not be on any medical program before the intervention and afterward they are usually prescribed medications that are completely inadequate in both the drugs given and the dosage. These surgical enthusiasts rarely attempt to address the issue of treatment of basic coronary artery disease and its complications. It should come as no surprise, therefore, that the patient's disease will progress, and that relief of symptoms is, at best, only temporary for the majority of individuals, and that heart failure may be the ultimate consequence.

Heart failure will continue to develop in the undertreated patient as well as in those overtreated with surgery or angioplasty, if they are not placed upon an appropriate medical program. This situation will persist until patients with heart disease assume more responsibility for their own treatment, they learn what medications and dosages are needed, and they understand why they are necessary. Most patients probably give their cars more attention than their disease. This must change.

REFERENCES

1. Grambow DW, Topol EJ. Effect of maximal medical therapy on refractoriness of unstable angina pectoris. Am J Cardiol 1992; 70:577-581.

8

WOMEN AND HEART DISEASE: IT ISN'T NEW

Each year, over 100,000 women die prematurely from cardiovascular disease. It is the leading cause of death for females. One out of every five women have heart disease, and half of all women above the age of 65 and 80% above age 75 have hypertension. In 1993, the last year for which figures are available, the mortality from cardiovascular disease was 500,387 for women, as compared to 447,211 for men. In contrast, breast cancer claims about 43,000 lives a year, while lung cancer claims about 56,000 women. Many women have their heart disease for years before it is recognized. Even then, they are not treated in the same way that men are treated. The following true story illustrates many of the problems regarding heart disease in women.

LORETTA'S STORY

Loretta Saunders well understood the meaning of "stress." A 36-year-old trial attorney who worked for a law firm with 75 other lawyers, Loretta had started out as a legal secretary, worked her way up to a paralegal, and finally was able to attend and finish law school. She had joined the firm five years before, and found herself overwhelmed with work from the start. She and her husband, also an attorney in the same firm, had started their family after she finished law school, and now they had two daughters, ages three and five. Trying to raise a family and keep up with her practice seemed impossible at times.

Because her husband was constantly travelling, Loretta wasn't always able to depend upon him for help. Most of the time, the responsibility for taking the children to and from school and day-care fell to Loretta. It was hardest in the mornings when she had to be in court early and her husband was away on a trip. Too many times, Loretta was ready to leave the house, only to discover that her three-year-old, who was not completely toilet-trained, had soiled her pants and had to be changed. And then there was the housework, shopping and meal preparation. As a woman, she was expected to "do it all." Although Loretta and her husband had tried to get a live-in housekeeper, it hadn't worked out.

Two years before, Loretta had started to smoke again. And after her second child, Loretta began taking birth control pills; they simply could not afford for her to become pregnant again. She had heard it might not be such a good idea to take the pill and continue to smoke, but she couldn't quit smoking now. The work load at the office continued to grow and the pressure just never let up. The firm's income had dropped in the past two years, and they couldn't afford to hire any new attorneys.

Then, the chest pains started. They did not last long at first, and Loretta wasn't worried, but since it was time for her annual physical examination she mentioned them to her internist anyway. He asked her a few questions and performed an electrocardiogram, an exam that creates a record of the electrical impulses that cause the heart to beat. At the end of the examination, her doctor reassured her it was not her heart. He explained that if there been hand been any damage to her heart it would have shown up on the electrocardiogram; but the test had been perfectly normal. Therefore, he said, these were not cardiac pains. Yet, the doctor was unable to explain why the chest pains occurred.

Unfortunately the pains continued, growing more frequent and prolonged. At first, Loretta noticed them only when she was climbing the stairs to the house, carrying in the groceries. Then she began to notice them during her lunch-time exercise class. Finally she began to get them in court, during difficult cases. Sometimes the pain lasted for hours.

Loretta began to worry. Her mother had developed high blood pressure when she was only 40, had a heart attack at 48, and died at 52, a few months after bypass surgery. Loretta also had a cousin who had died suddenly at the age of 49. She decided to make an appointment with a cardiologist.

The cardiologist listened to her story, briefly examined her, and had her return the following day for a stress thallium study. To Loretta's great relief, the study showed negative. She was surprised when the doctor said she would have to undergo an angiogram. He explained that stress imaging procedures with radioactive substances were not as sensitive as desired, especially for women. Reluctantly, Loretta agreed to have the angiogram.

The angiogram was performed the next day without complications. To her great relief, it, too, was negative. She was informed that her coronary arteries were normal, and that there was nothing wrong with her heart. Loretta was told that in all probability the pain was coming from her chest wall and was muscular in origin. She was not given any medicine.

When Loretta returned to work, the stress level was even greater than before. Cases, depositions and meetings, which had been put on hold while she was seeing the doctors, had piled up. But instead of disappearing, the chest pains increased and were of greater intensity. One day in court during a particularly stressful trial, Loretta was unable to continue because of the pain. She asked to be taken to an emergency room.

Once Loretta arrived she was quickly given medication for the pain while a technician did an electrocardiogram. When the emergency room doctor saw her hospital records, which showed that the results of her recent angiogram were negative, he became very flippant. The electrocardiogram that had just been taken was also considered normal. The doctor told Loretta her pain was psychosomatic and stress-induced, gave her a prescription for a tranquilizer, and sent her home. Now Loretta thought she was losing her mind. Could the pains really be psychosomatic?

And still the chest pains grew more severe. Sometimes it seemed as if the pain were present all day long. One night she had a nightmare and awoke in a sweat, and the pain was so intense that it felt as if someone were sitting on her chest. Fortunately her husband was home and took her to the emergency room immediately. This time, Loretta decided to go to another hospital.

When Loretta arrived at the hospital, another cardiologist was called. Loretta told this doctor nothing about her previous angiogram. The doctor took her electrocardiogram and seemed surprised that it was normal. He had blood tests taken and found that her enzymes also were normal. He still didn't seem satisfied, and said he was going to personally do an echocardiogram on her. But first he decided to check her blood pressure, both at rest and then during stress.

Loretta's resting blood pressure was 140/85; the upper limit of normal. Then the cardiologist had her squeeze what he called a hand gripper for a full minute and he took her blood pressure while she was still squeezing. She was shocked to find out that in less than a minute, her blood pressure had increased to 230/125. The doctor went on to do the echocardiogram, and she repeated the squeeze test while he watched the motion of the heart walls. "There it is!" he exclaimed, "Your entire ventricular septum stopped moving while you were squeezing. Although there is no evidence that you've had a heart attack yet, I'm going to admit you to the coronary care unit for observation." Loretta was relieved. Someone had finally found a real cause for her symptoms.

The following morning the cardiologist came to her bedside. "I checked your electrocardiogram this morning, and it shows that you have had what we call a non-Q wave heart attack. You were lucky. The medications I put you on provided you with protection. Without them you might have died. But you will have to give up smoking and birth control pills, because you also have hypertension."

The rest of Loretta's hospital stay was uneventful. She started taking medication for her blood pressure and her heart condition, and she had no further symptoms. She felt more relaxed about everything, and the stress didn't seem so bad. When she mentioned this to her doctor, he said it was because the effects of the stress were being buffered by the beta blocker medication she was taking. In addition, her blood pressure no longer rose precipitously when she was under stress.

IS HEART DISEASE DIFFERENT IN WOMEN?

Women are different from men. They think, react, behave and even have heart disease differently. They don't even get heart disease at the same age that men do —they get it 10 years later, and when they get it, it affects them differently, too. Being older, they are more likely to have hypertension, diabetes, impaired cardiac function and congestive heart failure.[1]

Not surprisingly, women's cumulative in-hospital and three-year mortality rates are significantly higher than men's. Even in the absence of a heart attack, they have a greater chance of dying than do men. Among women who have heart attacks, 44% die within one year compared to only 27% of men. Older women are twice as likely to die within a few weeks of a heart attack, as compared to men.[2,3]

For most men (60%), the initial manifestation of coronary artery disease is a heart attack. In contrast, the initial symptom in 80% of women who develop the disease is angina pectoris. Unfortunately, such chest pain is not acknowledged as angina in most of its victims.[4] Heart attacks also go unrecognized more often for women. While one out of four heart attacks go undiscovered in men, one out of three go undetected in women.[5]

Even a doctor's reaction to a women with chest pain is not the same as it would be if she were a man, nor is the way he would treat her. Often a doctor will ignore chest pain in women because it is not typical, or worse, will misdiagnose it as a symptom of depression or anxiety.[5]

Had Loretta been a man, her thallium stress test would have been abnormal, and obstructive coronary artery disease would, almost certainly, have been found on the angiograms. Angioplasty or coronary artery bypass surgery would have been recommended immediately. In contrast, up until relatively recently, the general attitude of the medical profession toward women getting heart disease was that it was quite rare, particularly below the age of 50 to 60 years old. There were several reasons for this sexist view. For one thing, it was believed to be uncommon. In addition, women seemed to have a different kind of pain than men. Doctors had traditionally been taught that angina pectoris was a heavy, squeezing, tightness in the middle of the chest that occurred only during exertion, and that it disappeared within a few minutes with rest. In contrast, women often would have their pain over their left breast, and instead of fading away with rest, it might last 30 minutes or several hours. Or they might only have their pain while asleep, or following stress. Doctors call this atypical chest pain.

In time, doctors came to recognize that the onset of symptoms of coronary artery disease typically begins with a heart attack in men, but with angina pectoris in women. Even with that information, women had long since muddied the waters by frequent episodes of noncardiac chest pain. It was common knowledge among all doctors who saw a large quota of females in their practice that noncardiac chest pain was a very prevalent symptom. Often such patients were anxious, tense, sometimes hysterical, and had many other complaints in addition to their chest pain. Usually their pain was atypical, occurring both at rest and during physical exertion, and almost always was accompanied by a normal electrocardiogram and chest x-ray. These women were usually told their symptoms were psychosomatic or muscular, and they were often given a tranquilizer. Since these female patients never died or had a heart attack, the doctor's opinion that only elderly women had heart attacks was reinforced. So imbedded were the views that younger women simply did not get heart disease, that when a patient with chest pain underwent a stress electrocardiogram, and it turned out to be abnormal, the information was discarded, and the test declared to be a false positive! This view was supported by the findings of normal angiograms in many such patients on whom this test was done.

I still remember the shock I experienced shortly after I started practice when a 41-year-old lady came to me because she had been having pain over a circumscribed area about the size of a quarter just beneath her left breast. It had been present for several hours. Because this lady did not look sick and because I had been taught that a common pain like this was never cardiac in origin, I was prepared to do no studies and simply give her a pain reliever. But it was the intensity of the pain that got my attention, and so I ordered an electrocardiogram. I was dumbfounded when the tracing showed that she had just had an acute heart attack!

Eventually, doctors became curious about these patients with atypical chest pain, normal electrocardiograms, abnormal stress tests, and normal angiograms, and they began to study them more carefully. Cardiac catheters were placed in the coronary sinus. This is reservoir-like area on the surface of the heart where coronary venous blood returns. Analysis of this blood following exercise revealed that it contained high concentrations of lactic acid, a substance that forms when there is a deficiency of blood flow to the heart muscle. In other words, it provides chemical proof that the heart muscle had become ischemic. This meant that the abnormal stress tests these patients had were not false positives but were truly positives. The term microvascular angina was applied to these women with chest pain and normal coronary arteries. No explanation was offered as to why they were having chest pain. Now, of course, we know that when someone has an increase in their blood pressure, that pressure is transmitted back to the cavity of the left ventricle. Such a rapid increase in pressure should cause the heart's chamber to expand like a balloon. Fortunately, it does not; it is protected by the thickness of the heart muscle and the pericardium. In much the same way that an inflated blood pressure cuff around one's arm transmits the pressure from the cuff to the tissues of the arm, causing the brachial artery to collapse, so does the increased pressure within the heart muscle cause the tiny, thin-walled arteries that nourish the muscle to collapse. In other words, when the blood pressure goes up, the microcirculation shuts down, the heart is deprived of oxygen, and chest pain occurs.

These studies played an important role in changing the way doctors thought about their female patients with chest pain. But something else happened that changed the rules. Women became liberated, or at least, partially so. In the past 25 years, women have appeared where none have gone before: at West Point, Annapolis and the Air Force; as astronauts, CEOs and business owners. There are more women attorneys and doctors than ever before. In short, women are being subjected to the same kind of job stresses that men have, but there is a difference. Most men still expect their wives to be the homemaker, even if the wives have a 40 to 50 hour-a-week job themselves.

In the past, women were always expected to make the meals, clean the house, do the laundry and shopping, and get the kids ready for school. Sounds stressful, doesn't it? Well, perhaps not the same kind of stress they have to face today. You see, doing all that homemaking years ago was truly hard work, especially without modern conveniences. But Mom wasn't also worried about being fired or laid off.

Where does all of this leave us in relation to heart disease? The stress level has increased enormously for women. And what do we know about stress? It is a major risk factor for heart disease. Stress increases the production of cortisol and this, in turn, increases the heart rate and blood pressure. This can cause more damage to the circulatory system and heart than any other risk factor. It can bring about hypertension, heart attacks, or sudden death, and it is responsible for major acceleration of coronary artery disease. The women of today are locked into what has happened to most families in our society; that is, both spouses must work, simply to make ends meet.

Clearly, women have increased their risk of developing heart disease with some special twists. Stress will produce menstrual irregularities in many women. If it is great enough, actual ovarian impairment will occur with psychogenic amenorrhea, i.e., their menstrual periods will simply stop. Population studies have shown that women with menstrual irregularities have a higher risk of coronary heart disease. Those with psychogenic amenorrhea produce increased amounts of cortisol which, as I have already indicated, causes the heart rate and blood pressure to increase. Animal experiments done on monkeys with stress-induced ovarian impairment have shown an increased development of arteriosclerotic plaque. However, it was observed that the administration of oral contraceptives reversed that tendency.[6]

While this seems to imply that taking modern oral contraceptives is perfectly safe, this is not actually the case for women who smoke. Research has shown that women who smoke and take oral contraceptives have a 40 times greater risk of heart disease than a woman who neither smokes nor takes birth control pills. Smoking enormously increases the risk of cardiovascular disease, and this may have been the reason that Loretta got into trouble. Fifty percent of the heart attacks in middle-aged women are attributable to tobacco. In addition, hysterectomy and especially oophorectomy (removal of one or both ovaries) are also associated with early heart disease. For this reason, gynecologists of today will make every effort to preserve a woman's ovaries when they are removing her uterus. Unfortunately, the blood supply of the ovaries may be damaged in the process creating an early menopause.

Many doctors are still not prepared for the fact that now women are experiencing their hypertension, angina and heart attacks in their thirties and forties, and that heart disease is the leading cause of death in women. The shocking fact is that *commonly* neither hypertension nor angina in women are recognized. Recall the chapter on hypertension where I pointed out that resting blood pressure may be normal for years, but under stress there may be a striking elevation, often to values in excess of 200 mm Hg. If the blood pressure is never checked under stress, neither the doctor nor the patient will be aware of its existence. As far as angina is concerned, in women it masquerades as atypical chest pain with a normal electrocardiogram. Even today, when the stress test is abnormal, all too often it is assumed to be a false positive. As I indicated earlier, one-third of heart attacks in women go unrecognized only to be discovered accidentally when an electrocardiogram is taken. The bottom line is a stunner: in 63% of the women who died suddenly from coronary heart disease, there was no previous evidence of disease.

There are multitude reasons why coronary artery disease may go undetected in women, some of which I have already touched upon such as the frequent presence of a normal electrocardiogram. Both stress imaging with radioactive thallium and echocardiography are compromised by breast tissue in women. This also interferes with coronary angiograms. In young women this is not a problem; however, women who are young are not apt to get coronary artery disease. But many older women have considerable breast tissue from the combined effects of both nursing and weight gain. Even doing angiograms is complicated because women are more likely to experience kidney and vascular complications from the x-ray opaque dye that is injected into the coronary arteries. Thus, the diagnosis of coronary artery disease is less than perfect for women.

Women also differ in how they can be treated and in their responses to treatment. Unlike men, women can easily be given estrogens after they reach the menopause. Over 30 studies have been carried out showing that estrogen replacement therapy will reduce the risk of coronary artery disease to nearly half of those without such therapy,[7] and death by one-third.[8,9] While in men the daily administration of aspirin has been shown to reduce the likelihood of future heart disease, no such proof has been established in women. Similarly, there is no evidence that lowering cholesterol reduces the risk of heart disease in women.[10,11]

Women also respond differently to surgical treatment of their heart disease than do men. Women who undergo coronary angioplasty are older, more likely to have hypertension, diabetes, congestive heart failure and other severe noncardiac diseases. They have more complications, including acute closure of a coronary artery and death.[12] With coronary artery bypass surgery, the mortality of women is higher than men, in some studies it is even two to four times as great.[13-15] They are more likely to experience complications such as heart attack, congestive heart failure and death. The reasons are thought to be smaller body size and coronary artery diameter, older age and the presence of other diseases.

It is high time that the medical discrimination against women stop. It is based not only on the ignorance of doctors but also on the lack of information among women. The diagnosis of coronary heart disease can be readily made in women, even if it is a little harder to do so. All that is required is awareness on the part of both patient and doctor that more effort will be involved in uncovering the source of the symptoms. The good news for women is that medically they can be treated more effectively than men. The remarkable benefit of estrogen replacement therapy is equal to or better than any of the drugs conventionally used in males. Unfortunately, such therapy cannot be practically used in men. Women should refuse treatments like angioplasty and coronary artery bypass surgery if they are offered as initial treatment, because of the poor response women have to these interventions. These treatments should be reserved for women who fail to respond to medical treatment. In my experience, such failures are rare.

Women who are under a great deal of stress should take special precautions to be on guard against the development of coronary heart disease. This is particularly true for those who have other risk factors, such as a family history of heart disease or hypertension. Smoking should be forbidden, and exercise should be part of the daily activities. Many studies have now established that the less exercise a woman engages in after the menopause, the greater her mortality from all diseases.[16-18] Consequently, regular exercise should be started as early as possible. Women deserve better treatment than they are getting. Perhaps the information in this chapter will help us reach that goal.

REFERENCES

1. Fiebach NJ, Viscoli CM, Horwitz RI. Differences between women and men in survival after myocardial infarction. Biology or methodology? JAMA 1990; 263:1092-1096.

2. Bush TL. Evidence for primary and secondary prevention of coronary artery disease in women taking estrogen replacement therapy. Eur Heart J 1996; 17:9-14.

3. Sonke GS, Beaglehole R, Stewart AW, *et al.* Sex differences in case fatality before and after admission to hospital after acute cardiac events: analysis of community based coronary heart disease register. BMJ 1996; 313:853-855.

4. Reunanen A, Suhonen O, Aromaa A, *et al.* Incidence of different manifestations of coronary heart disease in middle-aged Finnish men and women. Acta Med Scan 1985; 218:19-26.

5. Heart disease in women: How high is your risk? The Planned Parenthood Health Letter 1995; 2(3).

6. Kaplan, J. Vessel disease reduced in monkeys given oral contraceptives. Abstract #3007. Presented at the American Heart Association 68th Annual Scientific Sessions at Anaheim, California, November 15, 1995.

7. Sampfer MJ, Colditz GA, Willett WC, *et al.* Postmenopausal estrogen therapy and cardiovascular disease. Ten year followup from the Nurses Health Study. N Engl J Med 1991; 325:756.

8. Grady D, Rubin SN, Pettitti DB, *et al.* Hormone therapy to prevent disease and prolong life in post menopausal women. Ann Int Med 1992; 117:1016.

9. Sampfer MJ, Colditz GA. Estrogen replacement therapy and coronary heart disease. Prev Med 1991; 20:47.

10. Barrett-Conner E. Hypercholesterolemia predicts early death from coronary heart disease in elderly men but not women. The Rancho Bernardo Study. Ann Epidemiol 1992; 2:77-83.

11. Edmond MJ, Zareba W. Prognostic value of cholesterol in women of different ages. J Womens Health 1997; 6:295-307.

12. Keelan ET, Nunez BD, Grill DE, *et al.* Comparison of immediate and long term outcome of coronary angioplasty performed for unstable angina and rest pain in men and women. Mayo Clin Proc 1997; 72:5-12.

13. Farrer M, Skinner JS, Albers CJ. Outcome after coronary artery surgery in women and men in the north of England. QJM 1997; 90:203-211.

14. Simchen E, Israeli A, Merin G, *et al.* Israeli women were at a higher risk than men for mortality following coronary bypass surgery. Eur J Epidemiol 1997; 13:503-509.

15. Risum O, Abdelnoor M, Nitter-Hauge S, *et al.* Coronary artery bypass surgery in women and men; early and long-term results. A study of the Norwegian population adjusted by age and sex. Eur J Cardiothorac Surg 1997; 11:539-546.

16. Kushi LH, Fee RM, Folsom AR, *et al.* Physical activity and mortality in postmenopausal women. JAMA 1997, 277:1287-1292.

17. Eaton CB, Lapane KL, Garber CA, *et al.* Med Sci Sports Exerc 1995; 27:1535-1539.

18. Folsom AR, Arnett DK, Hutchinson RG, *et al.* Med Sci Sports Exerc 1997; 29:901-909.

Part II:
The Diagnosis & Treatment of Heart Disease

9

DIAGNOSING HEART DISEASE
THE MODERN WAY

U p until 1958, if someone were unfortunate enough to have obstructive coronary artery disease, there were only three ways to diagnose its presence. The first way depended upon the existence of symptoms. Mere chest pain was not enough. As discussed in Chapter 6, there are over 50 different medical conditions that will cause recurring chest pain. Accordingly, prior to 1958, for a doctor to be certain that his patient's chest pain was cardiac in origin, the pains must have had distinctive characteristics. It must have been brought on by specific triggers such as exertion, emotional stress, a cold wind, or physical activity shortly after eating. It must have been located in the center of the chest over an area about the size of one's hand; it must have come on gradually and become progressively worse if the activity was not stopped. And then, it must have disappeared within a few minutes of stopping the stress. Also, the quality of the pain must have been quite typical. For example, it couldn't have been a sharp shooting pain lasting only a second or two, nor could it have been a gas-like colicky pain that came and went. It had to be described as a steady heaviness, a tightness or a full feeling in the chest. The patient would describe more severe discomfort as feeling as if his or her chest were in a vice, or as if a heavy weight were sitting upon it. Finally, if the discomfort radiated, it could do so only to certain areas, such as the center of the neck, the jaw, shoulders and arms.

There was little doubt as to the source of a patient's symptoms when the description matched that just described. Unfortunately, a patient's disease didn't always cooperate. Many patients with obstructive coronary artery disease had few, if any, symptoms. In some cases, the primary symptoms were exertional shortness of breath or fatigue, and patients would deny any type of chest discomfort. Other patients simply would restrict those activities that produced symptoms, and would insist there were no symptoms at all.

The second way that coronary artery disease was able to be diagnosed prior to 1958 was if an electrocardiogram showed evidence of a previous heart attack. Alternatively, if the electrocardiogram showed distinctive changes that were characteristic of injury or ischemia to the heart muscle, then coronary artery disease was said to be present.

The third way that coronary artery disease was identified was when the resting electrocardiogram was normal, and if during or after an exercise stress test, the characteristic changes of ischemia developed in the electrocardiogram. This was acceptable proof that obstructive coronary artery disease was present.

These guidelines seem fairly straightforward. In the presence of severe coronary artery disease, there was rarely a problem in demonstrating at least two of the three conditions. Unfortunately, for early or moderate disease, none of the three conditions were usually evident. This meant that not until the disease was far advanced would anyone be aware of its presence. Since there was no higher authority (other than autopsy), large numbers of individuals either went undiagnosed and untreated, or were told their symptoms were psychosomatic and were prescribed tranquilizers.

Even if these people had been properly diagnosed, it may not have mattered, because other than nitroglycerin placed under the tongue for immediate relief of pain, there were no other medications available. Although aspirin was available, its use for patients with coronary artery disease had not yet been demonstrated and although other drugs known as nitrates (isosorbide dinitrate or Isordil) were known, they were thought to be ineffective. They are really quite effective, but at that time it was not known how to use them. Physicians were also unaware that tolerance to the medication would occur within days, unless there was a 12 hour interval between doses.

CORONARY ANGIOGRAMS

In 1958, the modern era of cardiology began. A pediatric cardiologist by the name of Dr. Mason Sones at the world-renowned Cleveland Clinic, while working in the heart catheterization laboratory, accidentally slipped a catheter in a coronary artery while injecting x-ray opaque dye. To his surprise, the vessel lit up, and he could immediately see the entire artery and its branches. Since no harm came to the patient from this therapeutic misadventure, Dr. Sones reasoned that if an injection were made into a patient with obstructive coronary artery disease, then he could see on the x-rays where the vessel was blocked. Soon Dr. Sones was regularly injecting dye into coronary arteries, and diagnosing the presence of coronary artery disease when it couldn't be diagnosed in any other way. It wasn't long before cardiologists from around the world were travelling to the Cleveland Clinic to learn the new technique of coronary arteriography. Now when a patient experienced chest pain and both resting and exercise electrocardiograms were not diagnostic, an angiogram could be used to determine the problem.

Doctors became intoxicated with the new technology. It was prestigious to do angiograms and many patients would be referred to them because few were capable of using this new technique. The patient was impressed with this new, high-tech test and doctors were paid a large fee for doing it.

Little thought was given to the possibility that the coronary artery disease found in patients with recent onset of chest pain might have been there for years in unchanged form. Nobody yet knew how long it took for an artery to become obstructed and there certainly were no prior angiograms to compare. Doctors quickly became mesmerized by the fact that the coronary arteries could be imaged in a living patient, for this had never been done before. Furthermore, the fact they could get rich doing angiograms didn't escape anyone. It was here that cardiologists and hospitals made their pact with the devil. Greed was the fuel that allowed angiograms to quickly spread throughout the United States. It wasn't long before every hospital of any reasonable size wanted to do their own angiograms. Besides bringing in money to the doctor, it also brought money and patients to the hospital.

So great was the impact of angiograms that its side effects were conveniently ignored. After all, only three or four out of a one thousand patients had a heart attack during the procedure... A similar number might die, another two would have a stroke, and several would have a miscellaneous assortment of complications, provided the cardiologist doing the procedure had been properly trained. For those cardiologists who were not trained well, the complication rate was much higher.

The limitations of the angiogram were not recognized during its rapid spread throughout the country. While they will be discussed in greater depth in a later chapter, in essence, the angiogram works to discover coronary artery blockages that may or may not be the source of the patient's symptoms. Patients with gastroesophageal reflux, gallbladder disease, peptic ulcer disease and countless other illnesses were told that coronary artery disease was the cause of their symptoms, just because of what was found on their angiogram. Like the innocent man who is convicted on the basis of circumstantial evidence, the case is closed, and nobody bothers checking further. That is, when coincidental coronary artery disease was found, both the doctor and patient stopped thinking. Other possible causes of the patient's symptoms were ignored.

For the next 10 years after the introduction of the angiogram, the consequences of an erroneous diagnosis of coronary artery disease were related primarily to the failure to find the true cause of the patient's symptoms. Bypass surgery for coronary artery disease had not yet been discovered. Not until 1968 when coronary artery bypass surgery was introduced, also at the Cleveland Clinic, would it make a difference; accurate diagnosis was important, otherwise a lot of patients would be undergoing bypass surgery for the wrong reasons.

RADIOACTIVE IMAGING

The next test to be introduced involved the use of radioactive imaging. If radioactive substances known as a radiopharmaceuticals were injected into the blood stream, it would find its way to the coronary circulation on the surface of the heart. If there were no restriction of blood flow to the heart muscle, then there would be equal distribution of the radioactive material, which then would be extracted by the heart muscle. The heart muscle now emits gamma rays which are collected by a special gamma or scintillation camera that is interfaced with a computer. The image that results reflects the amount and location of the radioactive material within the heart muscle; which, in turn, depends upon the integrity of the blood flow to the heart muscle. The two most common radiopharmaceuticals used for this purpose are thallium-201 and technetium-99m sestamibi, but there are others. Each have advantages and disadvantages.

Radioactive imaging has been a major advance in the field of noninvasive cardiology. Its true value depends upon a thorough under-standing of the strengths and weaknesses of the technique. This, in turn, requires a cardiologist or radiologist who is expert in its use, and this may take years of experience. Unfortunately, many cardiologists who use radioactive imaging are captivated by the images, believing them to be nearly one hundred percent accurate merely because they were produced by a highly sophisticated piece of equipment. Sadly, such images also may be highly inaccurate. Some of the limitations of radioactive imaging are as follows: if a major artery is obstructed and the adjacent coronary arteries are not diseased, there will be an easily discernable difference between the adjacent areas. This is because the images seen depend upon a *relative* difference in blood flow between the two areas. Suppose, however, all three major coronary arteries on the surface of the heart are severely narrowed. All three areas of heart muscle supplied by these arteries will be limited in the amount of the radiopharmaceutical that will be received. Accordingly, the amount of radioactivity emitted by each area will be similar and the image obtained by the gamma camera will show no blood flow or perfusion deficit. In short, even though there is severe disease, it will be interpreted as normal.

A second disadvantage of radioactive imaging is that the demonstration of ischemia usually requires that the patient undergo a stress test. This is similar to the procedure advised for patients with obstructive coronary artery disease who often have a normal resting electrocardiogram but an abnormal stress electrocardiogram. Experience has shown that in such circumstances, when ischemia does occur during or following exercise, its duration may be very brief, e.g., one or two minutes. When radioactive imaging is employed, the radiopharmaceutical is not injected until peak exercise, and several minutes must elapse before imaging is begun. Another several minutes must elapse before enough radioactive counts are acquired for an image to be obtained. By that time the ischemia may be gone.

A third disadvantage of radioactive imaging is that a before and after image must be compared. With any imaging procedure, the patient's position is critical. If the angle of view after exercise differs by more than a few degrees from the observed control image, it may result in a wrongful interpretation. This is, of course, true for any imaging procedure. However, the difference in positioning may not be as evident during image acquisition with radioactive imaging as it is with other imaging procedures.

A fourth disadvantage of radioactive imaging is the possible appearance of a type of an artifact in patients with large right or left ventricles. Obese individuals and women with large breasts may show an attenuation of radioactivity, resulting in a false positive test.

Finally, the immense cost of the equipment and the need for highly skilled technicians makes radioactive imaging very expensive and impractical to use for follow-up studies. In addition, one cannot get an immediate answer as to whether ischemia is present in the event of an emergency need for information.

ECHOCARDIOGRAPHY

Throughout the 1970s, as radioactive imaging was being developed, a new imaging technology was evolving. This type of imaging was based upon the wartime use of radar and sonar. In echocardiology, high frequency sound waves were directed toward the chest rather than at long distances, and were focused inside of the heart. These sound waves would be reflected back from whatever structures were encountered to the emitting sound wave transducer. The images would then be seen on an oscilloscope. The pictures received would show the muscular walls of the heart while they simultaneously thickened and contracted making the cavity of the heart much smaller. During this process, blood would be squeezed out of the heart much like air escaping from a balloon. Then, during relaxation, one could see the heart muscle thinning and expanding as well as the heart's chambers enlarging as blood entered. In addition, the opening and closing of all four of the heart's valves could be seen. One could precisely measure the thickness of the heart muscle at the end of contraction and relaxation. In this way, the amount of thickening of the muscle could be determined. Similarly, the dimensions of the heart's chambers could be ascertained at the beginning and end of contraction, allowing the determination of the ejection fraction.

One area where such information was extremely important was for patients with borderline blood pressures. Typically, doctors will tell such these patients to watch their pressures closely during the next year or two. Not until the pressure is clearly elevated will they begin treatment. In the interim, the patient may have a heart attack or stroke. However, an echocardiogram can determine the presence of thickened muscle or enlarged chambers that indicate that a patient's blood pressure has been elevated for a considerable period of time. Thus, treatment could be undertaken immediately. Similarly, if the motion of one muscular wall of the heart were impaired when compared to the opposite wall, this could indicate blockage of the blood supply to the impaired muscle. The doctor would not have to wait until the patient began having chest pain to start treatment. Also, if there were a heart murmur, direct visualization of the valve via echocardiography would allow the doctor to determine which valve was damaged (heart murmurs are like noises heard inside of a car— one cannot always tell from where they originate). In the past, these patients would have to undergo a heart catheterization to determine which valve was damaged and its severity. Finally, if heart failure were present, the echocardiogram would tell us the disease that was responsible for the failing heart.

In the 1980s, special applications of echocardiography were developed. Using a technique known as Doppler color flow imaging, it became possible to determine the direction of travel of blood within each of the heart's chambers. Echocardiogram machines were engineered so that blood entering the heart was red, while blood leaving the heart appeared blue. This allowed for the detection of leakage or obstruction of a valve when examination with a stethoscope was inconclusive. For example, if the color blue was found in the left atrium, it could only mean the valve between the left atrium and ventricle, the mitral valve, was leaking or incompetent.

Another technique known as spectral Doppler made it possible to calculate the velocity of blood traveling through the heart's valves. From this information, the degree of obstruction or leakage of a valve could be calculated. Spectral Doppler also provides special information about the function of the heart muscle during the relaxation phase of the cardiac cycle, known as diastole. This is particularly important, because relaxation abnormalities are often the first sign of impaired cardiac function. More recently, by injecting special preparations known as contrast agents into the blood stream, the blood flow through the heart muscle can be seen in order to determine whether it receives an adequate amount of blood.

In addition to being extremely sensitive in the detection of heart disease, echocardiograms are an affordable, noninvasive test that poses no danger to the patient and can be used to tract the progress of the patient's disease. For example, if a hypertensive patient with an enlarged heart were on a good medical program, a repeat echocardiogram at 6-12 months should show a reduction in heart size. If the dimensions of the heart were not appreciably different, it would mean the patient was not on an effective medical program. In another example, if an echocardiogram showed weakened contractions of the heart muscle on the original examination, but follow-up studies at six months showed it was no longer present, it would suggest that new vessels had grown into the ischemic area providing the muscle with a new blood supply.

The value of echocardiographic imaging can be greatly increased by performing the imaging study during any form of stress that increases the heart rate and work load. The degree of narrowing of a coronary artery required to decrease the resting blood flow to the heart muscle is approximately 75%. Consequently, if an artery is only 50% to 60% narrowed, there is no reduction in blood flow at rest. Wall motion will be normal and obstructive coronary artery disease will go undetected. There are several ways of getting around this limitation. All depend on speeding up the heart rate and increasing the work load of the heart. Since the heart muscle requires more blood under such conditions, the blood flow in the coronary arteries must increase. In much the same way that gridlock will occur on a narrowed freeway only during rush hour traffic, the extra blood flow cannot get through a narrowed artery as easily as it can through a nonobstructed artery. Accordingly, there will not be enough blood to supply the increased needs of the heart muscle. The ability of the heart muscle to contract will be impaired, its motion will be decreased, and the synchrony of contraction will be discordant with heart muscle that has an adequate blood supply.

The most common way of making the heart work harder is with the standard stress test. This is exactly the same as the traditional EKG stress test using a treadmill. Indeed, the stress echocardiogram and EKG stress test are usually done together. Unfortunately, when exercise is carried out on a treadmill, there is too much movement of the chest to obtain a satisfactory echocardiogram. Accordingly, many cardiologists prefer to have the patient perform their stress on a bicycle ergometer so that the echocardiogram may be performed during the stress as well as immediately afterwards.

Another increasingly popular method of performing a stress test is to intravenously infuse a drug that will speed up the heart rate. This test is referred to as a pharmacological stress echocardiogram, and most often uses the drug dobutamine. One advantage of such a test is that the patient is lying motionless on a bed, allowing for much better quality images to be obtained. The technician performing the echocardiogram has more time to get optimal echoes as compared to the brief period following an exercise test. Stress echoes greatly increase the ability of the echocardiogram to detect the effects of early obstructive coronary artery disease.

Because it is not possible to obtain satisfactory echoes on every patient with heart disease, there have been modifications to the way the test is done. Patients with very thick chests, those with severe lung disease such as emphysema in which there is a great deal of air filling the lungs between the heart and the chest wall, and women with very large breasts all make for very poor quality echocardiograms. By placing the imaging transducer at the end of a gastroscope, the probe can be inserted into the esophagus and stomach. High quality images may be obtained of the heart muscle and valves. In a sense it has now become a semi-invasive test and, as such, a description of it is out of place in this book. However, it is not a truly invasive test and is not associated with the kind of complications seen with invasive procedures.

The immensity of the information provided by the echocardiogram has revolutionized the diagnosis and treatment of heart disease by allowing access to information that had never been available before. Unfortunately, most patients with heart disease never have an echocardiogram. Often they are sent to the hospital only for an angiogram. When an obstructed coronary artery is found, the patient is automatically urged to undergo angioplasty with little regard to whether it is necessary. Perhaps those doctors who engage in this practice recognize that a good echocardiogram would probably eliminate the need for either of these procedures.

This point is illustrated in the following true case history. Sam was a 60-year-old engineer who had been told he must undergo urgent bypass surgery for his angina. An angiogram revealed that one coronary artery was obstructed 90% and another was obstructed 50%. He had been warned that unless this surgery was performed immediately, he would have a massive heart attack and might die. The only medications he was taking were aspirin, a cholesterol-lowering agent and nitroglycerin for his angina. He had not been told that noninvasive imaging tests could be done to determine whether there was truly a reduction in blood flow to the heart muscle, nor had he been advised that there were alternative forms of treatment.

Fortunately, Sam was well-informed and was aware that even though a coronary artery were obstructed, new blood vessels known as collateral vessels could form in and around the obstruction, thereby bypassing it. Accordingly, he decided to seek another opinion, and that is how Sam came under my care. Echocardiography demonstrated almost normal wall motion throughout the heart. Only in one area was the contraction of the heart muscle impaired, and then only mildly so. Administration of sublingual nitroglycerin restored that abnormal function to normal. A stress echocardiogram did demonstrate further impairment of motion, but not until the heart rate reached a level of 135. Sam was placed on a beta blocker, an ACE inhibitor, a diuretic and nitrates. A follow-up echocardiogram at 6 months showed wall motion had returned to normal not only at rest, but after exercise as well. He no longer had any angina. After 12-18 months, the nitrates were discontinued and Sam continued to do well.

Sam's case is exceedingly common. I have seen many patients who have been urged to undergo immediate surgery, and have yet to find one case where such surgery was necessary. To the carpenter, everything looks like a nail. To many surgeons and cardiologists, all patients with obstructive coronary artery disease must be treated in only one way. Whether this is because their knowledge is limited and their training very narrow (i.e., this is the only way they have been taught to treat the disease), or whether their standard of living is so high that they must make as much money as they can, we may never know. In either case, the situation is not serving the patient's best interest.

MAGNETIC RESONANCE IMAGING

Magnetic resonance imaging or MRI has been clinically available since the 1980s. While it has become a standard and valuable diagnostic tool for study of many areas of the body, only in the past few years has it been used to image the heart. Unlike other organs, joints and bones of the body, the heart is moving, and this made using the MRI trickier. Although images of the heart now provide striking views of its structure, anatomy, wall and chamber dimensions, and can reveal evidence of scarring from a prior heart attacks, MRI is used more in the field of research than it is in clinical cardiology. The length of time it takes to perform the test, and its inability to provide "on-line" functional information at the bedside make it impractical to use in clinical cardiology settings.

POSITRON EMISSION TOMOGRAPHY

Positron emission tomography (PET) is an imaging tool that allows one to observe metabolic activity. The usual metabolic substances employed are ammonia, glucose and nitrogen. These compounds are produced by living cells as a result of the metabolic breakdown of more complex products.

To find out whether an area of heart muscle is still functional, these metabolic substances are made radioactive, and then injected into the circulation. A portion of this radioactive material will find its way to the heart where it will be incorporated into heart muscle cells. If the cell is reasonably functional and accumulates enough radioactivity, then that activity can be detected by a PET scan. Failure to do so has been shown to mean that area of the heart is no longer alive.

Since the manufacture of these substances depends upon the cell being alive, PET studies have found use in so-called viability studies. Ordinary radioactive imaging studies require an adequate amount of blood flow to deliver the radioactive material, e.g., thallium. Often, there is so much restriction of blood flow that there will be an imaging defect on a thallium study. As a result, the heart muscle, or myocardium, is thought to be irreversibly injured or even dead. In fact, such muscle may be alive and well, but merely needs to have its blood supply restored. Muscle in this state has been called *hibernating myocardium*. At other times, after a heart attack or cardiac surgery, the muscle may be too injured to move, and in this case it has been called *stunned myocardium*. Whether the muscle is stunned or merely hibernating, the bottom line is if enough of heart muscle is damaged or if the patient has had previous, irreversible damage from multiple heart attacks and no reserve, then the heart functions poorly. In such circumstances, the ability to bring additional heart muscle back to life may make the difference between heart failure accompanied by death, or survival with a reasonable quality of life.

A substantial number of viability studies have been performed before and after revascularization with either angioplasty or coronary artery bypass surgery. It has been found that if a PET study is able to demonstrate that an area of heart muscle is alive, then there is a high probability that some function will return when blood flow is restored with these procedures. Conversely, if PET studies fail to demonstrate viability, then there is little likelihood that any revascularization procedure will make a difference because the heart muscle is dead. In such situations, the trauma to the heart caused by the surgery, as well as post-operative complications, are apt to do far more damage than good.

In theory, every patient who undergoes coronary artery bypass surgery or angioplasty should have these studies. In a perfect world, no patient would undergo any surgical intervention unless it had been demonstrated that there was a high probability of success. Conversely, those who failed to demonstrate viability would not have to undergo such procedures. The benefits are obvious. Unfortunately, a high percentage of cardiologists who do angioplasty and surgeons who perform coronary artery bypass surgery pay little or no attention to the advantages of having the patient undergo a preoperative imaging study.

OTHER IMAGING TECHNIQUES

A number of other imaging techniques can be used in the study of heart disease. These include ultrafast CT (computed tomography) scanning, cine magnetic resonance imaging, first-pass radionuclide angiocardiography and equilibrium radionuclide angiocardiography. These procedures are either primarily used for research purposes or with certain rare diseases (e.g., ultrafast CT scanning and cine MRI), or they are older procedures. None of them are used for routine clinical diagnostic purposes. Attempts have been made to use CT scanning to detect calcium in coronary arteries, but the sensitivity and specificity of this procedure is unacceptably low. Thus, the absence of calcium does not mean that obstructive coronary artery disease is not present. Conversely, the mere presence of calcium in a coronary artery in no way means there is serious disease.

HOW USEFUL ARE THE HIGH-TECH TOOLS?

Doctors have a love affair with technology. If there is a machine that will provide information about the function of our bodies, then there will be a company that will manufacture it, an advertising company that will market it, doctors who will use it, patients who are willing to have the "test" performed, and insurance companies that will pay for it. It doesn't matter if the information the "test" provides can be obtained in simpler, less expensive ways, or if the readout from the "test" is often inaccurate when performed by poorly trained technicians and read by unskilled doctors. We have become slaves to technology and believe blindly in its unerring accuracy.

Manufacturers of medical equipment fight furiously for their "market share" and try to justify selling their equipment by making it ever more complicated. Of course, doctors want the latest and the best in equipment for their patients. The more expensive the equipment, the more they can charge the patient, and the bigger will be their tax write off. Pretty soon, perfectly good equipment that can perform highly useful tests fall by the wayside. Doctors stop using such tests— after all, why do an older test on a patient when there are newer ones— even if the information is no better than that obtained with the older equipment. In time, insurance companies will declare the older test "obsolete" because it isn't being used any more. At this point, the new test will have officially replaced the older ones, although it will never have been proven that it is any better in terms of useful information provided.

Doctors are capable of obtaining a great deal of complex information about the patient's disease. The cardiologist can identify which portions of the heart have impaired function, whether the impairment is confined to systole or diastole, the percentage thickening of the muscle, the actual velocity of the movement of the muscle in the damaged area as compared to a healthy area, the percentage of reduction in blood flow, which arteries are diseased and where they are diseased, what the arteriosclerotic plaque looks like from the inside of the artery, which heart valve is damaged, the actual number of millimeters the valve opens, how much obstruction or leakage of a valve is present, and an endless assortment of other important and unimportant details.

Is all this information necessary to treat the patient, will it influence the treatment offered, and will it save lives? Unfortunately, we do not know as yet whether the acquisition of such detailed information is meaningful and cost effective. Yes, it is nice to know that Mrs. Jones' heart has disease of all three coronary arteries and is functioning poorly. It may have taken thousands of dollars to find this out. Will this knowledge improve the quality of her life and allow her to live longer? There is no evidence that it will. Often, patients like Mrs. Jones are made to undergo coronary artery bypass surgery on the misguided premise that it will be beneficial. Yet, there are no modern studies to prove this. However, there are many studies that show that appropriate use of beta blockers and ACE inhibitors, as well as other drugs, will prolong a patient's life and will reduce the frequency of hospitalization. Yet other studies have shown that most patients with poorly functioning hearts are not treated with these drugs. So, why spend thousands of dollars finding out how bad her heart is, if she isn't going to be correctly treated, or if it isn't known whether the treatment is going to do any good? Perhaps it would be best to resurrect older tests and use these to follow patients with heart disease.

OLDER TESTS THAT CAN STILL BE USED IN MODERN DIAGNOSIS

A number of older tests for heart disease can still provide a great deal of useful information in the detection, tracking, and assessment of cardiac function in patients with heart disease. These tests do not have the glamour or prestige of some of the new imaging procedures, nor can doctors charge several hundred or several thousand dollars for performing them. Insurance companies even consider some of them obsolete. In fact, such tests are anything but obsolete. They are still widely used in most other countries throughout the world that can't afford the kind of technology we have in America, and are used in most countries that do not have the kind of fee-for-service medicine practiced here.

The explosive development of technology in the diagnosis of heart disease has left an enormous void between high-tech evaluation in hospitals and large clinics, and follow-up evaluation in the average doctor's office with the EKG and stethoscope. The high-tech type of cardiac evaluation with sophisticated imaging procedures are quite capable of making a gross diagnosis of the disease, its location and severity. However, once treatment is started, such techniques are incapable of measuring the small, day-to-day changes in the way the disease behaves, nor can they accurately assess the response of the patient's disease to medications. To put it succinctly, expensive and prestigious tests are very good at providing qualitative information for initial diagnoses, but do not do as well in providing quantitative information about the progression or regression of the patient's disease. This is the "Achilles heel" of high tech tests.

Apexcardiography

Unlike the electrocardiogram which records only the electrical output of the heart and a measurement that correlates poorly with its mechanical function, the apexcardiogram records the relative changes in volume and pressure inside of the left ventricle on a moment-to-moment basis throughout the entire cardiac cycle. In addition, it also reflects the pattern of the muscular contraction and relaxation of the heart, and correlates very well with total cardiac function. Indeed, a far more appropriate name would be a muscle cardiogram. The apexcardiogram is recorded by placing a transducer over the impulse beat produced by the heart against the chest wall. This is called the cardiac or apex impulse, hence the name apexcardiogram. A transducer is a device that transforms mechanical motion into an analog recording that can be seen on an oscilloscope, and then permanently recorded on a recorder. It has been well established that if the transducer were placed directly upon the heart, the pattern of motion obtained would be identical to that obtained by an external recording from the apex impulse.

If one area of heart muscle is not working very well and the opposite muscular wall works normally, the apexcardiogram will not tell us which area of the heart is malfunctioning, only that such an area is present. The picture of the heart presented will be the combination of the two walls of the heart working together. If the diseased wall is severely damaged and is unable to contract at all, then the pressure created inside the heart's chamber will push the weakened wall out in a reverse motion. Imagine a balloon that is uniformly collapsing as air is let out. Suppose it were possible to isolate one portion of that balloon and blow air into it. That section would expand while the rest of the balloon were collapsing. This is exactly what happens with the heart when there is a scar or an ischemic area. We call such an area an aneurysm, and the motion of the muscular wall dyskinetic. Dyskinesis is not detected on a radioactive imaging test, although it can be seen on an echocardiogram.

In addition to the apexcardiogram's unique ability to reflect the pattern of contraction of the heart muscle, its ability to record relative changes in both volume and pressure simultaneously is unshared among all the noninvasive tests. Suppose a weakened heart is unable to contract forcefully enough to empty completely. Let's say of the 100 ml of blood within the left ventricle, 90% or 90 ml, exits from the heart. There will be 10 ml left over. During the next filling cycle another 100 ml of blood enters the heart from the lungs. Now there are 110 ml within the left ventricle. Again, only

142

90 % leaves the heart, but this time it is 90% of 110 or 99 ml Now there is 11 ml of blood left over. One can only guess how much blood will be left after 100,000 contractions in 24 hours. In actual practice, it may only be a fraction of a milliliter that remains behind, but even a small residual fraction adds up after 100,000 beats a day, and three million beats a month. In time, larger and larger amounts of blood accumulate within the left ventricle. At some point, a full quota of blood will no longer be able to enter the ventricle, and it will back up into the left atrium. If this goes on long enough, blood will back up all the way to the lungs, the lungs will fill with fluid, the patient will develop congestive heart failure and will die. Fortunately, the heart has a way of compensating. As blood accumulates within the left atrium, it begins to stretch. Like a rubber band that when stretched is released with great force, so does the stretched left atrium shrink with greater force. Now a relatively large volume of blood under great pressure is forced into the left ventricle. This chamber is compelled to accept the blood; it, too, expands like the left atrium, and contracts more forcefully, forcing the blood out into the circulation.

It is evident that the volumes and pressures within the left atrium and ventricle have increased in this scenario. Neither the echocardiogram, the electrocardiogram nor the radioactive imaging test will reflect or record the changing pressures. But the apexcardiogram reflects this very nicely. It records moment-to-moment changes in pressure, volume and the pattern of muscular contraction throughout the cardiac cycle. In the case of a muscular contraction, when the pressures and volumes within the left ventricle are normal, the pattern of contraction is also apt to be relatively normal, even if there is an ischemic area. However, when both the pressures and volumes are increased, the weakened wall can no longer handle the extra load and it will contract abnormally.

The apexcardiogram can be recorded continuously or intermittently daily, weekly, monthly, or as often as needed to track the progress of the patient's heart disease. Accordingly, it reflects directional changes in cardiac function. It is also invaluable in determining the optimal dosages of the various medications used to improve cardiac function. Since it is noninvasive and can be done quickly, safely, cheaply, and without a lot of complicated equipment, it's beautiful in its simplicity. Unfortunately, it is rarely used because it isn't high-tech enough, nor is the doctor able to charge much for doing it; it costs about the same as an electrocardiogram. Its value lies in the fact that it is highly sensitive and accurate in detecting and tracking heart disease.

Systolic And Diastolic Time Intervals

Modern day medical recorders are no longer limited to one channel of information as in times past. Multiple readouts can be obtained simultaneously. When an apexcardiogram is recorded, it is customary to record several other channels of information at the same time. For example, we might record one lead (a single channel) of the electrocardiogram, place a second transducer over the carotid artery (the main artery in the neck) for a pulse recording, and put a high fidelity microphone over the heart to record the various sounds that are produced.

The heart is an enormously complicated organ. It does far more than just pump blood around the body. Think about all that has to happen: an electrical impulse is generated from the upper corner of the right atrium, it spreads in wave like fashion throughout both atria. This causes both atria to contract and empty whatever blood there is into the ventricle. Normally, this does not result in any heart sounds. While the atria are contracting, the electrical impulse spreads throughout both ventricles activating the heart muscle. This causes the muscle to thicken and tense up. At this point the pressure within the heart's chambers begin to rise very rapidly. After about 40 milliseconds, the pressure is great enough to close the intake valve between the atrium and ventricle. This is called the mitral valve. If the valve did not close, blood would be regurgitated back into the left atrium. When the mitral valve closes, it creates a sound called the first heart sound.

In the normal heart, within approximately 75 milliseconds— i.e., well under a tenth of a second— the pressure is great enough to force open the exit valves known as the aortic valves. For the heart, this is blast-off time. As soon as the aortic valves open, the muscular walls of the left ventricle simultaneously begin to come together and squeeze blood into the aorta. This takes about 300 milliseconds, or nearly one-third of a second. Soon the pressure begins to decline within the ventricle as it relaxes. When the pressure in the ventricle falls below the pressure in the aorta, the aortic valves close, preventing the ejected blood from falling back into the ventricle. The pressure continues to decline within the ventricle and after another 75 milliseconds, it falls below the pressure in the left atrium. When this happens, the mitral valves open and all the blood that was filling the atrium while the heart was emptying now pours into the ventricle over the next 500-600 milliseconds.

It is evident that both the contraction and relaxation phases of the heart's cycle can be broken down into several parts: electrical activation, contraction of the atria, rise in pressure within the ventricle, ejection of blood, followed by early and late relaxation. Each of these phases takes a certain amount of time. It can be compared to riding in a car. We tend to think only about the driving part, but in reality, we have to turn the key in the ignition, turn it further to start the motor, back the car out of the garage, drive out of the driveway, accelerate the motor, etc. If we are entering a freeway, we must accelerate to freeway speeds. If the car you are driving takes 6 seconds to reach 60 miles per hour, it is a powerful, well-tuned car. If it takes 30 seconds to reach freeway speeds, it is an old clunker. Similarly, I indicated earlier it takes about 75 milliseconds for the pressure development in the left ventricle to reach a level where it can force open the aortic valves. If it takes 125 milliseconds then this is a diseased heart.

Measuring the duration of each of the phases of the cardiac cycle is called the systolic time interval if the time frame occurs during the contraction phase of the cardiac cycle, or diastolic time interval if it occurs during the heart's relaxation phase. These time intervals are enormously useful in studying component functions of the heart. Instead of waiting until the patient has a heart attack or heart failure, or suddenly dies because the heart no longer can function, measuring these time intervals might provide the initial clue that something is wrong.

For example, if instead of a heart's taking 300 milliseconds to empty, it now takes 350 milliseconds, then the patient's disease might have to be studied more carefully, even if the patient says, "I feel great." Careful studies might establish that an area of heart muscle has become ischemic and medication needs to be added to the patient's regimen that increases the blood flow to the muscle. Or a study may determine that the patient has an obstructed aortic valve, and that it takes longer for the blood to exit from the heart.

Tests that measure the systolic and diastolic time interval allow us to detect problems before they produce symptoms, and thus they give us a chance to correct them whenever possible. Heart attacks are like earthquakes: they may occur without warning and they have devastating effects, but the forces that go into creating them usually have been going on for years. There are many other uses for the systolic and diastolic time intervals measurements.

The Phonocardiogram

The simple recording of heart sounds is another procedure that can easily be performed at the same time as the recording of the apexcardiogram, and the systolic and diastolic time intervals. When a doctor listens to a patient's heart, there are two important limitations. The first is that there is no permanent record of what is heard. Accordingly, at a later date, when the doctor listens to the patient's heart again, he or she has no way of comparing what he or she has heard before with the patient's current heart sounds. The other limitation is that the human ear is unable to hear the low frequency sounds that the damaged heart emits. These sounds are generated whenever blood backs up into the left atrium, and it has to contract with greater force. As indicated earlier, normally the atrium doesn't make any sound when it contracts. Thus, when a low frequency sound can be detected during atrial contraction, it is a red flag that something is wrong. A similar low frequency sound may be heard when the ventricle is relaxing, and the pressure in the left atrium is elevated. Such sounds have been called fourth and third heart sounds, respectively. It should be apparent that if such sounds are present in a patient and they disappear with treatment, it is a guide to a successful response. Conversely, if they do not regress or if they become louder, the patient is not responding or is getting worse. Obviously, if these sounds can't be heard because the doctor is using an ordinary stethoscope, a valuable barometer of the patient's disease will be lost.

The Holter Monitor

One of the limitations of the electrocardiogram other than the facts that it is quite insensitive to the presence of damaged and ischemic heart muscle and that it does not reflect the heart's mechanical function, is the very brief period during which it is recorded. Current machines may only record 12 to 16 beats. This is hardly representative of the 100,000 or so beats each day the heart performs. A patient might demonstrate cardiac ischemia for only a few minutes a day. Even if a patient had a total period of ischemia lasting for an hour, which would be considered a great deal of ischemia, there is little chance it would be detected with a standard electrocardiogram. In contrast, a Holter monitor records all of the heart beats in a 24 hour period. Thus, if an ischemic episode lasted only a few minutes on a given day, the test will record the ischemic event.

The appeal of a Holter monitor test is that patients can be studied during their normal activities, and especially when they are under any form of stress. Emotional stress, which cannot be easily reproduced in a doctor's office, is far more likely to cause ischemia than physical stress.

The limitation of the Holter technique is the same as the basic limitation of the electrocardiogram. That is, it is relatively insensitive to the detection of ischemia. Also, whether or not ischemia is detected is almost totally dependent upon environmental factors. In other words, if there is no stress, then there may be no ischemia. A third limitation of the Holter technique is that the patient must wear multiple electrodes across the chest for a 24-hour period, and carry around a cumbersome battery pack. Finally, it is not a test that can provide an immediate answer. It takes 24 hours to collect the information, the patient must return to the office to return the recording tape or computer disc, and often the tape must be sent to a special center for reading, which takes another day or two. Nevertheless, the Holter technique is a very useful noninvasive test that can provide valuable information that might not be obtained in any other way.

The Stress Test

For most of this century, some form of stress test has been used by doctors to help diagnose heart disease. The earliest test was developed by Dr. Arthur Master, and was known as the Master Two Step Test. Patients would climb two steps, and then go down two steps for a period of three minutes. An electrocardiogram was recorded immediately afterwards. The number of steps the patient would climb depended upon his age and sex. The idea was to increase the patient's heart rate to a predetermined amount. If the stress electrocardiogram did not show evidence of ischemia, then the patient was told he or she did not have heart disease. Doctors of that time had little awareness of how insensitive the electrocardiogram really was in detecting ischemia. Another major limitation of the test was that the electrocardiogram could not be recorded while the test was being performed.

In the late fifties, the treadmill and bicycle ergometer came into use and it was much more effective in detecting the presence of coronary artery disease. With these devices, monitoring could be carried out while the patient was exercising. The work load on either the treadmill or bike was adjusted so that patients would achieve a given heart rate for age. The formula generally used was 220 - age x 85%. Thus, a 60-year-old patient would be expected to achieve a heart rate of 136.

The conventional stress test is a valuable addition to the diagnosis and tracking of patients with heart disease. It is particularly useful because the exercise work load can be quantified very precisely. This allows for a comparison of cardiac performance over a period of years. Like the Master's test which preceded it, cardiologists came to have a unquestioning belief in its accuracy. If it were abnormal, you had obstructive coronary artery disease and were dangerously close to having a heart attack. In contrast, if it failed to demonstrate ischemia, the patient was told no heart disease was present.

As with all tests that are developed for the detection of disease, early research studies are always performed in patients with known severe disease. This makes sense. You collect a lot of patients whom you know already have the disease. Perhaps they already have had a heart attack or two, or maybe an angiogram has unearthed evidence of severe coronary artery disease. These are the patients you put on a treadmill to see how many will have an abnormal test. When you do this, about 95% will be abnormal. The sensitivity of the test is then said to be 95%. However, one also would like to know how specific the test is; that is, if an individual does not have coronary artery disease, and undergoes a treadmill test, how often will it become positive? The problem here is that you do not know beforehand if the subject has coronary artery disease. Since you can't just go up to a healthy individual and say, "I want to do an angiogram on you. It will cost you $4,000 and you might die, have a heart attack or a stroke while I'm doing it." Who, then, can you do the test on? Patients who come to you because of chest pain. But, if they have chest pain, they are not normal. Obviously, we have a dilemma. In addition, the angiogram has severe limitations in being able to detect coronary artery disease. It has long been known that it grossly underestimates the amount of disease present. Well, let me shortcut through 40 years of research to straighten this problem out. If a stress test is performed on an average patient who has only mild or even moderate disease, in my experience the test will be abnormal in only 25-30% of cases even when there is evidence of significant coronary artery disease using other diagnostic procedures. Consequently, like the electro-cardiogram that forms the basis of the test, it is not a reliable procedure for diagnostic purposes. Nevertheless, it has a great deal of value when used in other ways. For example, if the test is negative, although a patient may have coronary artery disease, it is unlikely that the patient has severe disease. Accordingly, his prognosis would be very favorable. Also, since the amount of exercise the patient must undergo can be measured, the test may be used to track the functional capabilities of the heart over a period of time.

The danger of the exercise test is that it has been transformed from a diagnostic test to a procedure that is being used to recommend angioplasty or coronary artery bypass surgery. That might be appropriate if it had been established that the degree of abnormality of the test was a prognostic indicator of impending heart attacks or survival, but this is not the case. Indeed, the opposite is true— an abnormal test has little relation to outcome.

The second limitation of the test is the unrealistic way in which it is performed. As a result, there is a lack of correlation between the results of the test and the prognosis of the patient's disease. I mentioned that there is a formula for determining the maximal heart rate a patient should achieve while doing a stress test. For a 60-year-old male that number would be 136. To subject someone of that age to a heart rate that high is hardly relevant to any activities someone of this age would do. Probably anyone above the age of 50 who got their heart rate high enough would develop ischemia. But that doesn't mean that the person is at risk of dying or having a heart attack. The reason the test becomes abnormal at those high heart rates is because the patient's backup blood supply through his tiny collateral vessels are not capable of carrying the same volume of blood flow that can be carried by the larger arteries. At rest, and with only mild increases in heart rate, the amount of blood that collateral vessels can carry is entirely adequate. Under these circumstances, the heart muscle receives plenty of blood, and the patient is neither ischemic nor is he or she in danger of a heart attack or death. At high heart rates, the heart muscle needs more blood, but it can't get through fast enough, and the test becomes abnormal.

It is here that the stress test may be easily abused. At this point, the cardiologist informs the patient that his or her test is abnormal, and that he or she is in grave danger of having a massive heart attack or dying. The patient simply does not have the background knowledge to challenge the cardiologist's opinion although the patient is, in fact, in no such danger. The patient might be if he or she were stupid enough to increase his or her heart rate to 136. But that itself might be hard to do, unless the patient were running from danger.

If you are asked to undergo a stress test, you should find out in advance what heart rate you will be expected to achieve. If it is above 110, and you are above the age of 50, refuse. Agree to do the test only if the doctor agrees you can stop whenever you wish, and that you do not wish to exceed a heart rate of 110. If you do have a strongly positive test at a heart rate of less than 100-110, you probably are at greater risk, *if you are not treated appropriately*. Above these numbers, in my view, the prognostic capabilities of the test are meaningless. Appropriate treatment, however, essentially neutralizes your excessive risk when your test is abnormal at very low heart rates.

The same recommendations hold true if you are advised to undergo a stress test during radioactive imaging, or if you are asked to do a stress echocardiogram. The doctor will be very unhappy about this. The issue here should not be whether you do or do not have obstructive coronary artery disease. Assume you do— everyone above the age of 40 probably does. The question is: will the amount of disease you do have affect your life in any way? Will it shorten it, produce symptoms, or cause a premature heart attack? That question cannot be answered by doing a test— any test, including an angiogram. The point is that if you have to be subjected to extremes of testing to uncover a disease, it's hardly likely to be at a stage where it is serious. It makes much better sense to say to the doctor, "Look, I'm perfectly willing to come back every year and undergo a resting evaluation by echocardiogram, radioactive imaging or whatever. If the resting tests show no evidence of disease, then leave me alone. If, at some point, you begin to find evidence that I have ischemia, then I will agree to nonsurgical treatment at that point." It is highly likely that you will live much longer than someone who is found to have ischemia at a heart rate of 160, and is made to undergo prophylactic angioplasty or coronary artery bypass surgery on the mistaken belief that it will prevent future heart attacks and premature death. No such evidence exists.

This chapter has touched upon only some of the diagnostic methods used to detect heart disease. Since the focus of this book is primarily the diagnosis and treatment of obstructive coronary artery disease, diagnostic procedures for other cardiac conditions, such as valve disorders, congenital heart defects, cardiac tumors, and diseases known as dilated cardio-myopathy, have been left out. The diagnosis and treatment of these other diseases are fairly standard. There is no controversy for most of these conditions. Consequently, patients are not apt to become the accidental victim of an unnecessary surgical procedure, and this is not where public education is needed. On the other hand, how a patient with coronary artery disease should be treated shows enormous variation, not only throughout the world but from state to state in our own country. Patients should be aware that the rush to use technology to diagnosis and treat their disease does not mean this approach is correct. All too often, this technology is used not for the benefit of the patient but for the doctor or institution for whom he works. Rarely is the patient aware that, in reality, he or is being used as a guinea pig. This is not a new observation, and has been made by many other physicians over the years. But it must be constantly brought to the forefront, not only because it continues to be true, but because every year new ways are found to practice the latest in medical experimentation on the patient.

10

INACCURATE AND UNRELIABLE

Tests That Won't Diagnose
Coronary Artery Disease

The Holy Grail for cardiologists is the angiogram. It is worshipped with a religious fervor unlike any test in medicine. Go to any invasive or interventional cardiologist, and he or she will invariably recommend an angiogram either the same day or the next day— and will often become upset if you refuse. Frequently my patients tell me how a cardiologist they had just seen kept calling them at home, urging them to undergo a study immediately. Many were told they would die or have a massive heart attack if the test were not done immediately and followed by treatment (usually angioplasty or coronary artery bypass surgery).

Is the cardiologist's faith in this procedure justified? Is the information the angiogram provides that reliable? Can it tell the doctor how his or her patients should best be treated, and if they are likely to have a heart attack or die? Will it provide information that can't be obtained in any other way? And, most importantly, is it even necessary to know whether and where an artery is narrowed to treat the patient? In simple terms, is the angiogram recommended for the patient's— or for the doctor's— benefit? Let's examine the evidence available to find out.

IS THE CORONARY ARTERY DISEASE FOUND ON AN ANGIOGRAM NEW OR OLD?

When a patient develops symptoms of an illness, it is usual for both the patient and the doctor to assume that this is indication of a new development. In most cases, such assumptions are correct. However, a number of chronic diseases may exist in silent form for years before symptoms appear. Hypertension, tuberculosis, cancer, arthritis, cirrhosis, valvular heart disease, AIDS, syphilis and coronary artery disease are just a few of the many disorders that may be present for decades before anyone is aware of them. For many of these diseases, when symptoms do appear, they are quite specific. For example, if a long-time cigarette smoker develops severe pain in the upper back, and an x-ray shows partial destruction of a rib, there is little doubt the victim has lung cancer and that it has spread to the bones. If a middle-aged runner begins having knee pain and an x-ray shows degenerative changes, one can be certain that it is arthritis. However, chest pain is another matter.

Chapter 6 discussed over 50 reasons why chest pain may occur. Knowing this, and also recognizing that coronary artery disease may exist for most of a person's life without symptoms, you can easily understand that both chest pain and coronary artery disease can exist independently of one another. Thus, when coronary artery disease is found on an angiogram, the cardiologist cannot be sure whether it is causing the patient's symptoms, or if the disease is has been present for years without problems and there is no danger of its becoming worse; that is, if its presence is merely coincidental. In most cases, there is no prior angiogram with which to compare.

IS THERE A CORRELATION BETWEEN A PATIENT'S SYMPTOMS AND THE SEVERITY OF CORONARY ARTERY NARROWING?

The co-existence of chest pain and coronary artery disease does not mean that angiograms should not be done, only that whatever the angiogram shows should be interpreted with caution. This brings us to a second dilemma encountered when interpreting angiograms. If a patient has experienced recent recurring chest pain and the angiogram shows marked narrowing of one coronary artery, and moderate narrowing of one or two other arteries, it seems reasonable for the cardiologist to assume that the most narrowed vessel is responsible for the patient's symptoms. But a cardiologist who has been trained not to jump to conclusions might say to himself or herself, "Hmmn, this artery is severely narrowed, and it looks as if it has been that way for years, but my patient has only had symptoms for one week. Why did his symptoms start at this time? Let's check out a few other things."

Our cautious cardiologist is well aware that there is a very poor correlation between the anatomical amount of coronary artery disease and the presence or absence of symptoms. For example, 40% of women and 10-15% of men with recurring chest pain have normal or nearly normal coronary arteries when angiograms are done. Why, then, are they having chest pain? Conversely, a large number of patients with extensive coronary artery disease never have chest pain. Often they have completely occluded arteries and have never experienced chest pain or had a heart attack. Why not?

Another disconcerting finding that questions the relationship between symptoms and disease is the poor correlation between the severity of the disease found on an angiogram and at autopsy. Many studies have documented that patients with mild disease on a coronary angiogram are found to have severe disease at autopsy. Thus, many of those patients with "nearly normal" coronary arteries may actually have fairly severe obstructive coronary artery disease that is not detected by the coronary angiogram. Yet such patients are usually told that their chest pain is not due to heart disease.

Frequently patients will come to me with stories of having undergone three, four and even more angiograms each time their chest pain returns, or every year or two as a follow-up test. If doing an angiogram were free from complications and low in cost, and if progression of a patient's symptoms correlated closely with angiographic evidence that the patient's disease was getting worse, repetitive angiograms might be justified. But this is not the case. Cost and complications aside, there is a very poor correlation between symptomatic progression and anatomic progression of their coronary artery disease. Many patients will have progression of their symptoms, but do not have progression of their coronary artery narrowing. Conversely, many have progression of their obstructive coronary artery disease, but no change in symptoms. In view of the fact that there are several excellent noninvasive tests to determine whether a patient's disease is progressing, one can only conclude that the practice of repeating angiograms is motivated by economic gain.

IF NONINVASIVE TESTS HAVE BEEN DONE, IS AN ANGIOGRAM ALSO NECESSARY?

Many patients who have been told they needed to have an angiogram, already will have had a radioactive imaging procedure and an echocardiogram. Even if these imaging studies show that all the muscular walls of the heart are functioning normally, angiograms still will be advised. The truth is that such imaging tests provide all the information the cardiologist needs to know to treat the patient. Angiograms in such instances are completely unnecessary. The disturbing fact is that even though heart function is normal in these patients, angioplasty or coronary artery bypass surgery is usually recommended immediately. It has been known for nearly 20 years that neither surgery nor angioplasty are any better than medical treatment for these patients. Indeed, in Europe where revascularization is done with far less frequency than in the United States, survival is actually better without surgery— and that's often with medical treatment that is less than optimal.

At other times, the imaging tests will show one or more areas of ischemia; that is, areas of heart muscle where the blood flow is reduced. Angiograms are then recommended to "confirm" what the noninvasive test shows. This statement implies that the cause of the abnormal tests may not be obstructive coronary artery disease. However, this is highly unlikely. Noninvasive tests have been well validated over the past 20 years. They are not only highly reliable for detecting the presence of obstructive coronary artery disease, but also for determining its severity and location. To expose the patient to a potentially hazardous test merely to confirm what is already known is unwarranted.

CAN AN ANGIOGRAM DETERMINE THE CAUSE OF A PATIENT'S CHEST PAIN?

Still another reason why patients with coronary artery disease are urged to undergo angiograms is to determine the cause of their chest pain. If this were the case, it would imply that there is some magical distinguishing characteristic that appears on an angiogram and allows the cardiologist to make a clinical diagnosis. But this is wishful thinking. If I were to take the angiograms of 50 patients without chest pain who had undergone this procedure because of an abnormal stress test, and the angiograms from another 50 patients with chest pain, and gave the video tapes of both groups to a cardiologist, asking him or her to identify which angiograms came from patients with chest pain, the cardiologist would not be able to do this.

CAN AN ANGIOGRAM PREDICT A HEART ATTACK?

Sometimes patients are told that angiograms must be done to find out if they are at risk of having a heart attack. Other patients who have had an angiogram have been warned that a massive heart attack will soon take place. Can the angiogram tell us this information? No way! No test can allow us to predict the future. Many studies have now been done where angiograms were performed before and after a heart attack. The goal was to determine which artery was going to close off. It had always been assumed that the coronary artery that was the most severely narrowed before a heart attack would be the artery most likely to be found blocked after the heart attack. Again, this theory was not supported by the study. In most cases, the coronary artery that was only mildly narrowed, or not even diseased, was the artery that shut down. Coronary arteries that were nearly closed (90% narrowed or greater) were calcified and fixed because they were so old— it takes years for an artery to become this narrowed. Even when an artery that was 90% narrowed did close off, usually nothing happened because there were already enough collateral blood vessels in place to allow adequate amounts of blood to reach the heart muscle. Thus, when the artery finally did close off, it had no effect and no symptoms. In spite of this information being widely known among cardiologists, many patients are still subjected to emergency bypass procedures. It should be obvious that prognostic conclusions from angiograms are unreliable because heart attacks may occur in patients with mild disease, while patients with severe disease may never have a heart attack.

DO THE FINDINGS ON AN ANGIOGRAM RELATE TO THE CLINICAL COURSE OF THE PATIENT WITH CORONARY ARTERY DISEASE?

Another disturbing limitation of angiography is that if we were to divide patients into several groups, it would be impossible to distinguish one group from another based on the angiogram results. Doctors can not use angiograms to differentiate from the following five groups of patients: patients with stable angina pectoris and stable coronary artery disease; patients with unstable angina; patients who have recently had a heart attack; patients who have had a heart attack in the past; and patients who are about to have a heart attack.

FINDINGS ON ANGIOGRAMS BEFORE AND AFTER SURGERY

Many patients who already have had coronary artery bypass surgery or angioplasty may continue to have chest pain, or experience only temporary relief. But if their obstructed arteries have been bypassed, then why do they continue to have chest pain? Studies have been done before and after coronary artery bypass surgery to determine whether the amount of heart muscle ischemia seen preoperatively disappears postoperatively. A variety of different noninvasive tests have been performed in addition to angiograms. The angiograms usually show that most of the bypasses put in are functioning. In contrast, the noninvasive tests show that although there may be some improvement in 30% to 40% of patients, significant ischemia is still present in the majority. Stated another way, normal blood flow is not restored when an obstructed coronary artery is bypassed. The reason for this will be explained in a later chapter.

At the opposite end of the spectrum are the group of patients who have undergone bypass surgery and who have had repeat angiograms not long after surgery. Incredibly, the angiograms revealed that all of their bypass grafts were closed, yet they no longer had chest pain. Similarly, patients with recurring chest pain were taken to the operating room, anesthetized, and although skin incisions were made on their chests, their chest cavities were not entered and their hearts were not exposed. Their skin incisions were sewn and they were returned to their rooms. Guess what? Their chest pain disappeared.[1,2]

MORE ON THE DISCORDANCE BETWEEN SYMPTOMS AND DEGREE OF CORONARY ARTERY OBSTRUCTION

Among my patients with angina pectoris, there are some in whom it has not been possible to completely eliminate their symptoms. For some unknown reason, there seems to be more engineers in this group. Perhaps it is because they are more analytical about their symptoms. They will tell me that some days they can only walk one quarter of a mile before chest pain occurs, while on other days they can walk a mile or more. They ask, "Why should there be so much variability in the onset of chest pain?" While I cannot provide them with a direct answer, I can explain to them that obstruction of a coronary artery is only partially responsible for their symptoms. What those other factors are will be described in a later chapter.

I often see patients who have undergone angiograms and have been told that one of their coronary arteries is severely narrowed, another is moderately narrowed, and that one or two others are merely diseased without narrowing. A quadruple bypass has been advised. More and more patients are seeking second opinions. While I will usually find evidence of impaired blood flow on one or more noninvasive tests, I will just as often find that the heart muscle is functioning normally. Clearly, if the artery is obstructed, but muscle function is normal, there must be an alternate route of blood supply. If there is, why destroy it by doing a bypass procedure?

WHY CORONARY ANGIOGRAMS DO NOT CORRELATE WITH SYMPTOMS, PROGNOSIS, CARDIAC FUNCTION, AND BLOOD FLOW TO THE HEART MUSCLE

All technologies have limitations. The Hubble Telescope was created because of the inability of Earthbound telescopes to penetrate the atmosphere. This limited the distance land-based instruments could image and, therefore, the number of stars that could be seen. The angiogram also is also limited in what it can see; specifically, the size of the blood vessels that can be detected on an x-ray film or video image. That size happens to be about 0.5 millimeter, or the size of the lead in a mechanical pencil. While this may not appear to be large, 90% of all of the heart's vessels are smaller than 0.5 millimeter. These small vessels collectively are referred to as the heart's microcirculation. There is a vast network of these small vessels, and they are responsible for supplying blood to all of the heart. In a sense, the heart's microcirculation can be likened to looking at a city from a plane at a high altitude. We may see the freeways quite easily, but the city streets are invisible, even though we know they are there. This, then, accounts for the fact that we will often find that a coronary artery is completely obstructed, but the patient has never had any symptoms and there is no evidence that a heart attack has ever taken place. In addition, it's common to observe an area of the heart that seems to be nourished by a completely obstructed artery but which, nonetheless, is functioning normally. Obviously, the muscle is getting blood from some source, and that source is the microcirculation. However, on the angiogram, it appears that no blood is getting through.

In addition to the microcirculation, blood can reach the muscle directly from an obstructed artery. Chapter 1 describes the growth of collateral vessels and the process of angiogenesis, that is, the formation of new blood vessels. Recall that these new vessels will grow out from an obstructed artery and connect with either a healthy artery, or reconnect up with the obstructed artery downstream from the obstruction. In other words, the heart has put in its own bypasses.

It is evident that these other sources of blood, collectively referred to as collateral vessels, explain the failure of the angiogram to provide information on the cause of a patient's symptoms, which artery is responsible, whether or not the patient will have a heart attack and when, what the function of the heart is, how the patient should be treated, and a host of other variables. It is unfortunate that these tiny collateral vessels cannot transport the volume of blood carried by the large coronary arteries, much like city streets can't handle the traffic carried by a freeway. As a result, when the heart has to work harder or faster, and the muscle requires more blood to supply the nutrients so that it can work harder, if it is unable to get blood quickly enough it will become ischemic. To the modern day, over-reactive, invasive cardiologist, this means immediate angioplasty or bypass surgery.

RELEVANT ISCHEMIA

It is important to understand the concept of relevant ischemia. That a heart becomea ischemic when it is beating at a rate of 140 to 160 bpm is insignificant. Yet this is usually the heart rate a cardiologist tries to achieve when he or she has a patient undergo a stress test. This can be called irrelevant ischemia. In daily life, heart rates rarely reaches these levels, even during exercise. Indeed, with modern usage of beta blockers for the treatment of coronary artery disease, it's hard to get the heart rate above 100. It is significant, however, if your heart becomes ischemic at a heart rate of 60-80. This would be relevant ischemia. In the former instance you are not at an increased risk of a heart attack; in the latter example, while you still may not have a heart attack, you are at a higher risk. In other words, what really matters is whether or not you are at increased risk at normal heart rates.

Finally, another disturbing feature regarding the interpretation of angiograms is the variability of the interpretation. One cardiologist might say that a given artery is 40% narrowed, while another may say it is 75% narrowed. Even the same cardiologist reading the same angiogram at two different times, but unaware that it was a repeat interpretation, may show such discrepancy.

A patient with recent onset of chest pain who knows all of the facts and uncertainties just described ought to be highly suspicious when urged by a cardiologist to have an immediate angiogram. Cardiologists who practice this way are determined to perform an angiogram on every patient they see as soon as possible, unless that patient is moribund or has no insurance. Such angiograms are never necessary as an initial test. These cardiologists rarely provide the patient with information about other tests that will provide the same data. During or after the angiogram, they will invariably recommend that they perform an angioplasty immediately. Sometimes they will recommend bypass surgery if they think angioplasty will not work. Once more, the patient is not informed of other forms of treatment. Obviously, if the patient were to be advised that there were alternatives for both the diagnosis and treatment of their disease, the cardiologist would lose the $5,000 to $10,000 he or she would receive for doing these procedures. It is difficult to avoid the conclusion that the economic benefits of these interventions are more important to the cardiologist than the potential harmful effects that might happen to the patient because of the aggressive surgical treatment. The surgical risk might be justified if medical treatment were ineffective or unpredictable, but in my experience, the opposite is the case. Medical treatment is highly effective and predictable. Angioplasty and coronary artery bypass surgery are unpredictable, and accompanied by an unacceptably high incidence of complications.

It is worth noting that many doctors and patients confuse high technology diagnosis and treatment with good medical care. Often they do correlate. But just as often such technology is over-used because there is a blind faith in its accuracy that it doesn't deserve. For example, just because a high tech test provides more information about a patient's disease than an older or simpler test, it doesn't necessarily mean the abnormalities found are the cause of the patient's symptoms. Without having prior tests to compare with, the abnormal findings may be merely coincidental. In other words, if there are no previous tests, there is no way of proving whether any abnormalities present are new or old. An inability to recognize limitations in the high-tech tests frequently results in an incorrect diagnosis that leads to unnecessary surgery. Commonly there are post-operative complications that make the treatment worse than the disease.

Invasive treatments such as angioplasty, coronary artery bypass surgery, stents, and cardiac transplantation are heroic forms of medical care. They are not medical triumphs but represent medical failures in day to day care. Just as the helicopter evacuation at the scene of an automobile accident does nothing to prevent the accident, neither do heroic forms of medical care do anything to prevent the patient's disease or its complications.

It cannot be emphasized strongly enough that the coronary angiogram is one of the most inaccurate and unreliable tests in all of cardiology. More often than not it leads to the wrong diagnosis, and results in appropriate and unnecessary treatment. It has little relationship to symptoms, it does not relate to the cause of the patient's symptoms, it correlates poorly with the function of the heart, and it cannot accurately predict the occurrence of a heart attack. Immediate angiograms are done solely for economic reasons, not medical, reasons. Lest the reader think my views are too harsh, a list of references that will document what I have said has been added to the end of this chapter.

REFERENCES

1. Dimond EG, Kittle CF, Crockett JE. Evaluation of internal mammary ligation and sham procedure in angina pectoris. Circulation 1958; 18:712.
2. Cobb LA, Thomas GI, Dillard DH, *et al.* An evaluation of internal mammary ligation by a double-blind technic. N Engl J Med 1959; 260:1115-1118.
3. Topol EJ, Nissen SE, Our preoccupation of coronary luminology: The dissociation between clinical and angiographic findings in ischemic heart disease. Circulation 1995; 92:2333-2342.
4. Rosenschein U, Topol EJ, Uncoupling clinical outcomes and coronary angiography: A review and perspective of recent trials in coronary artery disease. Am Heart J 1996; 132:910-920.
5. Zir LM, Miller SW, Dinsmore RE, *et al.* Interobserver variability in coronary angiography. Circulation 1976; 53:627-632.
6. Galbraith JE, Murphey ML, Desoyza N. Coronary angiogram interpretation: interobserver variability. JAMA 1981; 240:2053-2059.
7. Arnett EN, Isner JN, Redwood CR, *et al.* Coronary artery narrowing in coronary heart disease: comparison of cineangiographic and necropsy findings. Ann Intern Med 1979:91:350-356.
8. Grondin CM, Dyrda I, Pasternac A, *et al.* Discrepancies between cineangiographic and post-mortem findings in patients with coronary artery disease and recent myocardial revascularization. Circulation 1974; 49:703-708.
9. Isner JM, Kishel J, Kent KM. Accuracy of angiographic determination of left main arterial narrowing. Circulation 1981; 63:1056-1061.

10. Vlodaver Z, Frech R, van Tassel RA, *et al.* Correlation of the antemortem coronary angiogram and the postmortem specimen. Circulation 1973; 47:162-168.
11. White CW, Wright CB, Doty DB, *et al.* Does visual interpretation of the coronary arteriogram predict the physiological importance of a coronary stenosis? N Engl J Med 1984; 310:819-824.
12. Kern MJ, Donohue TJ, Aguirre FV, *et al.* Assessment of angiographic intermediate coronary artery stenosis using the Doppler flow wire. Am J Cardiol 1993; 71:26D-33D.
13. Ito H, Tomooka T, Sakai N, *et al.* Lack of myocardial perfusion immediately after successful thrombolysis: a predictor of poor recovery of left ventricular function in anterior myocardial infarction. Circulation 1992; 85:1699-1705.
14. Folland ED, Vogal RA, Hartigan P, *et al.* Relationship between coronary artery stenosis assessed by visual, caliper and computer methods and exercise capacity in patients with single vessel coronary artery disease. Circulation 1994; 89:2005-2014.
15. Karnegis JN, Matts JP, Tuna N, *et al.* Relation between changes in severity of coronary artery stenosis and anginal pattern. Cathet Cardiovasc Diagn 1994; 32:324-329.
16. Liclen PR, Nikutta P, Jost S. *et al.* Anatomical progression of coronary artery disease in humans as seen by prospective, repeat, quantitated coronary angiography. Circulation 1992; 86:828-838.
17. De Feyter PJ, Serruys PW, Davies MJ, *et al.* Quantitative coronary angiography to measure progression and regression of coronary atherosclerosis: value, limitations and implications for clinical trials. Circulation 1991; 84: 412-423.
18. Gould KL, Kelley KO. Experimental validation of quantitative coronary arteriography for determining pressure-flow characteristics of coronary stenosis. Circulation 1982; 66:930-937.
19. Donohue TJ, Kern MJ, Aguirre FV, *et al.* Assessing the hemodynamic significance of coronary artery stenosis: analysis of translesional pressure flow velocity in patients. J Am Coll Cardiol 1993; 22: 449-458.

20. Peterson RJ, King SB III, Fjman WA, *et al.* Relation of coronary artery stenosis and pressure gradient to exercise induced ischemia before and after angioplasty. J Am Coll Cardiol 1987; 10:253-260.

21. Ambrose, JA, Tannenbaum MA, Alexoupoulous D, *et al.* Angiographic progression of coronary artery disease and the development of myocardial infarction. J Am Coll Cardiol 1988; 12:56-62.

22. Beauman GJ, Vogel RA. Accuracy of individual and panel visual interpretation of coronary arteriograms: implications for clinical decisions. J Am Coll Cardiol 1990; 16:108-113.

23. Cianflone D, Ciccrillo F, Buffon A, *et al.* Comparison of coronary angiographic narrowing in stable angina pectoris, unstable angina pectoris, and in acute myocardial infarction. Am J Cardiol 1995; 76:215-219.

11

TREATMENT OF CORONARY HEART DISEASE

W hen blood flow to the heart muscle is reduced and it becomes ischemic, there are a number of approaches other than medication or surgery that can be used to improve the situation. Among the first things to be done is to eliminate or reduce the influence of those risk factors that speed up the progression of obstructive coronary artery disease. The most important of these are hypertension, stress and smoking, all of which have been discussed in previous chapters. Although medication is required for the treatment of hypertension, and will be discussed in more detail in the next chapter, non-drug approaches also may be effective. For example, if a patient with obstructive coronary artery disease is grossly overweight, major weight loss will not only help reduce an elevated blood pressure, it also will decrease the work load on the heart, making it easier to contract. Similarly, cigarette smoking increases the blood pressure, heart rate and work the heart has to do. Obviously, avoidance of smoking will allow the blood pressure to remain at a lower level and the heart to function more efficiently. Not smoking also means more oxygen will be delivered to the heart because the portion of the hemoglobin molecule that carries the oxygen to the tissues will not be occupied by carbon monoxide.

Stress can have a major impact on the progression of both hypertension and heart disease. The next chapter discusses beta blockers, which are highly effective in neutralizing the effects of stress upon the heart. Unfortunately, such drugs may not completely block the effects of stress. Accordingly, attempts to control the amount of stress the patient has to deal with can be very successful. A number of books are available on stress relaxation techniques which can be moderately successful in reducing the effects of stress on the cardiovascular system and the body as a whole.

Another important issue is the amount of exercise regularly performed by patients with obstructive coronary artery disease. Most of these patients have never bothered to undertake a daily exercise program. Once exercise-induced chest pain begins, physical activity tends to be avoided. While the very young can quickly adapt to an exercise program after prolonged inactivity, as we get older it becomes more difficult to get back into shape. Also, the older you are, the more quickly you will become deconditioned if you stop exercising. Many a patient has experienced the onset of angina after a vacation or some other hiatus from their regular exercise. Not exercising, more than anything else, is responsible for weight gain in most patients. In my practice, all patients are weighed at every visit. Whenever I see a weight gain of more than a few pounds, I inquire whether the patient has changed his or her eating habits, or whether there has been a reduction in physical activities. Rarely does the patient state that he or she is eating more food. Almost always, the cause is less physical activity.

In addition to weight gain and deconditioning with lack of exercise, there is a more serious impairment of adaptive mechanisms on the part of the body. Briefly, certain changes take place in the coronary circulation and elsewhere in the cardiovascular system when exercise is undertaken. The nature of these changes are not fully understood at the present time. How they operate, however, is well known. For example, a patient with angina pectoris regularly induced by a particular activity will often say that his chest pain occurs when he first starts exercising. If he stops and allows the discomfort to disappear, and repeats the same activity, he will no longer have chest pain. One may say that engaging in physical activity begets more physical activity. If a patient is unaware that this response to exercise occurs only initially, he or she might be discouraged from proceeding further.

While many patients have chest pain as a limiting symptom, a substantial number will deny having chest pain but will admit to exhaustion when any sustained exercise is performed. Some also will note mild shortness of breath. If there is added weight to carry from their physical inactivity, these symptoms will become even more noticeable. In the beginning, it is the symptom of chest pain that gets the attention of subjects who develop angina as a result of their coronary artery disease. The chest pain creates a certain apprehension of a heart attack or even a fear of death. In time, as was described in the previous chapter, the heart adapts by forming new blood vessels in the region of the obstructed coronary artery that detour the obstruction. As a result, the blood supply of the endangered heart muscle is preserved. The new blood supply may not be equal to the old blood supply, but it is adequate to allow partial return of function to the previously ischemic cardiac muscle. Consequently, at least 75% of such patients will have an improvement or disappearance of their angina. We know this from placebo studies. Experiments carried out on patients with recent onset of angina, who are treated with only sugar pills, show significant improvement in 75% at six months. Incidentally, this is one of the reasons why so many therapies— be they for the heart, arthritic pain, stomach, or other pains— result in the patient's getting better. A favorite trick of the advertising industry is to get testimonials from subjects who have improved. The hope is that the viewer, listener or reader will assume that it was the advertised product that was responsible for that recovery. In fact, such improvement often has nothing to do with the use of the product.

In the case of the heart, the eventual outcome is one in which the chest pain usually disappears. In its place there is now exercise-induced fatigue. While sometimes the reason for exertional fatigue may be failure of the heart muscle to fully recover, more often than not, the fatigue is due to the effects of deconditioning. Unfortunately, there is no good way to identify the source of the fatigue. The patient usually assumes it is due to his heart and refrains from further activities. This only makes matters worse.

One way to identify whether fatigue is due to deconditioning or to reduced blood flow to the heart muscle is to measure the subject's heart rate. Angina patients whose symptoms are due to their disease will have only a slight increase in heart rate, or no increase at all. If the heart rate is 65 before exercise, it might go up to 70. In contrast, the deconditioned patient is likely to have a higher heart rate to begin with— usually in the 70s. Physical activity will rapidly make it go up to more than 100 beats per minute. A stress test in the patient with fatigue due to true ischemia will usually be quite abnormal. If the fatigue is due to deconditioning, then it is unlikely to be abnormal. Where differentiation becomes difficult is when there are components of both involved. In other words, the exercise-induced fatigue is due to combined ischemia and deconditioning. In this circumstance, the only option is to encourage the patient to begin an exercise program anyway, and hope that there will be improvement.

WEIGHT LOSS

This is not a book about weight loss. Bookstores have shelves and whole sections devoted to this subject. Clearly there are a variety of techniques, diets and weight reduction plans, and theories to incur weight loss. Therefore, I will offer only a few general guidelines regarding what one eats.

In my view, to lose weight involves understanding certain principles of nutrition and metabolism. It is obvious that many overweight people do not know these principles because, if they did, when they lost weight they would not promptly gain it back. Obese people will often confess they have lost hundreds of pounds over the years. When they are off of their diet, their weight not only returns to its former level, but often it will become even higher.

The most popular weight loss programs are the structured ones that replace regular foods with a food substitute, usually in the form of a liquid. The dieter is not allowed to eat food at all. For those who have the fortitude and the dedication required to endure such torture, considerable weight loss invariably occurs. Usually the sensation of hunger disappears after the first week or two, making the ordeal somewhat more tolerable. But at some point these diets must end. If the dieter returns to his or her former eating habits, even if this occurs gradually, then it is only a matter of time before the lost weight returns. This leads to the conclusion that one's eating habits must hold the key to weight gain or loss.

As I have already indicated, lack of adequate exercise is probably the most important factor contributing to obesity. However, another contributing factor is not that the individual eats too much or too frequently, it is that he or she eats the wrong foods. Most diets are high in carbohydrates and low in protein and fat. Significant weight loss and, in particular, loss of body fat, will not occur with this kind of diet. High carbohydrate intake causes the body to secrete excessive amounts of insulin. The insulin will store the excess carbohydrates as fat, and at the same time will prevent the fat from being converted back into sugar. Dr. Barry Sears, in his book *Enter The Zone*,[1] states that the key to weight loss is not restriction of calories, but eating the proper combination of carbohydrates, proteins and fat. He advises people who wish to lose weight to eat a ratio of 40% carbohydrates, 30% protein and 30% fat and to eat about five times a day. Protein should be eaten at every meal. This diet will result in both a loss of weight and a loss of fat.

Another type of diet that is often recommended for individuals concerned with the health of their heart is the so-called Mediterranean Diet. This diet is modeled on the eating patterns of residents of Southern Italy, Crete and Greece, who are often said to have the lowest incidence of coronary heart disease in the world. Their diet is high in fruits and vegetables, and contains moderate amounts of fish, chicken and dairy products such as cheese and yogurt. In addition, moderate amounts of breads, cereals, and red wine are advised, and about four tablespoons of olive oil a day. Red meat is eaten only occasionally.

While it may be true that there are less reported incidences of coronary disease in these regions, it is unlikely that this is because of their diet. These areas are all quite rural and there are relatively few doctors. Accordingly, the accuracy of the medical diagnoses listed on death certificates is open to question. In addition, there is a notable absence of stress in the life-styles of these people, and this might play a major role in the low death rate from coronary heart disease.

One side effect of diets that have a heavy concentration of carbo-hydrates along with inadequate amounts of protein is the frequent occurrence of hypoglycemia, or low blood sugar. Usually this occurs three to four hours after the last meal, and it is characterized by profound fatigue and sometimes chest pain. When this happens, patients usually assume their symptoms are due to their coronary heart disease, and they will lay down and rest. But, as indicated in the previous paragraph, excessive carbohydrate intake results in an increased production of insulin. Depending upon the amount of carbohydrates ingested, at some point the blood sugar drops to very low levels. This can cause a rapid heart rate, a low blood pressure, dizziness, weakness, trembling, profound fatigue and chest pain. If the subject has engaged in a lot of physical activity, its onset will occur sooner. It can be recognized by the rapid disappearance of symptoms with eating.

While some of the effects of lack of exercise have been discussed, the effects of exercise upon the heart is a subject all by itself and will be discussed in a later chapter. The amount and duration of exercise has to be individualized for each patient. A rule of thumb that I use for my patients is that they can do as much exercise as they are able to, as long as it doesn't cause symptoms such as chest pain, shortness of breath or fatigue. I prefer they do at least 30 minutes of exercise a day, five days a week. Walking, treadmills, rowing machines and swimming are all acceptable forms of exercise.

For example, I might suggest that a patient exercise using a stationary bike. To keep from getting bored, he or she can read or watch television while pedaling. I recommend that there be no tension on the wheel during the first mile. Then, with each subsequent mile, the tension should be increased a detectable amount. Finally, during the last mile the tension should be reduced to zero to allow the subject to cool off. This program is vigorous enough so that if the patient's disease were to get worse, initial symptoms would probably appear at the higher levels of exercise, forewarning the patient. It is also possible for patients with an advanced degrees of coronary heart disease to safely maintain a reasonable exercise program.

DIABETES

Patients who have diabetes often have severe vascular disease in the heart, kidney, peripheral blood vessels and the brain. As a general rule, the cardiovascular system of a diabetic is 10 to 15 years older than a nondiabetic's. Thus, a 40-year-old diabetic woman, who we ordinarily think of as being too young for vascular disease, may have heart and blood vessels that are similar to a 55-year-old woman's. How and why diabetics develop such severe vascular disease is not truly known; however, that it exists is common knowledge among both the lay public and the medical profession. While it is generally assumed that tight control of the diabetic's blood sugar will protect the diabetic patient with coronary artery disease, that benefit is not very great, and is only seen in type 1 diabetes that is insulin-dependent. On the other hand, the absence of control does appear to increase the risk of cardiovascular events. Of great interest is the fact that in type 2 diabetics (that is, individuals with noninsulin-dependent diabetes that can be controlled with oral medication), the use of oral medication is associated with an increased risk of heart attacks and premature death. While no study has been able to explain this phenomena satisfactorily, one possible reason is that the oral medications for lowering the blood sugar may induce hypoglycemia if the patient has delayed eating, or if he or she is engaged in a vigorous exercise program that may do the same thing. The hypoglycemic patient is much more susceptible to an arrhythmia or irregular cardiac rhythm.

DEPRESSION, HOSTILITY AND ANGER

These subjects have already been discussed. Numerous studies have established the increased risk of heart attacks and death in patients who exhibits excessive hostility and anger. Depression lasting for more than a few days after a heart attack is a highly reliable indicator that the patient will have another cardiovascular event such as a repeat heart attack, recurring chest pain, congestive heart failure or death in the year after the initial heart attack. I feel that it is worth placing such patients on antidepressant medication, although I am unaware of any formal studies that have been done on this subject.

HOMOCYSTEINE

As was previously discussed under risk factors, increased levels of homocysteine will result in an increased tendency of blood to clot because of its effects on the blood platelets, clotting factors and the endothelial lining of the blood vessels. Because vitamin B_6 and folate will cause the metabolic breakdown of homocysteine and render it harmless, it is important for patients with coronary artery disease to eat adequate amounts of these vitamins.

DISEASE TRIGGERS

Some diseases may trigger previously silent coronary artery disease. In addition, there are many causes of chest pain that may be difficult to differentiate from angina pectoris due to cardiac disease. Chapter 6 offers a full list of all of these conditions. The list includes gallbladder disease, gastroesophageal reflux disease (GERD), disorders of the colon, and hyperventilation syndrome, all of which cause angina-like chest pain. In these cases, other diseases work to trigger previously silent coronary artery disease. Either disease by itself was not enough to cause symptoms, but together symptoms readily occur. Examples are hypertension, aortic valve disease with obstruction, anemia, hyperthyroidism, hypothyroidism and prostate disease with obstruction to urinary flow. At other times, the drugs used to treat a disease are the trigger. For example, the use of nonsteroidal antiinflammatory drugs (NSAIDS) for arthritis may cause fluid retention. It should be apparent that optimal treatment of obstructive coronary artery disease requires elimination, if possible, of those disorders that cause coronary artery disease to be more symptomatic.

MISCELLANEOUS FACTORS

Finally, it is worth noting that relatively minor factors can assume importance. It is common for patients who have angina to have it only after eating. Simply not exercising sooner than two hours after a meal is usually all that is necessary to prevent symptoms. Also, cold weather and not dressing warmly enough in cool weather may cause angina by triggering constriction of the coronary vessels. Each winter, deaths from coronary artery disease are reported in people who have been shoveling snow. Another miscellaneous factor that may trigger chest pain is hypoglycemia. While significant hypoglycemia is not likely to occur with ordinary activities, it will often occur during leisure activities involving exercise. A common occurrence is the individual who has an early breakfast and then engages in golf or tennis later in the morning. By late morning the blood sugar becomes very low, particularly if the victim has had fruit, cereal and no protein for breakfast. Still another minor reason for the occurrence of

174

chest pain is the patient who does his morning exercises before taking his morning medication.

At times, it may not be possible to eliminate symptoms completely. In such cases, the patient must learn to avoid the activity that is responsible for the symptoms.

REFERENCES

1. Sears B. Enter the Zone. New York: Regan Books, 1995.

12

HEART DISEASE MEDICATIONS

A wide variety of drugs have been used over the years to treat the symptoms of obstructive coronary artery disease. Few have stood the test of time, and most have slipped into oblivion. One of the reasons why so many drugs and treatments have been thought to be beneficial in the treatment of coronary artery disease is that their psychological effects can have a major impact on the relief of symptoms. For this reason, it is appropriate to begin the discussion on drugs used for the treatment of coronary heart disease with the effects of placebos.

PLACEBOS

A placebo may be defined as an inert preparation such as a sugar pill or a procedure that is known not to have an effect on a patient's disease. The patient receiving a placebo is not aware that it has no direct therapeutic effect, nor that it is a placebo. He or she is led to believe that it is a powerful drug. The mechanism of the placebo effect is not known, but it may have something to do with the release of neurohormones which can have a profound effect upon a patient's symptoms.

One night when I was an intern working in the emergency room of a large hospital in Cleveland, the police brought in a 19-year-old girl who was said to have collapsed and was unable to walk. Attempts to make the girl stand were unsuccessful. Both legs gave way and she would fall to the floor. An examination did not reveal any disease that might be producing her problems, and I felt her symptoms were psychosomatic. Accordingly, I informed the young lady that I was going to inject medication into her blood stream that would make her symptoms disappear immediately, and that would also give her a very warm feeling throughout her body. I then proceeded to inject a solution of nicotinic acid intravenously. This is a harmless preparation that dilates blood vessels, causing a slight drop in blood pressure and giving one a warm glow. Two minutes later, she was able to stand up, and she walked out of the emergency room. The police looked at me as if I were God, but I didn't bother to explain that this was a placebo effect. For if the nerves to both of her legs were damaged and the patient truly had been paralyzed, nicotinic acid could not possibly have had such an effect.

Dr. Henry K. Beecher, one of the outstanding anesthesiologists at Harvard during the middle of this century, was one of the earliest investigators to uncover the effects of placebos. He found that placebos would relieve severe pain after surgery, cough, the pain of angina pectoris, the common cold, seasickness, headache and anxiety. Not only was a placebo effective in relieving symptoms, but patients taking placebos reported a long list of side effects. They included dry mouth in 9%, nausea in 10%, headache in 25%, a sensation of heaviness in 18%, difficulty concentrating in 15%, drowsiness in 50%, fatigue in 18%, insomnia in 10%, relaxation in 9%, and a warm glow in 8%. In Beecher's review of over 1000 patients who had received placebo therapy, an average of 35% benefitted. It has been suggested that if a placebo were submitted to the FDA as a new drug, they would accept the drug based upon therapeutic efficacy, but it would be rejected because of the high incidence of side effects.

Studies using placebos in patients with cardiovascular diseases have shown a therapeutic effect in 30% to 80%. One such therapy was sham coronary artery bypass surgery with relief of angina pectoris. Patients with congestive heart failure, a very difficult disease to treat, have also shown improvement in 25% to 35% of cases. There even has been objective evidence of improvement in patients with coronary heart disease. This includes an increase in exercise time on a treadmill, an increase in the ejection fraction, an improvement in irregular cardiac rhythms, a reduction in the amount ischemia measured by the electrocardiogram, and a reduction in the amount of silent ischemia on a Holter monitor.

It is essential to understand the placebo effects of medication. Countless testimonials have proclaimed the success of treatments such as chelation therapy, vitamins, minerals, antioxidants, acupuncture, and even meditation. Such procedures probably owe their "success" to the placebo effect. Scientific studies that have been done have not shown any of these preparations to be any more effective than a placebo.

Unless treatment with a drug has been approved by the Food and Drug Administration, claims as to efficacy in the treatment of coronary artery disease should be viewed with suspicion. Don't be mislead by statements that claim a treatment is under investigation but hasn't been released yet. It is illegal for someone to make such a statement.

All drugs mentioned in the discussion below have been approved for treatment of patients with obstructive coronary artery disease. In general, these drugs act in one of two ways. Either they reduce the work load of the heart, thereby reducing the heart's need for extra blood, or they increase the blood flow to the heart muscle directly by dilating the coronary arteries and allowing those arteries to carry more blood to the muscle.

DRUGS WHICH DECREASE THE WORK LOAD OF THE HEART

Beta Blockers

When the body is subjected to stress of any kind, a variety of physiological changes will take place. The cardiovascular changes include an increase in the heart rate and the force with which the heart contracts; a constriction of blood vessels in certain areas of the body such as the skin, intestine and kidney; a decrease in urine formation to increase the blood volume; and a rise in blood pressure. Part of this response is due to the release of the neurotransmitters norepinephrine and epinephrine from the brain and adrenal gland, and of the hormone vasopressin from the pituitary gland.

The normal subject can tolerate these changes quite well. In contrast, individuals with underlying heart disease or hypertension may respond negatively. If coronary artery disease is present, the blood flow required by the heart muscle may not adequately increase to support the heightened work load the heart must perform. As a result, the victim may develop angina, shortness of breath, cardiac arrhythmias, or excessive fatigue. If the stress is great enough, a heart attack or sudden death may even occur. And if hypertension is present, a precipitous rise in blood pressure may cause a stroke.

Although these various hormones and neurotransmitters may be secreted during periods of stress, in order for the heart, blood vessels and kidneys to respond, the neurochemical substances must first interact with specific cellular receptors on the surface of the target organ. The receptors on the surface of the heart are called beta$_1$ receptors, and those on blood vessels beta$_2$ receptors.

About 30 years ago, Inderal, the first beta blocker medication, was approved by the FDA for clinical use. The generic name is propranolol. This was an entirely new class of drug to be used and it represented a major advancement in the treatment of heart disease. Inderal interacts with the beta$_1$ receptors on the surface of the heart and prevents norepinephrine and epinephrine from increasing the heart rate and blood pressure. It also helps to prevent the increase in blood volume due to decreased urine formation. Thus, not only is the work load of the heart decreased, but the amount of blood required by the heart muscle is also lowered. The net result is that an activity or stress that formerly caused the patient to experience chest pain, shortness of breath, fatigue or arrhythmias no longer does so.

Not only does Inderal prevent the acute increases that are seen, but it is also highly effective for the relief of pain in patients with chronic angina pectoris and in the lowering of blood pressure in patients with hypertension. The number and duration of anginal episodes decreases, as does the number of arrhythmias. In addition, cardiac function improves and exercise tolerance increases as well.

Patients who develop unstable angina, a form of angina occurring at rest or at low levels of activity, are well known to be at increased risk of a heart attack. But when such patients were treated with beta blockers, fewer heart attacks developed.

When beta blockers were given intravenously to patients with an acute heart attack, mortality was lowered by 43%, there were fewer episodes of cardiac arrest, the amount of the damaged muscle was reduced and patients were less likely to have a repeat heart attack. Approximately 27 clinical trials have been carried out in over 27,000 patients who were chronically treated with beta blockers, and almost all have shown a significant reduction in mortality.[1-3]

More recently, beta blockers have been found to be highly effective for patients with congestive heart failure. Heart failure is the end result of all forms of heart disease, regardless of the cause. Sooner or later, all of the many forms of heart disease will result in a reduced output by the heart. It does not matter whether the heart disease is an obstructed or leaky valve, ischemic heart disease with damage to the heart muscle from multiple heart attacks, or damage to the heart muscle from an infection. In order to compensate, signals are sent to the brain to release norepinephrine and epinephrine, and to the kidney and adrenal gland to release the other hormones of the renin-angiotensin system. The heart begins to enlarge because it is easier for a large heart to pump out blood than it is for a small heart. Ultimately, however, this proves to be toxic to the heart. As a result, there is an overproduction of calcium, an increased death of the heart muscle cells, and loss of elasticity until the heart can no longer function effectively as a pump.

When the output of the heart is unable to meet the body's needs, the patient is considered to be in heart failure. The patient experiences symptoms such as extreme shortness of breath at rest or with minimal exertion, fluid in the lungs, bluish discoloration of the skin, known as cyanosis, enlargement of the liver, and swelling of the legs and abdomen. Once heart failure occurs, the outlook is extremely poor: the mortality rate within the first few years is as high as 50%. The only treatment for congestive heart failure is a heart transplant. Medication is not as effective for treating congestive heart failure as it is for treating coronary artery disease. Thus, the recent finding that beta blockers can reduce mortality and symptoms is major news.

Initial observations about the therapeutic efficacy of beta blockers was made over 20 years ago. Why hasn't it been used in patients with coronary artery disease? Unfortunately, beta blockers are also known to depress cardiac function, and may actually make patients with congestive heart failure worse when administered in conventional doses. For this reason, most cardiologists have been reluctant to use this class of drugs in the treatment of heart disease. A recent study of 3,737 Medicare patients with heart disease found that only 21% were given beta blocker therapy, and that these patients were three times as likely to receive a calcium channel blocker. Those who received calcium channel blockers had a two-fold increase in the risk of death. Calcium channel blockers will be discused later in this chapter.

Studies show that when beta blockers are given in very low doses, and only gradually increased over a period of months, the heart has a chance to adjust. Technically, there will be an increase in the number of beta$_1$ receptors on the surface of the heart that results in an improvement in cardiac function. In spite of the extensive dissemination of this information, study after study has revealed beta blockers are underused in the treatment of heart disease. Less than half of all heart patients are on this medication, but almost every patient with heart disease should be taking it on regularly.

A disadvantage of the use of beta blockers have been their side effects. Although side effects are limited to only 10% to 15% of the patients taking them, the publicity they have received has made them appear to be far more common than that. Side effects include fatigue, low blood pressure, flare-up of asthma, slow heart rate, decreased sexual function, depression, hair loss, low blood sugar, vivid dreams, insomnia, cold hands and feet, and a worsening of congestive heart failure, if it is present. Usually such side effects occur when the beta blocker dosage is too high or if the dosage has been increased too rapidly. In the majority of patients, simply reducing the dosage will eliminate the side effect. Also, keep in mind that many of these side effects are identical to the side effects claimed to arise with administration of placebo medications. Unfortunately, knowledge of this basic medical fact seems to be lacking among the doctors who will not use this class of drug in the treatment of heart disease. It is the most important drug that we have for the treatment of heart disease.

The most common beta blockers are Inderal (propranolol), Lopressor (metoprolol), Tenormin (atenolol), and Corgard (Nadolol). The average dose of Inderal needed for heart disease patients is 160 mg each day, administered as a long-acting preparation once a day, or in divided doses of 80 mg twice each day. However, occasionally, a total of 80 mg each day is all that is required. Rarely, and in patients who have cardiac side effects,

TABLE III: BETA BLOCKERS		
Brand Name	Generic Name	Average Dosage
Inderal	Propranolol	80-160 mg/day
Lopressor*	Metoprolol	100-200 mg/day
Tenormin*	Atenolol	100-200 mg/day
Corgard	Nadolol	80-160 mg/day
Normodyne, Trandate	Labetalol	400-800 mg/day
Sectral*	Acebutolol	200-800 mg/day
Coreg	Carvedilol	25-50 mg/day
Visken	Pindolol	20-60 mg/day
*Cardioselective acting preferentially on the heart		

40 mg each day may be given. At the other extreme, some patients require as much as 320 mg each day.

Tenormin is much weaker than Inderal, but it can be effective when administered in doses of 150 to 200 mg each day. Although it is the standard dose, 50 to 100 mg administered once daily generally does not relieve symptoms as effectively as when larger amounts are given twice each day. Tenormin is particularly useful when a patient has a serious side effect from Inderal such as hair loss or depression.

Lopressor is an excellent drug, and is especially useful in patients who have a history of asthma, and who are unable to tolerate therapeutic doses of Inderal. It is effective when given in a dose of 50-100 mg twice each day.

Corgard needs to be given only once daily, in a dose of 80-160 mg. It is similar to Inderal in its effects. Carvedilol (brand name Coreg) is the newest beta blocker that has been approved specifically for the treatment of heart failure. Dosages for this drug are still being established. There are a number of other beta blockers available, and they are listed in Table III.

ACE Inhibitors

Another class of drugs used in the treatment of coronary heart disease are the ACE inhibitors. ACE stands for angiotensin converting enzyme. Angiotensin is a powerful vasoconstrictor (i.e., it narrows blood vessels) produced by a complex hormonal system involving the kidneys, adrenal glands and liver known as the renin-angiotensin system. One form of angiotensin, angiotensin II, contributes to the development of the arteriosclerotic plaque within blood vessels, as well as to the enlargement and remodeling of the heart after an acute heart attack, and to the activation of the sympathetic nervous system (which has an adverse impact upon the heart). It also reduces the diameter of the coronary arteries, makes the heart muscle stiffer and less compliant, interferes with the relaxation and contraction of the heart causing impairment of cardiac function, and has a major impact on increasing both morbidity and mortality from heart disease.

In the past 10 years, an entirely new class of drugs has evolved that blocks the formation of angiotensin. These are the angiotensin converting enzyme inhibitors and they inhibit the enzyme that is the catalyst for the conversion of angiotensin I to angiotensin II. The formation of angiotensin II is blocked, and so are the effects it has on the cardiovascular system.

Initially ACE inhibitors were introduced as a new treatment for high blood pressure, for which they are highly effective. Prior to their introduction, hypertension treatment was complicated by the frequent occurrence of side effects by drugs that acted primarily of the brain. The ACE inhibitors changed all of that, and not only made the treatment of hypertension much easier but safer because of fewer side effects.

In the decade following the introduction of the ACE inhibitors, research has established that these drugs have actions far beyond merely lowering the blood pressure. The use of ACE inhibitors has resulted in improved cardiac function and survival in heart failure— an important accomplishment for a disease whose only effective treatment is cardiac transplantation. Following a heart attack, treatment with ACE inhibitors has been shown to limit the amount of damage that occurs, prevent enlargement and remodeling of the heart, improve cardiac function and metabolism, and increase the number of blood vessels in the damaged heart muscle. These drugs also increase the amount of nitric oxide produced by the heart's microcirculation, improve the compliance of blood vessels within the heart muscle so that they are more expansive, and improve survival. Long-term treatment with ACE inhibitor drugs reverses previous cardiac enlargement and improves coronary blood flow. On a cellular level, these drugs inhibit the changes that make the heart stiffer and harder to fill. If not corrected,

TABLE IV: ACE INHIBITORS		
Brand Name	**Generic Name**	**Usual Dosage**
Capoten	Captopril	25-50 mg; 2-3x/day
Vasotec	Enalapril	10-20 mg; 1-2x/day
Lotensin	Benazepril	10-20 mg; 1-2x/day
Monopril	Fosinopril	10-20 mg; 1-2x/day
Prinivil, Zestril	Lisinopril	10-20 mg; 1-2x/day

this leads to cardiac enlargement, impaired function and increased mortality. ACE inhibitors also increase the diameter of the arterioles and veins, which not only lower the resistance against which the heart must work, but also increases blood flow to the kidneys.

The side effect profile of the ACE inhibitors reveals that they are among the safest of all the cardiac drugs that we use. The most serious side effect is apt to occur in patients who have unsuspected narrowing of their renal artery, that is, narrowing of the artery that supplies the kidney with blood. If this artery is narrowed significantly, then the drop in blood pressure that may occur after the administration of an ACE inhibitor may be just enough to reduce the flow of blood to the kidney, causing acute kidney failure. This, of course, may happen with any drug that lowers the blood pressure. Usually, when blood pressure drops, the kidney is able to produce a substance called renin. Renin acts through the renin-angiotensin-aldosterone system to cause the production of more aldosterone, a powerful hormone from the adrenal gland that makes the kidney retain more water, increasing the volume of fluid in the cardiovascular system and causing the blood pressure to rise back up. Thus, the blood pressure lowering effects are counteracted. However, the ACE inhibitors prevent this counter-reaction from happening. Once the blood pressure is lowered, it won't come back up, and if the renal artery is narrow enough, kidney failure will follow. Fortunately this particular side effect is extremely rare.

Another side effect which, although annoying, is benign, is a dry, hacking cough. It may take several weeks before it appears and it is usually not recognized by the patient as a side effect. Consequently, it may be present for months before anyone is aware that something is wrong. It usually stops several weeks after the ACE inhibitor is discontinued. Rarely, patients will develop a rash or a loss of taste on using these medications.

ACE inhibitors are an important advance in the medical treatment of coronary artery disease. Reversing the effects of coronary artery disease is complex, and does not occur following angioplasty or coronary artery bypass surgery. These procedures restore the blood flow only temporarily, and do nothing to correct the underlying process that causes heart attacks and premature death.Table IV provides a list of the more common ACE inhibitors and their dosages.

Angiotensin II Receptor Antagonists

The newest class of drugs available for the treatment of hypertension and coronary heart disease are the angiotensin II receptor antagonists. In contrast to the ACE inhibitors, which inhibit the enzyme that catalyzes the formation of angiotensin II from angiotensin I, the angiotensin II receptor antagonists block the effects of angiotensin II on the angiotensin II receptors. This is similar to how the beta blockers intervene to block the effects of norepinephrine and epinephrine on the cardiac tissue. The pharmacological effects of the angiotensin II receptor antagonists are the same as the ACE inhibitors but they are accomplished by a different mechanism.

Because the drugs in this class are new, at the time of this writing they may be capable of certain actions on the cardiovascular system of which we are unaware.* The drugs in this class will be useful for treatment of patients who are unable to tolerate the ACE inhibitors because of side effects.

At the present time, there are only three drugs in this class that have been approved by the FDA. The first is losartan, known by the brand name of Cozaar. The usual dose is 50 to 100 mg each day. The second drug is valsartan, brand name Diovan. The recommended dose for Diovan is 80 to

---

* Author's Note: Almost all drugs are found to have a mechanism of action that is different from the mechanism of action believed to be present when the drug is released. ACE inhibitors are a classic example. Originally, it was thought to inhibit the formation of angiotensin II. Now we know it has many other actions. Angiotensin II receptor antagonists should follow the same pathway.

160 mg each day. The third and newest drug in this category is irbesartan, brand name Avapro. It is similar to the other two drugs in this group. The usual dose is 150 to 300 mg once daily. Side effects of these medications are minor and include leg pain, muscle cramps, dizziness, insomnia and gastrointestinal upset.

DIURETICS

Diuretics are a class of drugs that promote the formation of urine by the kidney by increasing the excretion of sodium. In so doing, there is a reduction in the volume of fluids circulating within the vascular system. This leads to dilatation of the small arteries and arterioles by the body, which lowers the resistance to blood flow. The net result is a a lower blood pressure.

Most cardiologists do not use diuretics in the treatment of coronary heart disease. Indeed, the majority of cardiologists do not even use diuretics for the treatment of high blood pressure, although it has been officially recommended as one of the first drugs to use. This is particularly worrisome for many patients who are urged to undergo immediate angioplasty or bypass surgery because they have not had relief from their chest pain caused by hypertension. This kind of pain may be called hypertensive angina. In my experience, diuretics are the linchpin without which beta blockers, nitrates, and ACE inhibitors would be far less effective.

Until a few years ago, misinformation about diuretics made doctors reluctant to use them. Drug advertisements and academic doctors, who know a lot about theory but often have little practical experience, claimed that diuretics were harmful. They were said to elevate cholesterol and triglyceride levels, as well as blood sugar, calcium, and uric acid levels, and to cause a loss of potassium. The pharmaceutical industry managed to see to it that this half-truth was widely disseminated. So effective were diuretics in lowering blood pressure that if they were used popularly, pharmaceutical companies would have lost their market share of their own drugs. It is true that diuretics do the things they stated, but the metabolic elevations are mild, and the elevated cholesterol, blood sugar, calcium and uric acid levels return to their former levels within a few months. Potassium loss was initially a concern, but it can be easily counteracted by the simultaneous administration of a potassium-blocking drug that prevents potassium loss. In fact, more than one company markets a combination of a diuretic and a potassium blocker in the same pill. When this is used, potassium loss is rare. Nevertheless, so effective was the negative publicity that, to this day, many doctors are extremely reluctant to use diuretics in the treatment of either heart disease or high blood pressure.

There are sound reasons for using diuretics in the treatment of both hypertension and coronary heart disease. In both conditions, it is not possible to lower the blood pressure to an optimal level without a diuretic. If diuretics are not used in the treatment of hypertension, although blood pressure will be lower, it will still be mildly elevated, particularly when the patient is under stress. Maintenance at such a level will eventually be harmful. In coronary artery disease, the cornerstone of treatment is to lower the blood pressure as low as possible, as long as there are no side effects. A normal blood pressure is too high for someone with significant coronary heart disease. By lowering the blood pressure, the heart's work load is reduced, and with it the heart's need for oxygen. Therefore, the amount of blood that must go through the narrowed coronary arteries is reduced. Since the amount of blood that can get through the narrowed artery is already less than is needed, reducing the heart's need to what one can get through the artery allows the heart muscle's demand for blood to equal the supply that is available.

Another reason for the need for diuretics is related to the fluid retention and fluid shifts brought about by the very medications used to treat the disease. Beta blockers and nitrates are often responsible for a significant increase in the volume of fluid within the circulatory system. Were it not for diuretics, the therapeutic effects of these medications would be seriously compromised.

There are several classes of diuretics. The most commonly used and mildest are the thiazide diuretics, listed in Table V. Far more potent are the loop diuretics. These differ from the thiazide diuretics in where they act in the kidney and in their length of action. Thiazide diuretics last about 12 hours if only one pill is taken; two pills taken at the same time will last 24 hours. In contrast, the more commonly used loop diuretics such as Bumex

TABLE V: COMMONLY USED DIURETICS		
Brand Name	**Generic Name**	**Usual Dosage**
Thiazide Diuretics:		
Diuril	Chlorothiazide	0.5-1.0 g; 1-2x/day
HydroDiuril	Hydrochlorothiazide	50 mg; 1-2x/day
Enduron	Methychlothiazide	2.5-10 mg; 1x/day
Esiderix	Hydrochlorothiazide	50 mg; 1-2x/day
Oretic	Hydrochlorothiazide	50 mg; 1-2x/day
Potassium Blocking Agents:		
Midamor	Amiloride	5 mg; 2x/day
Aldactone	Spironolactone	50 mg; 2x/day
Dyrenium	Triamterene	100 mg; 2x/day
Combined Thiazide and Potassium Blocker:		
Moduretic	Hydrochlorothiazide+Amiloride	1; 2x/day
Dyazide	Hydrochlorothiazide+Triamterene	2; 2x/day
Aldactazide	Spironolactone+Hydrochlorothiazide	2; 2x/day
Maxide	Hydrochlorothiazide + Triamterene	2; 2x/day
Loop Diuretics:		
Lasix	Furosemide	40-80 mg; 2x/day
Bumex	Bumetanide	1-2 mg; 2x/day
Edecrin	Ethacrynic Acid	50-100 mg; 2x/day
Demadex	Torsemide	50-200 mg; 1x/day
Miscellaneous Diuretics:		
Lozol	Indapamide	2.5-5.0 mg; 1x/day
Zaroxolyn	Metolazone	5-20 mg; 1x/day

and Lasix last about four hours. Demadex, a newer loop diuretic, lasts about 8 to 10 hours.

Yet another difference is what is referred to as the dose response curve. For thiazides, the curve is flat, which means increasing the dosage does not increase the response. For loop diuretics, the curve is linear, i.e., increasing the dose of a loop diuretic increases the response proportionately.

The main side effects of diuretics are related to a depletion of fluid volume. This can lower the blood pressure and cause dizziness, weakness, and fainting. It also will cause chemical changes in the blood and make it appear as if the kidneys are failing. Actually, they are not failing— the body is merely showing the effects of dehydration. It is rare for this to happen unless higher doses of the loop diuretics are use. Even then, experience has shown that the side effects seen are due less to the medication than the fact that the patient typically has gone on a diet and has lost a significant amount of weight. Alternatively, the patient has developed a febrile illness with dehydration resulting from the fever or from diarrhea. These side effects are never serious, but can cause significant weakness and fatigue over a period of a few days. Temporarily stopping the medication and resuming it a few days later at a lower dose will correct these side effects.

Diuretics have also been blamed for causing gout. It is more likely that patients who must take diuretics naturally have elevated uric acid levels and are therefore predisposed to gout. The most serious side effect of diuretics occurs in patients who are allergic to sulfur, because most diuretics contain sulfur in one of their molecules. Many of these patients are able to tolerate the loop diuretic Edecrin.

Listed in Table V are the most commonly used diuretics.

DRUGS WHICH INCREASE THE BLOOD FLOW THROUGH THE CORONARY ARTERIES

Calcium Channel Blockers

Calcium channel blockers are a group of drugs that have the ability to block the movement of calcium into both cardiac muscle cells and the smooth muscle cells that make up the muscular wall of arteries, thereby causing them to relax. As a result, the main effect of calcium channel blockers is the dilation of both peripheral arteries and the coronary arteries on the surface of the heart. This causes an increase in blood flow in these arteries, along with a decrease in blood pressure. Whether the increase in blood flow in the coronary arteries is a direct effect of the drugs or an indirect effect of the drop in blood pressure is not known. Patients with chest pain due to coronary artery disease find that calcium channel blockers are effective agents for pain relief, and they have achieved widespread popularity. In my own personal view, this popularity is due less to their therapeutic effect than it is to the mass marketing techniques and media blitzes put on by the pharmaceutical companies who manufacture these drugs. Nevertheless, these drugs have proven to be effective against anginal pain. A few of them also are able to improve the filling of the heart with blood during diastole by relaxing the heart muscle.

Calcium channel blockers are made up of a heterogeneous group of drugs having major differences in both their mechanism of action and side effects (see table following). They vary in their affinity for vascular and cardiac muscle, but share an ability to interfere with the movement of calcium inside of the muscle cell. They do not have metabolic effects such as an increase in uric acid, blood sugar, or cholesterol, nor do they cause fluid or sodium retention. They also can be used in patients with asthma, reduced blood flow to the kidney, and circulatory problems of the extremities. They are not affected by the use of nonsteroidal anti-inflammatory drugs that interfere with the function of diuretics. Thus, they fill the empty niche that occurs when the side effects of beta blockers, ACE inhibitors or diuretics prevent them from being used at a dose high enough to achieve maximal therapeutic efficacy.

The down side of the calcium channel blockers are their side effects. The side effects common with dihydropyridines (e.g., Procardia) include peripheral edema, headache, flushing, palpitation and a rapid heart rate. Side effects from diphenylalkylamine drugs include headaches, low blood pressure, peripheral edema, and constipation. Fortunately, these side effects are less likely to occur with the newer, longer-acting dihydropyridines such as Norvasc. The major problem with the dihydropyridines, particularly the shorter-acting ones like Procardia, have been the reported increase in heart attacks and mortality in patients with coronary artery disease. In part, this may be because this group of drugs, as well as the diphenylalkylamines and the benzothiazepines, are capable of depressing heart muscle and interfering with the heart's contraction. The dihydropyridines also stimulate the sympathetic nervous system which increases both the heart rate and force of contraction of the heart muscle. Unfortunately, this predisposes the heart to malignant irregular cardiac rhythms. Accordingly, these drugs cannot be used in patients who are in heart failure. The diphenylalkylamines and the benzothiazepines also are capable of interfering with the conduction of electrical impulses within the heart, and may cause heart block.

TABLE VI: CALCIUM CHANNEL BLOCKERS		
Brand Name	Generic Name	Average Dosage
Diphenylalkylamines:		
Calan	Verapamil	240-360 mg/day
Isoptin	Verapamil	240-360 mg/day
Covera-HS	Verapamil	240-360 mg/day
Verelan	Verapamil	240-360 mg/day
Dihydropyridines:		
Norvasc	Amlodipine	5-10 mg/day
Plendil	Felodipine	5-10 mg/day
DynaCirc	Isradipine	10-20 mg/day
Cardene	Nicardipine	60-120 mg/day
Procardia	Nifedipine	30-60 mg/day
Adalat	Nifedipine	30-60 mg/day
Sular	Nisoldipine	20-40 mg/day
Benzothiazepines:		
Cardizem	Diltiazam	240-360 mg/day
Dilacor	Diltiazam	240-360 mg/day
Tiazac	Diltiazam	240-360 mg/day
Tetralol:		
Posicor	Mibefradil	50-100 mg/day

Since there is an increased risk of both heart attacks and death with the use of calcium channel blockers, in the past few years there has been a marked decrease in the use of these medications, in spite of a massive publicity and marketing campaign by the pharmaceutical companies. The newer preparations such as Norvasc, Sular, Plendil, and Posicor appear to be safer. Please see Table VI for a list of calcium channel blockers.

NITRATES

Second only to beta blockers in therapeutic efficacy in patients with coronary artery disease, are the nitrates. In one form or another, nitrates have been available for the relief of symptoms from coronary heart disease for well over 100 years, and have very powerful effects. No other drug acts so quickly and effectively to relieve chest pain as well as nitroglycerin.

Sublingual nitroglycerin is one fast-acting form of this drug. It is available as a tiny tablet that can be placed beneath the tongue, where it will dissolve and be pharmacologically effective after about two minutes. These effects will disappear in approximately 10 minutes. Nitroglycerin is also is available as an aerosol that can be sprayed beneath the tongue, a method that works even faster.

Of the various classes of drugs used for the treatment of obstructive coronary artery disease, nitrates are one of the few that both increase the blood supply to the heart muscle and reduces its demand for more blood. Thus, it effectively treats both of the major causes of chest pain— increased need for blood caused by an increased work load, and a decrease in coronary blood flow due to narrowed arteries.

Nitrates cause a blood vessel to dilate by supplying a substance known as nitric oxide (NO). Normally this chemical is produced by the endothelium, the cellular layer that coats the inner surface of all blood vessels. This endothelial layer regularly produces NO which controls the diameter of the vessel. It accomplishes this by causing the smooth muscle cells that encircle the blood vessel to relax, and in so doing, allows the vessel to carry more blood. Coronary artery disease interferes with the production of NO and causes the artery to constrict, reducing the amount of blood going to the heart muscle. However, by replacing NO with nitrates, the coronary artery increases its diameter sufficiently to allow more blood to reach the heart muscle.

The reason nitrates are able to both reduce the need of the heart for blood and increase the blood flow to the heart muscle, is because they have the ability to relax the muscular walls of blood vessels on both the arterial and venous sides of the circulation. This will cause the blood vessel to dilate but with entirely different effects, depending upon whether the vessel is an artery or a vein. To understand how it works, some background anatomy is helpful. Arteries branch into smaller and smaller arteries. When they are small enough they are called arterioles. After they become arterioles they become capillaries, and the capillaries, in turn, become venules. Venules initiate the venous side of the circulation, and these vessels become larger and larger till eventually they are the veins that we see. Venules are able to dilate, and when they do, they can hold an enormous amount of blood. For reasons that are not well understood, nitrates preferentially act on venules. In larger doses they also will dilate small and large arteries.

On the venous side of the circulation, NO from the nitrates causes the venules to enlarge. In so doing, they trap a large amount of venous blood without changing the blood pressure. Accordingly, there is a reduction in the amount of blood returning to the heart. This will reduce the volume of blood entering the ventricles, as well as the pressure within these chambers. Less pressure inside of the heart's chamber means less pressure exerted against the heart muscle and less pressure within the tissues. These tissues surround the tiny, thin-walled collateral vessels that develop after an artery becomes obstructed. Excessive pressure within those tissues, i.e., when there is hypertension, compresses the small vessels, thus reducing the flow to the heart muscle and causing angina. Conversely, a reduction in the pressure within the tissues will allow the collateral vessels to expand, and allow the blood flow to increase. This is more likely to happen when the ventricle is already enlarged to compensate for impaired cardiac function due to prior damage from a heart attack.

Thus, nitrates will cause relaxation of surface coronary arteries, even the narrowed ones, as well as collateral vessels. The result is an increase blood flow to the heart muscle that needs more blood to function normally. Allowing the heart to become smaller because of the entrapment of blood within the venules reduces the volume of blood returning to the heart and also, therefore, the work load of the heart. A reduced work load means less oxygen and less blood is required by the heart muscle. Also, the reduced volume of blood returning to the heart means there is a fall in pressure within the heart's chambers making it easier for it to contract.

Nitrates have one other ability that has only recently been discovered. They have an aspirin-like effect that reduces the ability of platelets to agglutinate. You may recall that in a region of an arteriosclerotic plaque, or a clot that has formed upon such a plaque, one of the cellular components of the blood has a tendency to cling together or agglutinate. This results in a cascade of changes within the blood that eventually causes it to clot. Aspirin— and now nitrates— tend to inhibit those changes from taking place, thus preventing the blood from clotting.

Because of all these marvelous effects upon the heart, it should come as no surprise that during a heart attack, early treatment with nitrates prevents the heart from becoming larger, improves the overall pumping function of the heart, and reduces the risk of dangerous cardiac rhythms, the frequency of chest pain, and the number of patients dying. When used in proper doses on a chronic basis in patients with recurrent angina, it essentially prevents most episodes of pain, it reduces the amount of cardiac-induced fatigue, and it improves exercise tolerance. While formal studies have not yet established that regular usage of nitrates will prolong survival in patients with coronary artery disease, I am convinced from my own experience that it does. Formal studies have established that when nitrates are combined with another drug known as hydralazine, and administered to patients with chronic congestive heart failure, survival is improved.

In spite of the well-documented efficacy of nitrates for the treatment of coronary heart disease, acute heart attacks and congestive heart failure, only a minority of patients are treated with these medications. There are several reasons for this. Doctors like to use new drugs to treat their patients for the same reasons all of us like to drive a newer car or wear the latest fashions. Because nitrates have been around for so long, there is this mistaken belief that the newer drugs are better. Indeed, the newer drugs, to be discussed below, are not nearly as effective as the older ones such as nitrates and beta blockers.

A second important reason why nitrates are often not used is because of the rapid development by the cardiovascular system of tolerance to the effects of the medication. Tolerance can develop in one to two days, resulting in a decrease or loss of therapeutic effect. It only has been in the past 5 to 10 years that we have become aware of such tolerance, and have learned how to compensate for it. It is not known why such tolerance develops, although there are many theories to account for it. I believe it may be because nitrates, as well as beta blockers, will cause fluid shifts within the body and retention of fluid by the kidney. This will increase the volume of fluid not only within the circulatory system, but within the body tissues as well. A boil or an infection is painful because of the swelling surrounding the infection. There is an increase in fluid within infected tissues, and the increased pressure that results puts pressure on the nerve endings resulting in pain. Increased pressure within the tissue also can compress the tiny venules within the tissues. This reduces the reservoir function used so successfully by nitrates to decrease the flow of blood back to the heart. Thus, all of the beneficial effects of reduced blood flow back to the heart will be lost. Fluid retention can be rapidly overcome with diuretics, and the therapeutic efficacy of nitrates is rapidly restored. This subject will be discussed in greater detail shortly.

The third reason why nitrates tend to be underused is because of their side effects, the most common of which is a headache. Initially, many patients develop headaches when they start to use nitrates. If a low dosage is used at onset, then a headache usually will not occur. If one does, it is most often mild, and disappears within a week or so. When this is explained, patients recognize that probably a mild headache is preferable to a heart attack, and they are able to tolerate the pain. Occasionally, however, someone will have an unusual sensitivity to nitrates and experience severe discomfort. When this happens, using very small doses of nitrates will overcome the problem. Only rarely can oral preparations of the drug not be used at all. In these cases, the use of nitroglycerin patches on the surface of the skin will minimize the side effects.

Another side effect that may occur with nitrates, particularly with higher doses, or when there is too long a delay between ingestion of the drug and eating, is the development of hypotension or low blood pressure. When this happens, the patient will feel dizzy upon standing, and occasionally may even faint. Typically, such events occur in patients who have been doing well but then lose weight, or develop a flu-like illness that lowers their blood pressure additionally. In these situations, the nitrates may cause their blood pressure to drop too low. Treatment is simple: reduce the dose of the medication.

In all, side effects to nitrates are uncommon when the dosage is started low and is gradually increased. None of the side effects are serious or life-threatening. The problem of tolerance has been avoided in the past few years by using incremental doses, and by allowing a 12-hour free period between the last dose taken in the evening, and the first dose taken in the morning.

Incremental doses can be used in the following way: if the initial dose is 10 mg, then six hours later it should be increased to 15 mg and, six hours after that, 20 mg. If the initial dose is 20 mg, then the next dose should be 30 mg, then 40 mg. If the first dose is 30 mg, then it should be increased to 45 mg, then 60 mg. Finally, if the initial dose is 40 mg, then the next two doses should be 60 mg, and then 80 mg. Patients who require yet higher doses to prevent chest pain may follow one of these incremental patterns: 20 mg, 40 mg and 60 mg; 30 mg, 60 mg and 90 mg; or 40 mg, 80 mg and 120 mg. The bottom line is that this therapy does work very well. Doctors who have been unsuccessful treating patients with nitrates usually use grossly inadequate doses, such as 10 mg two or three times each day. Most of the time the initial dose should be 20 to 30 mg with incremental increased doses to follow.

Nitrates are available in a variety of preparations. The sublingual nitroglycerin tablet dosage that is most often used is 0.4 mg, although it is also available in the 0.3 mg and 0.6 mg doses. The brand name for sublingual nitroglycerin is Nitrostat. The dosage of the sublingul form of nitroglycerin is low because this form of administration allows the drug to be absorbed directly into the blood stream. A sublingual tablet is also available as Sorbitrate in doses of 2.5 and 5.0 mg. These have the advantage of lasting for nearly an hour. Sorbitrate is also available as an oral tablet in a variety of doses, and as a chewable tablet. Sublingual nitroglycerin also can be obtained as an aerosol called Nitrolingual Spray at 0.4 mg per metered dose. An oral tablet known as Isordil (isosorbide dinitrate) is available in strengths of 5 mg, 10 mg, 20 mg, 30 mg and 40 mg that are taken three times every day. There also is a long-acting form of this that is taken only once each day. I do not recommend its use because it is more likely to cause tolerance.

The breakdown product of isosorbide dinitrate known as isosorbide 5-mononitrate is the metabolically active portion that is responsible for relief of angina pectoris. It is available as two relatively new drugs known as Imdur and Ismo. These drugs are used only twice each day, but they are no more effective than Isordil and are a lot more expensive than the generically available isosorbide dinitrate. Finally, there is a topical ointment called Nitrol that can be placed upon the skin where it is absorbed beginning at about 30 minutes. It, too, is available is a variety of strengths. I generally

TABLE VII: NITRATE PREPARATIONS			
Brand Name	**Generic Name**	**Method of Administration**	**Usual Dosage**
Indur	Isosorbide Mononitrate	Oral; 1x/day	120-240 mg
Ismo, Monoket	Isosorbide Mononitrate	Oral; 2x/day	20 mg
Isordil, Sorbitrate	Isosorbide Dinitrate	Oral; 3x/day in incremental dose	45-240 mg/day
Nitrobid	Nitroglycerin	Oral	19.5-39 mg/day
Sorbitrate	Isosorbide Dinitrate	Chewable	5-10 mg chewed prior to activity
Sorbitrate	Isosorbide Dinitrate	Sublingual	2.5-5 mg for pain
Nitrostat	Nitroglycerin	Sublingual	0.4 mg for pain
Nitrolingual	Nitroglycerin	Sublingual spray	1-2 squirts
Minitran, Nitrodur, Nitrodisc, & Transderm Nitro	Nitroglycerin	Skin patch	0.4 mg for 12 hr.; patch removed after 12 hrs.
Nitrol	Nitroglycerin	Ointment	1/2 to 1 inch on skin

do not use the nitroglycerin patches because tolerance is more likely to occur, as well as skin irritation from the patches. Table VII lists the various forms of nitrates and how they are administered.

ESTROGENS

A large number of studies have now shown that the use of estrogens in postmenopausal women reduces subsequent heart attacks and mortality when compared to women who do not take estrogens. The problem with this observation is that women who take estrogens tend to be more health conscious, better educated, healthier in general, and are often able to afford and have better access to medical care. The distinction between those who do and do not use estrogens may be due more to these characteristics than they are to the actual effect of the estrogen. However, some studies have shown such a marked difference, i.e., more than a 60% reduction in heart attacks and mortality, that it would indicate that the estrogen is responsible, not simply the subject's healthier life-style. Compounding the problem is the increased risk from both uterine and breast cancer in women who take estrogens, although simultaneous use of progestins eliminates the risk of the uterine cancer.

There are good reasons for believing that benefits from estrogen administration are real, based upon the changes that accompany their use. For example, estrogens have the ability to dilate blood vessels and increase coronary blood flow which will enhance the heart's performance. In part this is because estrogens enhance the production of nitric oxide, the substance responsible for controlling the diameter of the coronary arteries. Estrogens also inhibit the synthesis and release of agents within the circulation that cause the blood vessels to constrict or become narrower. Finally, estrogens are able to inhibit the proliferation of vascular smooth muscle cells which are involved in the formation of the arteriosclerotic plaque.

Estrogens have a favorable effect on coronary blood flow in men as well. Acetylcholine, a substance usually produced by the parasympathetic nervous system, will increase the flow of blood in patients without coronary artery disease, but will cause coronary blood flow to decrease in patients with coronary artery disease. In a recent study, 20 men with coronary artery disease were given an acetylcholine injection in their coronary arteries. All showed a decrease in coronary blood flow. Twelve men were then given an infusion of estrogens followed by a repeat injection of acetylcholine. Now coronary blood flow increased. In contrast, the remaining eight patients were given a placebo infusion instead of estrogens. When acetylcholine was given to these patients again, coronary blood flow decreased. Currently research is being done to find estrogen compounds which do not have feminizing effects and which could be given safely to men. Because of the many preparations that are available, if estrogens are to be taken, they should be done so under the supervision of a gynecologist.

ASPIRIN

When an arteriosclerotic plaque ruptures, the contents of the plaque are exposed to blood within the coronary artery. The cellular debris and other material within the arteriosclerotic plaque are thrombogenic; that is, they set into motion a cascade of changes that involve the blood platelets and other substances that eventually result in the formation of a blood clot on the surface of the plaque. If the clot is large enough, it will block the flow of blood within the coronary artery. If there are no collateral blood vessels in the area to compensate for the reduction in blood flow, then the heart muscle will become ischemic and the victim will have a heart attack, or myocardial infarction. Key players in the development of this clot are the blood platelets. When activated by the material from within the arteriosclerotic plaque, they release various factors that cause the blood to clot, and at the same time they begin to aggregate, or clump together, to provide a foundation for the clot that is to develop. The complex interactions between the lining of the blood vessel wall, the arteriosclerotic plaque, and the cellular and other components involved in the formation of the clot are beyond the scope of this book. Suffice to say that aspirin interferes with the formation of the clot by preventing the aggregation of platelets.

A very large number of studies have established that when aspirin is used by patients undergoing a heart attack or who have unstable angina (a prelude to a heart attack), there is a significant reduction in the number of heart attacks, as well as the mortality and frequency of recurrent heart attacks. Similarly, patients with chronic stable coronary artery disease who take aspirin are not likely to have a future heart attack. Aspirin only seems to be effective in individuals who already have heart disease. Therefore, there is no benefit to taking aspirin on a prophylactic basis merely because you don't want to develop heart disease. However, aspirin will benefit subjects who have silent ischemia.

Most of the research studying aspirin's effect on heart disease have been relatively short-term, and centered around acute episodes. Furthermore, probably 95% of those taking the drug will not receive any long-term benefit. While taking aspirin for a short period of time— or even for a few years— is not apt to create any problems, it starts to become a problem when the patient continues to take aspirin over a 5 to 10 years or longer.

The main drawback of aspirin administration is the increased tendency for the patient to develop bruising and bleeding. In younger patients, this is not a major problem. In older patients, however, who already have fragile blood vessels and who have an increased likelihood of falling or having a stroke, it can be a major problem.

Aspirin should not be given to patients with coronary artery disease if they also have hypertension. A minor stroke, a frequent occurrence in both the elderly and in those with hypertension, can become a major or fatal stroke if the victim is on aspirin therapy. Similarly, a simple fall with a minor injury can become a major problem if there is a fracture or internal bleeding. Elderly patients not infrequently must undergo unexpected surgery. It takes about 10 days for the effects of aspirin to wear off, which means a greatly increased risk if surgery is performed.

Obviously, aspirin should not be given to patients with a prior stroke, nor should it be given to those with a history of an ulcer, as it might cause the ulcer to bleed. Thus, while I favor the use of aspirin for patients with a recent heart attack, unstable angina or simply frequent chest pain for a reasonable period of time (e.g., 1 to 2 years), I believe it should be discontinued after that period, particularly if the patient is elderly.

MISCELLANEOUS DRUGS

The drugs discussed in this chapter are commonly used by all doctors for the treatment of coronary artery disease. There are new drugs currently under investigation that may radically change the way we treat patients with obstructive coronary artery disease. There are also older drugs which may occasionally benefit patients with hypertension, coronary artery disease or congestive heart failure. Including all of these drugs here would be out of place. Instead, it would be more appropriate to discuss non-medical forms of treatment for coronary artery disease. Finally, cholesterol-lowering agents were not addressed in this chapter because they are of no use in the treatment of symptomatic coronary artery disease. While drug manufacturers claim they will lower the risk of developing coronary artery disease, this is a matter of controversy and ot will be covered in a future chapter.

REFERENCES

1. Deedwania PC, Carbajal EV. Role of beta blockade in the treatment of myocardial ischemia. Am J Cardiol 1997; 80:23J-28J.
2. Pepine CJ, Hill JA, Imperi GA, Norvell N. Beta-adrenergic blockers in myocardial ischemia. Am J Cardiol 1988; 61:18B-21B.
3. Braunwald E, Kloner RA, Maroko PR. Role of beta-adrenergic blockade in the therapy of myocardial infarction. Am J Med 74:113-123.

13

INVASIVE TREATMENTS OF HEART DISEASE

Caroline was 55 years old, the wife of a small town dentist and the mother of three children. The three children were grown and had been out on their own for the past few years. Consequently, Caroline had been less active physically, and as a result had put on about 25 pounds. Since she had already gained about 25 pounds during her marriage, she was clearly overweight. Nevertheless, other than having to wear loose-fitting clothes and experiencing some mild shortness of breath and fatigue when she climbed hills or stairs, Caroline had adjusted to her weight gain and was content. She was careful to see the local family doctor at least once a year for a check up. Blood tests, heart rate and electrocardiogram results were always normal. Although her blood pressure was normal, she did notice that on the past two examinations it was higher than when she was younger. This concerned her because her sister, brother and mother all had elevated blood pressures. However, the doctor reassured her that medication was not necessary.

Caroline and her husband were looking forward to a vacation in Denver where their oldest son, his wife, and their newest grandchild lived. The baby was six months old now, and they had not seen him since he was born. Immediately after their arrival in Denver, Caroline's first action was to hold the baby while they were leaving the airport. Right away she began experiencing chest pain. As she continued to walk with the baby, it became worse until finally she had to stop and give the baby back to her daughter-in-law. It felt as if her chest were in a vise. Although she had never had pain like this before, she remembered that when her mother used to have similar pain, she had been told it was angina. Soon the pain disappeared and Caroline felt better. She decided that it might have been caused by the anxiety of the trip, or that possibly she had pulled some chest muscles while carrying her luggage. She forgot about it until the next morning when she again began to carry the baby and experienced an identical pain. This time she set the baby down as soon as the pain began, and was relieved when it quickly disappeared. Her husband was concerned, and insisted that she not pick up the baby, and that she see the doctor when they returned. He reminded her that they were at 5,000 feet.

Upon her return, Caroline did go to see the doctor. He said her blood pressure, heart and electrocardiogram were still normal, but he strongly urged her to see a cardiologist. Since there were none in the town where she lived, she made arrangements to see a cardiologist in a nearby city. The receptionist reassured her she was in good hands. The doctor was very popular and had quite a few patients in the hospital that kept him very busy. A physician's assistant took her blood pressure, listened to her heart, and took an electrocardiogram. Only then did she see the cardiologist. As soon as he heard her symptoms he said he was admitting her to the hospital that afternoon, and that she would have to undergo an angiogram. Caroline was too upset to ask about alternative tests, or about what would happen after the angiogram. The cardiologist solemnly told her that her coronary arteries must be blocked, and that one of them could close off at any time and cause a massive heart attack. Consequently, he had to perform the angiogram immediately.

Caroline was admitted to the hospital, and the angiogram was performed by the cardiologist without any complications. A few hours later he appeared in her room with another doctor dressed in a surgical scrub suit. Fortunately, her husband was there to listen and give her support. They told her she had two severe blockages and needed bypass surgery immediately. They had already placed her on the schedule for the following morning. The surgeon showed her pictures of her angiogram and pointed out where the blockages were. There was no question that they were there. The cardiologist explained that this was the reason for her chest pain. She was very lucky that she had gone to Denver. The combination of lifting a heavy baby at 5,000 feet was enough to cause her chest pain to appear. Otherwise, her first symptom back at home might have been a major heart attack, or even death. The surgeon promised her she would be just fine after the bypass surgery. Not only would she no longer have the pain but she would not get as tired as she had been. After both doctors left, Caroline felt somewhat relieved. After all, they were going to save her life.

Caroline underwent her bypass surgery the following morning. The surgeon had said that he was going to use the internal mammary artery from the undersurface of the breastbone for one of the bypasses, and the other would be a vein graft from her leg. The operation took about four hours and was uneventful. Her recovery proceeded slowly because of a wound infection in her chest, and the swelling in her leg where the vein graft had been taken. For the next six weeks she was in a great deal of pain, but gradually it began to subside, and she was able to be more active. Three months later she was essentially back to normal and felt capable of beginning an exercise program. All that inactivity had resulted in her gaining another 10 pounds. As she increased her activity, to her horror she began to have the chest pain again. It was identical to the pain she had initially experienced in Denver, but this time she wasn't carrying a baby. At first she noticed it only walking up a hill or climbing stairs. Then she began having it walking on level ground.

She returned to the cardiologist and he arranged for her to be admitted to the hospital for repeat angiograms. During the angiogram he informed her that the vein graft had closed off, and that he was going to do an angioplasty to see if it could be unclogged. The procedure was accomplished without any complications, and Caroline was allowed to return to her home the following day.

Two weeks later the chest pains returned. Caroline returned to the cardiologist, feeling increasingly frustrated. This time he informed her that he didn't think the pain was from her heart. It was muscular pain from the operation. When she told him it was the same pain as before, and asked why they had operated if the pain wasn't her heart, she didn't receive an answer.

By this time Caroline was angry, in pain, frustrated, and nearly in tears. But she was determined to find an answer. Unfortunately, there were no other cardiologists in the area. She started to visit the library, book stores and even learned how to use the Internet. Before long she learned that many things could cause chest pain, among which was high blood pressure. Knowing her strong family history of hypertension, she purchased a blood pressure cuff and began checking her pressures whenever she had chest pain. Although her blood pressure was normal at rest and even with mild activity, when the chest pain occurred her blood pressure was invariably elevated to 170-180/100-110. On one occasion it even went up to 200! She began to take voluminous notes about where and when chest pain would occur, and even the time of the day. There was one particular hill that caused her to have chest pain only sometimes. Soon she discovered that if she climbed that hill in the morning she would have chest pain, but if she did it in the mid afternoon, it did not occur. Yet, if she climbed it in the evening after dinner, chest pain would occur once more. It didn't take her long to discover that her blood pressure was elevated in the morning and after dinner, but not in the afternoon. Now she was convinced her chest pain was due to her elevated blood pressure and not directly due to her heart.

Caroline knew that the cardiologist would never admit he had made the wrong diagnosis, and that her own family doctor hadn't even been aware that her blood pressure had been elevated. She was going to have to treat herself. She knew her weight was a key factor, so back to the library and bookstores she went. She found many books and diets dealing with weight loss, but the one that appealed to her the most was *Enter The Zone* by Dr. Barry Sears, because it was suggested a high protein diet.

For the next four months, rigorously adhering to the dietary instructions, Caroline lost 40 pounds. In the following four months she lost 20 more pounds. Gradually her blood pressure began to decline. In time it was no longer elevated in the morning or after meals. Slowly the chest pain began to diminish. By the time she had lost 60 pounds, there had been no episodes of chest pain for three months. Now she felt terrific. Her fatigue, chest pain, and even the shortness of breath she had learned to live with were gone. She was determined to go back to Denver and pick that baby up again. When she did, even though the baby weighed twice as much, Caroline had not a twinge of chest pain. Her only regrets were the scar on her chest, the swelling that remained in her leg, and all the money and anguish the doctors had caused her. She vowed never again to believe any cardiologist who urged her to undergo angioplasty or coronary artery bypass surgery.

Caroline's story is true. The only thing unusual about it is not the way she was rushed in for angiograms and surgery, but her determination to find a solution to her problem on her own. She learned that it was her hypertension that caused her chest pain, aided in no small part by all the extra weight she was carrying. One can ask, "Why didn't the cardiologist recommend blood pressure medication and weight loss first, rather than angiograms and surgery?" If the patient continued to have pain after these treatments, then more aggressive forms of treatment could be recommended. It might have been that the cardiologist did not know the patient had elevated blood pressure and did not believe she could lose weight. However, if an echocardiogram had been done first, an enlarged heart would have been found which would have led to the diagnosis of hypertension. Thus, the cardiologist would only have been negligent. But, I doubt this is the explanation. I believe that a more rational view would be that if her obesity and hypertension were treated, her chest pain would have disappeared, and there would have been no need for either an angiogram or bypass surgery. This would have meant the loss of a sizable amount of money for the cardiologist.

HOW COMMON IS CAROLINE'S STORY?

Anecdotal reports from hundreds of people throughout the country who have written, telephoned, or e-mailed me repeat a similar story. Some had recent onset of exertional chest pain, and some had no symptoms whatsoever, but had merely had an abnormal stress test at a very high heart rate. Some were found to have an abnormal electrocardiogram on a routine examination. Whatever the reason the patient came to the cardiologist, angiograms were immediately scheduled and carried out. Only rarely were noninvasive tests performed. When coronary artery disease was found, the patient was urged to undergo surgery or angioplasty as soon as possible as the first treatment. The patient is almost never informed that there are other options either for diagnosis or treatment. If medical treatment is provided to the patient, it is often totally inadequate in terms of the number of drugs prescribed, and is equally inadequate in terms of dosages. In all cases, the uninformed patient is led to believe that coronary artery bypass surgery will prevent his or her approaching heart attack, and imminent death. Is this true? Is the morbidity and mortality following these interventions significantly less than might occur on an adequate medical program?

DO MOST PATIENTS WITH CORONARY ARTERY DISEASE RECEIVE ADEQUATE MEDICAL TREATMENT?

If we are to compare either angioplasty or coronary artery bypass surgery with medical treatment, we need to define what adequate medical treatment is. The drugs that are used to treat heart disease have been described in Chapter 12. To reiterate, adequate medical treatment consists of beta blockers, nitrates (nitroglycerin-like drugs), ACE inhibitors, aspirin and diuretics. Calcium channel blockers also may be used, but are not as safe, nor are they as protective as the others. All these drugs must be given in *adequate* dosages.

Unfortunately, the great majority of such patients are not receiving anywhere near the appropriate medications. If they are, it is almost always in doses that are too low to be beneficial. Numerous studies have established this beyond any reasonable doubt. For example, a study of patients referred to the University of Michigan for angioplasty or bypass surgery found that only 17% were receiving adequate medications.[1] In a multicenter study from the Cleveland Clinic and Duke University[2] of 878 patients, aspirin was being taken by only 57% of patients, beta blockers by 32%, nitrates 40%, calcium channel blockers 48%, and combination therapy by only 53%.

- A study of beta blocker usage from the University of California, San Francisco reviewed multiple reports that listed the number of patients taking the medication and found that of patients being discharged from a hospital following a heart attack, only 41-58% were given beta blockers.[3] Of those receiving beta blockers, only 6% received an adequate dosage. It was estimated that more than 3,000 victims could be saved annually by increasing the number of patients on beta blockers from 50% to 70%.

- In a study comparing angioplasty, coronary artery bypass surgery, and medical treatment for the suppression of cardiac ischemia,[4] the 204 patients on medications were divided into two groups. In one group, 70% were taking beta blockers, the dosage of which was grossly inadequate, and only 20% were taking a calcium channel blocker, the type of which that has been found to increase mortality in patients with coronary artery disease. Seventeen percent of this group were taking no medication at all. In the second group, only 40% were taking nitrates. No patients were taking aspirin or diuretics. As an aside, 45% of the patients assigned to angioplasty or bypass surgery continued to have ischemia and needed medications. Forty percent of the medically-treated patients had relief of their ischemia in spite of a remarkably inadequate medical program.[5,6] My own experience reveals that 90-95% of patients would have had relief with adequate medication.

- In a Veterans Administration study[7] of 328 patients in which angioplasty of either one or two coronary arteries was compared to medical treatment, there was no significant benefit of angioplasty when two arteries were treated. When only one coronary artery had angioplasty, the mortality in the angioplasty-treated patients was nearly twice that of the medically-treated patients. The difference between the two forms of treatment would have been very much greater had the medically-treated patients received a full quota of drugs in appropriate doses. Only 50% received beta blockers and nitrates and 70% calcium channel blockers. Apparently, neither aspirin nor diuretics were used at all.

Study after study shows the same thing. It would appear that many cardiologists simply do not know how to use medication to treat patients with chest pain due to coronary artery disease, and especially do not know how to treat their patients who have silent ischemia. They can't possibly all be uninformed. There are too many studies, editorials and lectures that repeat the same message about how most patients with heart disease are shockingly undertreated.

Another example that shows how inadequate treatment is, is the admission rate to hospitals for patients with congestive heart failure. While this is not the same as coronary artery disease, it is the end result of coronary artery disease, and has a very high mortality rate. Twenty years ago, the annual number of patients with congestive heart failure admitted to hospitals was about 200,000. Today the number is 400,000. While a small percentage of this increase is due to the increase in the number of older patients, it should be offset by the striking increase in the amount of effective cardiac medications that are available. There are two possible explanations for this increase in hospital admissions, and probably both are true.

The first explanation is based upon the fact that both coronary artery bypass surgery and angioplasty are followed by accelerated progression of the patient's coronary artery disease. This means that coronary artery narrowing that might take 20 years to develop is occurring within a few years. As a result, bypass grafts may close off very quickly. This happened to Caroline, whose situation was described earlier in this chapter. In the case of angioplasty, the artery renarrows (restenosis is the term used) in 50% of patients within 6 months. Ultimately, so much damage occurs to the heart muscle that heart failure is the final outcome. Since there are 400,000 bypass surgeries and 400,000 angioplasties done each year, it's not hard to understand why there are so many more patients who develop heart failure than there were 20 years ago.

A second explanation for the increased frequency of congestive heart failure is that the undertreatment of the patient's coronary artery disease, over a period of years, results in progressive enlargement of the heart. Eventually, it becomes so stretched out that the heart finally fails. Another observation also supports the fact that most heart patients are undertreated: of the 400,000 patients who are discharged from the hospital each year, 50% are readmitted with the same diagnosis within just a few months. While a small percentage of such readmissions are because of end stage heart disease, it may be concluded that this is due to the continuation of the same undertreatment that was the original cause of the patient's congestive heart failure.

Doctors are uninformed because they are poorly trained in the basics of cardiology. They have spent too much time learning how to do angiograms and angioplasty, and in learning how to care for surgically-treated patients. This is by far the most glamorous area of cardiology, as well as the most profitable. As a result, they are poorly trained in the basics of medical treatment and the use of drugs. Almost all of the patients they deal with go directly to the surgeon. In Europe, where the rate of revascularization is far below what it is here in the United States, patients are much more likely to receive adequate medication in appropriate doses.[2]

COMPARISON OF MEDICAL TREATMENT WITH SURGERY OR ANGIOPLASTY

Unfortunately, the few modern studies that attempt to compare interventional treatment with medical treatment are like comparing apples with oranges. Nevertheless, a few good studies that have been done, and several reports have shown the remarkable ability of the heart to spontaneously recover as a result of the growth of new blood vessels into the damaged area after a heart attack. As a result, subsequent mortality with medical treatment is significantly less than we are seeing now with either angioplasty or coronary artery bypass surgery.

In the 1970s, major studies were done comparing bypass surgery to medical treatment. These studies are described in detail in my previous book, *How To Protect Your Heart From Your Doctor*.[8] The studies showed that when bypass surgery was compared to medical treatment, there was no difference in survival in patients with good left ventricular function. Surgery seemed to improve survival only in those patients with poor cardiac function. Before extrapolating these results to today, keep in mind that the medical treatment of that era was almost non-existent. Beta blockers were used in only 30% of patients. Aspirin was used for pain and fever, but not in patients with heart disease. Nitrates were available but considered ineffective (no one yet knew about the problem of tolerance to nitrates and how to counteract it). Calcium channel blockers and ACE inhibitors were unknown, and diuretics were only used for hypertension and congestive heart failure. In addition, the age of the surgery patients at that time was much lower than the average age of today's patients. Yet today's cardiologists are constantly assuring patients and their families that surgical treatment is better and safer than medical treatment, even though the medications used were from 20 years ago, and the patient is 75 years old (operative mortality 7%) compared to the results of studies from 20 years ago that were done on patients whose average age was 55 to 60 years (operative mortality 2%).

- Among the earliest of studies to establish the efficacy of medical treatment and that patients with good cardiac function had an excellent prognosis, was that of Dr. Bernard Lown and his co-workers at Harvard University. Patients with significant coronary artery disease with abnormal stress tests, and with stable symptoms had an annual mortality of only 1.5%.[9] This was quite remarkable considering the paucity of adequate medical therapy at that time. A 1987 follow-up study from the same group was done on 88 patients who had undergone angiograms and were considered candidates for surgery. The study revealed that only 20% of these surgeries were justified. After a 2.5 year follow-up, there were no deaths among the patients who were treated medically.[10]

- In a 1987 study of approximately 170 patients with major coronary artery disease treated with angioplasty, bypass surgery or medical treatment, and followed for three years, there were no differences in the frequency of heart attacks or in mortality.[11]

- Dr. Thomas Graboys of Harvard recently studied a group of 123 patients who had been advised to undergo angioplasty or bypass surgery by another physician.[12] Instead, Dr. Graboys started them on medication. With optimal medical therapy over a period of 28 months, the annual mortality rate for this group of patients was only 1%, and only 5% had heart attacks.

- In 1995, Dr. C. Richard Conti from the University of Florida reported on 111 patients with chest pain who were treated medically. 90% had excellent relief of symptoms. 6.6% had a heart attack and 3.6% died.[13] In his editorial on a review of medical therapy in comparison to surgical treatment and angioplasty, Dr. Conti concluded that emergency angioplasty or coronary artery bypass surgery is rarely necessary when the patient is treated with multiple drug therapy.

- In a ten-year study of 5,121 patients between the ages of 25 and 60 who suffered a heart attack and were treated medically, the 28-day fatality rate was only 4.6%.[14] In a smaller series of 44 patients with an acute heart attack, all were treated medically with a death rate of only 4%.[15]

- Even patients with severe heart disease show remarkable benefits from medical treatment. Of 18 patients who originally were scheduled for cardiac transplant, but who were removed from the transplant list and treated with medication, only one patient died over the two year study period.[16]

- Dr. Morton Kern from St. Louis University Medical Center carried out a very interesting study in order to determine the consequences of delaying angioplasty in a group of 88 patients with 100 areas of stenosis.[17] Ordinarily these patients would have been urged to undergo immediate angioplasty. Instead they were treated medically and followed for a period of 6 to 30 months, with a mean of 10 months. No patient developed a heart attack and only two patients died.

These investigations suggest that patients who are fortunate enough to come under the care of a cardiologist who is skilled in the used of modern drug therapy will have an excellent prognosis.

What is the outcome when either bypass surgery or angioplasty is used? The reader may judge for himself from the following studies found in the most recent medical literature. It is important to understand that the claims of medical researchers are often not supported by the facts they present. Frequently a research study is flawed by poor experimental design and by the inflated claims of the treatment or procedure used. At first reading, the "success" of the treatment may seem to be astonishingly good. Closer scrutiny reveals a selection bias that guarantees good results. The following two studies illustrate this point.

- The first is a widely quoted study by cardiologists who quickly do angioplasties on almost every patient they see who is having a heart attack. They quote this study because they think it will justify their aggressive treatment. The study is known as The Primary Angioplasty in Myocardial Infarction Trial, or PAMI trial.[18] In this study, 395 patients from a number of medical centers were treated with either medication or angioplasty. The hospital mortality rate for the angioplasty-treated patients was only about 2% while it was about 6% for the medically-treated patients. On the surface, these results support the use of angioplasty. However, a careful reading shows that patients who had severe coronary artery disease, or those with obstructive disease known to not be successfully treated with angioplasty, were sent to the surgeons for bypass surgery. In other words, angioplasty was done only on the patients who had fairly healthy coronary arteries. In addition, in this particular study, once again the medically-treated patients were grossly undertreated. Although this study is blatantly inadequate, it continues to be popularly quoted by aggressive cardiologists.

- A second study illustrating selection bias was one in which coronary artery bypass surgery was done within 24 hours of a heart attack, after the patient had been treated with thrombolytic therapy to dissolve the clot that was thought to be the cause of the heart attack.[19] The perioperative mortality was nearly 17%, as compared to the expected 4% mortality. In the year following the surgery, mortality was only 2%, compared to about 10% without such surgery. The authors state that the post-operative prognosis was excellent for the bypass surgery patients. Had the 17% who died following surgery had a later death, their conclusions would have been different. The only reason the survivors did so well was because the sick patients died early.

REVIEW OF CURRENT LITERATURE ON ANGIOPLASTY AND BYPASS SURGERY

The following series of reports are presented in chronological order. A common method of describing results is either mortality or freedom from a cardiovascular event such as death, heart attack, stroke, or repeat bypass surgery or angioplasty. Mortality figures are presented in a variety of formats, such as 3, 5, and 10 year mortality; and so are cardiovascular events. I have modified these figures so that they are on a yearly basis, in order to make comparison easier.

- Dr. Salem Yusuf from McMaster University in Hamilton, Canada, reviewed the medical literature from 1972 to 1984 and compared the mortality of medical and surgical treatment.[20] While three of these studies have been described previously, the remaining four involved a total of 416 patients. At 10 years, the mortality of the surgically-treated patients was 33%— or 3.3% per year. The mortality of the medically-treated patients at 10 years was 34%, or 3.4% per year. Again, this reflects the status of medical treatment in the 1970's. Advances in both surgical and medical treatment would reduce the mortality for both treatments, more so for medical treatment. However, that is not the point. What these studies show is that surgical treatment was no better than medical treatment in that era.

- Dr. Spencer King of Emory University compared 194 bypass surgery patients with 198 angioplasty patients. The annual mortality for the bypass surgery patients was 2.1% per year and that for the angioplasty patients, 2.4% per year.[21] These numbers are higher than the 1.0-1.5% annual mortality expected for medical treatment.

- In a study of mortality rates in different age groups in Medicare patients undergoing either bypass surgery or angioplasty, Dr. Eric Peterson and his associates at Duke University Medical Center found the following results which are summarized in table format:[22]

TABLE VIII: THE NATIONAL MEDICARE EXPERIENCE				
Age Range	Mortality after Angioplasty 225,915 patients		Mortality after Bypass Surgery 357,885 patients	
	30 day (%)	1 year (%)	30 day (%)	1 year (%)
65-69	2.1	5.2	4.3	8.0
70-74	3.0	7.3	5.7	10.9
75-79	4.6	10.9	7.4	14.2
>80	7.8	17.3	10.6	19.5

The study shows that mortality rate is clearly related to age. Unfortunately, rarely are these figures quoted to elderly patients when they are urged to undergo these procedures. Surgeons and cardiologists like to tell patients that the mortality for bypass surgery or angioplasty is only 1% to lure them into the operating room, but obviously such claims are not true.

- In a study of 591 patients from nine medical centers in North America, the in-hospital complication rate after angioplasty was: death 1.5%, heart attack 4.2%, emergency bypass 3.2% and total complications 15.4%.[23] This does not include complication rates after discharge.

- Another study from the University of Washington was done on the 15-year survival rate following the Coronary Artery Surgery's study of 6,018 men and 1,095 women who originally underwent treatment between 1974 and 1979.[24] For those who received medical treatment, the 15-year survival rate was 50% for men and 49% for women. For those with initial surgical treatment, the survival was 52% for men and 48% for women. Thus, there was no significant difference in survival between the two treatments, and annual mortality was 3.3%.

- Another interesting study was the CAVEAT Trial (Coronary Angioplasty Versus Excisional Atherectomy Trial).[25] Atherectomy refers to the use of a rotor rooter type of catheter that is inserted into a coronary artery and used to cut up and scoop out the arteriosclerotic plaque. In this study, only the frequency of a myocardial infarction (heart attack) was studied in 500 patients who underwent angioplasty and 512 who underwent atherectomy. The incidence of myocardial infarction in the atherectomy patients was 15.2% and it was 6.8% in the angioplasty patients. The high incidence of heart attacks with both groups was because cardiac enzymes were measured rather than merely getting an electrocardiogram after the procedure.

This study illustrates a common tactic that is used to minimize the complications of an interventional procedure such as angioplasty, atherectomy or bypass surgery. The frequency of a heart attack after an intervention is one of the complications that is measured. If the patients who have one of these procedures are only tested with follow-up electrocardiograms, then the frequency of a heart attack will be quite low, simply because the electrocardiogram is so insensitive that it will not detect damage to the heart muscle unless the damage is very great.

In contrast, if cardiac enzymes are measured after an intervention, as was done in the study quoted above, then the true incidence of post-procedural complications will be evident. For example, cardiologists like to tell their patients that the heart attack rate after angioplasty is no more than 1-2%. Yet, as we see from this study, when cardiac enzymes are measured, the heart attack rate goes up to nearly 7%.

- Another report dealing with the mortality rate of elderly patients undergoing cardiac surgery comes from Cedars-Sinai Medical Center in Los Angeles.[26] In a study of 528 patients over 80, the 30-day mortality was 8.3%. At one year it was 18% and at 5 years it was 38%. These figures are very similar to the Duke study.

- A review from St. Louis University Health Sciences Center[27] of 250 patients undergoing coronary artery bypass surgery found that the annual mortality for patients between 60 and 79 was about 7% per year, and that for patients above the age of 80 it was 13% per year.

- From the National Registry of Myocardial Infarction, a study showed that for 3,648 patients undergoing angioplasty, all of whom had this procedure done initially as the primary treatment, the in-hospital mortality for patients who were treated under one hour was 6.9%, from 1-2 hours 5.7%, from 2-3 hours 9.1%, and after three hours 9.4%.[28] These are large numbers. In my experience, the mortality rate of a heart attack patient after he or she reaches the hospital is excellent. There is a better than 95% chance of recovery, an an even better chance if the patient gets to the hospital early. Thus, the mortality rate for patients treated with angioplasty in this study is twice as high as with conservative medical treatment. A recent Veterans Administration Study showed similar findings in a group of 500 patients with an acute heart attack. At nine days, 21 patients in the group treated with surgery or angioplasty had died, but only 6 patients who were medically treated died during the same time period.[29,30]

Looking at mortality figures alone doesn't tell the complete story. Perhaps a better way to evaluate the outcome of these procedures is to combine all of the cardiovascular events, including death, on an annual basis. It is known, for example, that after angioplasty, the coronary artery that was dilated will usually become narrowed again and may close off. The frequency with which this happens is about 50%. How often this will result in repeat symptoms is not precisely known. The following reports describe recurrences of cardiovascular events including death, heart attack, unstable angina, repeat angioplasty and coronary artery bypass surgery.

- A Massachusetts General Hospital trial of 127 patients undergoing angioplasty or coronary artery bypass surgery resulted in an annual cardiovascular event rate of 7.7% per year for the surgery patients, and 17.7% per year for the angioplasty patients.[31]

- A 10-year study from the Thoraxcenter at Erasmus University in Rotterdam, on 856 patients undergoing angioplasty reported an annual mortality rate of 2.2%, and an annual cardiovascular event rate of 8.6%.[32]

- In the BARI trial (Bypass Angioplasty Revascularization Investigation), 1829 patients were followed for 5.4 years.[33] Annual mortality was 2.1% per year for bypass surgery and 2.7% per year for angioplasty. Event rate was 4% per year for surgery and 4.3% per year for angioplasty.

- Another 10-year study from St. Antonius Hospital in the Netherlands followed 351 patients who had angioplasty.[34] Annual mortality was 2% per year and cardiovascular event rate 10% per year.

- At the University of North Carolina at Greensboro, 633 patients were treated with primary angioplasty for their heart attack. The in-hospital mortality was 9%. Considering the fact that only patients who are still in good condition during their heart attack and/or that otherwise have healthy vessels will qualify for angioplasty, a mortality rate of 9% is two or three times higher than what it should be with standard medical treatment.[35]

- A 25-year study from the University of Ottawa Heart Institute in Ontario, Canada, followed 1,388 patients who underwent bypass surgery at an average age of only 48 years. It revealed an annual mortality of 2%. Eighteen percent had to undergo repeat surgery during this period.[36] The annual mortality for patients in this age group should be well under 1%.

- The Veterans Affairs Medical Center and the University of Colorado Health Sciences Center in Denver studied 131 patients above the age of 70 with unstable angina who underwent coronary angioplasty for their symptoms. The mortality at 30 days for this group was a striking 13%.[37] The mortality for this group of patients on optimal medical treatment should be only 3-4%.

- In a comparison of medical treatment versus angioplasty for patients with stable coronary artery disease, 20 centers from the United Kingdom and Ireland treated 1,018 patients. The risk of death or a heart attack was 2.3% per year for angioplasty-treated patients but only 1.2% per year for patients treated medically.[38]

- In a recent Veterans Administration study known as the VANQWISH trial, 920 patients who suffered from an acute heart attack and came from 15 different medical centers were randomized to treatment with revascularization (angioplasty or coronary artery bypass surgery) or conservative medical treatment. At the time of discharge from the hospital, 21 (4.6%) patients who had undergone revascularization had died versus only 6 (1.3%) of those patients who had been treated medically. At 2.5 years there were 80 deaths (17.4%) in the aggressively-treated group, versus only 59 deaths (12.8%) in the conservatively-treated patients.[29,30] This translates into an annual mortality of 5.1% for the medically-treated patients, a figure which is high for this group. Keep in mind, however, that about 75% of medically-treated patients are *not* on optimal medical treatment. Also, it is well known in the medical community that patients treated by the Veterans Administration are much sicker than patients treated elsewhere.

Obviously, the results of this study were completely opposite from what was expected, and it illustrates a major problem when a new treatment is introduced for the treatment of disease. If a new drug is developed, it must go through years of investigation, first on animals and then on a very select group of patients. After many years of study, usually on thousands of patients, the data is presented to the FDA and it is carefully scrutinized. Even after a drug is approved and is marketed, if the frequency of side effects is higher than anticipated, then the drug is promptly withdrawn from the market.

No such strict controls exist for the development of a new procedure or surgery. For example, both coronary artery bypass surgery and angioplasty were introduced for the treatment of patients with coronary artery disease whose symptoms could not be controlled by medical treatment. Quite properly, comparison studies between bypass surgery and medical treatment were undertaken in the 1970's. While those comparisons showing that surgery was no better than medical treatment in most patients are no longer relevant because of the many drugs that are now available, at least several studies were done to compare the two methods of treatment. No such study has ever been published for angioplasty. My instinct tells me that in all probability, a number of such studies have been performed in the 20 years or so that angioplasty has been available. They have not been published because, as in the Veterans Administration VANQUISH Trial, the results were opposite to what was expected. And that would have a negative impact on the income of all those cardiologists whose life styles depend upon doing large numbers of these procedures.

There are also no controls in place when the use of a surgical treatment for a disease is extended to include other indications. For example, any cardiologist can arbitrarily decide that instead of treating his or her heart attack patients with conventional medical therapy, he or she is going to have them all undergo either immediate angioplasty, or, if their coronary arteries do not qualify for such angioplasty, then they will undergo coronary artery bypass surgery. The cardiologist doesn't even have to compare this new treatment for a heart attack to another group of patients who are treated medically. He or she can use the expected survival rate that is known from the medical literature.

What has happened over the past several years, therefore, is that cardiologists and surgeons are treating all patients with heart attacks this way, without ever knowing whether it is better or worse than medical treatment. The patient is never told that this is really experimental treatment, and that in reality he or she is a form of guinea pig. For that matter, most patients are never really informed that medical treatment is an option. All they are told is that most cardiologists are now recommending immediate angioplasty, or even the insertion of stents as a new treatment for heart attacks. Obviously, this can be very profitable.

Thus, when a study comes along like the Veterans Administration VANQUISH Trial, everyone is shocked, for it wasn't what they expected. The sad part is that so great is the economic renumeration to both cardiologist and hospital that mere scientific evidence will not stop them. The only way these travesties can be stopped is for the patient and public to become aware of what is happening, and to refuse to allow these interventional and invasive treatments when they enter the hospital.

Only a few reports deal with the use of stents placed within a coronary artery. A stent is a metal tube that can be expanded when placed within a coronary artery. When it is fully expanded, it becomes a scaffolding that helps to keep the artery from closing. Typically, when an artery is dilated with balloon angioplasty, a delayed complication is collapse of the walls of the blood vessel, causing the artery to become blocked. Stents were developed to prevent this from happening. While a stent does help to keep the vessel walls apart, the inside of the stent may become filled with tissue that grows into the stent. Thus, stents often become occluded and the vessel still closes off.

- Harvard University researchers reported on 175 patients who had stents inserted. The annual mortality of this group was 2.7% and the annual cardiovascular event rate was 10%.[39] Long-term complication rates with stents are not known at this time because the procedure is too new.

- The Cardiovascular Division of the University of Pennsylvania studied the three-year outcome of 65 patients who underwent stenting. Mortality was 4% per year, and cardiovascular event rate was 14.7% per year.[40]

- A detailed analysis of 300 patients who underwent primary angioplasty for an acute myocardial infarction was done by researchers at the University of Giessen in Germany.[41] Their findings are described in the following table:

	1 Month	6 Months	1 Year	2 Years	3 Years
All Cardiac Events	13%	22%	34%	42%	51%
Cardiac Mortality	4%	5%	6%	7%	9%
Total Mortality	5%	6%	9%	10%	13%
Repeat Angioplasty		20%	23%	25%	31%

TABLE IX: FOLLOW-UP OF PRIMARY ANGIOPLASTY FOLLOWING ACUTE MYOCARDIAL INFARCTION (N=300) FROM THE UNIVERSITY OF GIESSEN, GERMANY

These cardiac event rates and mortality are extremely high in comparison with medically-treated patients.

IS THE PATIENT BETTER OR WORSE OFF AFTER BYPASS SURGERY OR ANGIOPLASTY?

It is apparent from the reports cited that the mortality rate, as well as incidence of other complications for both coronary artery bypass surgery and angioplasty, vary considerably. Outcome depends in large measure upon the patient's age, how much heart disease is present, the skill of the doctor who is treating the patient, and a host of other factors. A patient may be better off in the hands of a highly skilled surgeon than a cardiologist who has never learned how to medically treat coronary artery disease. *What is clear, at the very least, is that neither surgery nor angioplasty has an advantage over medical treatment. No studies have shown that either of these two interventions will prevent heart attacks or premature death.*

If revascularization does not prevent future heart attacks or death, what do these procedures accomplish? And, more importantly, do they cause any harm? These questions are cause for speculation. A sizable number of studies have been done using a variety of imaging procedures to determine whether there has been improvement in cardiac function after revascularization. When the echocardiogram was used, the focus was on the motion of the heart muscle before and after revascularization. With radioactive imaging, the focus was on the blood flow to the heart muscle, and with positron emission tomography (PET), the focus has been on metabolic function. Unfortunately, each of these procedures provide different answers. For example, a radioactive thallium study might show there is no blood flow to a given area of the heart. In contrast, A PET study might find presence of metabolic activity. In the former instance, the prediction might be that there will be no functional recovery after revascularization; however, results from the PET study would predict that recovery can take place.

To complicate matters, imaging studies done immediately after revascularization will usually show more impaired function simply due to the trauma of the procedure used to restore function. If, however, the imaging study is delayed for several months, recovery will often be seen. It is here that the waters become even muddier. There is solid evidence that recovery will occur without any treatment whatsoever, although medical treatment will speed the healing process up and will increase the chance of recovery. This occurs through the heart's own revascularization process, i.e., the development of new vessels into the area where the coronary arteries are narrowed or blocked.

While there are many reports that study the natural revascularization process, a recent study from the Department of Cardiology at the Academic Hospital in Leiden in The Netherlands is of particular interest. Researchers reviewed 37 studies that compared cardiac function before and after revascularization with angioplasty or bypass surgery, using a variety of imaging procedures.[42] Improvement after revascularization occurred only 37% to 55% of the time. The remainder of the hearts studied were either the same or worse following revascularization. The discouraging finding was that there was no reliable way to predict in the individual patient the likelihood of recovery from a revascularization procedure. Subjects who showed no viable heart muscle after a heart attack were less likely to show improvement, and those with viable muscle more often than not did show recovery. Unfortunately, a high percentage of patients with viable muscle did not get better, and some of the hearts that appeared to be not viable did recover.

Both coronary artery bypass surgery and angioplasty will relieve recurring chest pains in subjects with coronary artery disease. In the case of bypass surgery, 10% to 20% do not get effective relief, while 40% to 50% of patients who receive angioplasty have a return of their symptoms. However, relief from pain will occur in 75% of patients without any treatment within 3 to 6 months, simply because of the growth of new vessels. Treatment with medication will speed things up, and relieves pain in an additional 20% with a far lower complication rate than accompanies mechanical revascularization, as shown by the numerous studies cited in this chapter.

Aside from the acute and subacute complications of angioplasty and bypass surgery, a major concern is the acceleration of the arteriosclerotic process in the coronary arteries that are treated. For example, vessels that are bypassed often show rapid progression of the occlusive process which led to the patient's symptoms. More importantly, collateral vessels that had developed over a period of time to compensate for a narrowed artery will usually disappear following bypass surgery. Thus, the ischemic heart muscle may actually be worse off following such surgery. The importance of these collateral vessels is illustrated by the fact that when a coronary artery is severely narrowed and then becomes completely occluded, it has little effect on cardiac function. This is because there are enough collateral vessels to make up for the deficit in blood flow. In contrast, when a coronary artery is only mildly narrowed and closes off suddenly, it is likely that the patient will have a myocardial infarction or even die because new collateral vessels have not yet had a chance to develop. Because of these facts, the common practice of rushing patients in for emergency or urgent surgery because of a severely narrowed coronary artery is completely unnecessary, and needlessly frightens the patient and his or her family.

GEOGRAPHICAL VARIATION IN THE FREQUENCY OF CORONARY ARTERY BYPASS SURGERY AND ANGIOPLASTY

One of the facts that emerges from a review of the medical literature about bypass surgery and angioplasty is the enormous variation in the frequency with which these procedures are done. Such variation might be understandable if controversy existed over which patients should have such interventions, and when they should be done. The official guidelines of the American College of Cardiology and the American Heart Association recommend that symptomatic patients with good cardiac function initially be treated medically.[43] Surgery should be reserved for patients who fail to respond to medical treatment. The guidelines suggest that patients with poor cardiac function might fare better with revascularization. However, this latter recommendation is based upon studies from 20 years ago, when younger patients were operated upon by skilled surgeons and compared to the medical therapy of that day. It may no longer be true with older patients who are being operated upon by less skilled surgeons when compared to modern medical treatment.

The matter of skill is worth commenting upon at this point. Whenever a new surgical procedure is introduced into the field of medicine, it tends to be confined for many years to major medical centers where they have only the best of surgeons. Such was the case when coronary artery bypass surgery was introduced in the 1970's. Soon the new surgical technique was spread to all hospitals and every surgeon wanted to learn how it was done. Naturally, some surgeons are better than others. It would not be fair to apply the surgical results of a highly-skilled surgeon who performs many hundreds of bypass procedures each year with a surgeon who does only a few dozen. How much variation can take place in the mortality after bypass surgery was dramatically illustrated ten years ago when the *Los Angeles Times* studied the mortality associated with bypass surgery in nearly 17,000 patients in California (*Los Angeles Times*, March 27, 1988). The mortality ranged from 1.6% to almost 15% with the average being about 5.5%.

These recommendations are straightforward enough. Thus, it is of interest to compare the frequency with which bypass surgery and angioplasty are used in different regions. In a recent study from

Minneapolis-St. Paul and Göteborg, Sweden, the medical records of all patients hospitalized for a heart attack were compared.[44] Minneapolis-St. Paul was selected because its residents are primarily of Northern European origin. All 25 hospitals in Minneapolis-St. Paul and two large hospitals in Göteborg participated in the study. A total of 2,460 hospital discharges from Minneapolis-St. Paul and 1,189 from Göteborg were reviewed. Coronary angiograms were done for 10% of the Göteborg heart attack patients. In contrast, 49% of the male patients and 39% of the women from Minneapolis-St. Paul had angiograms. Angioplasty was done on 5% of the men and 3% of the women from Göteborg, while it was done on 20% of the men and 15% of the women from Minneapolis-St. Paul. Bypass surgery was done on only 1% of the men and women from Göteborg, but on 12% of the men and 10% of the women from Minneapolis-St. Paul. In spite of these wide variations in the use of these procedures, there was no significant difference in the mortality at either 28 days or one year.

The Minneapolis-St. Paul and Göteborg study is quite illuminating in that it demonstrates the marked overuse of technology and surgery in the United States as compared to a modern country in Europe with a medical system equal to ours. The indications for having a patient undergo angiograms after admission to the hospital for a heart attack are no different in Sweden than they are in the United States, or at least there should be no difference. Similarly, the indications for doing angioplasty or bypass surgery should be the same. Yet 44% of American patients versus only 10% of Göteborg patients had angiograms. Similarly, bypass surgery was done eleven times more often and angioplasty four times more often in Minneapolis-St. Paul as compared to Göteborg. Could the reason for this difference be due to the economic reimbursement? The higher use of technology and surgery in this country might be understandable if there were a considerable difference in the mortality after discharge from the hospital. But such was not the case; there was no difference. There is no reason to believe that this lack of difference was because American cardiologists and surgeons are better. The cardiologists and surgeons from both countries are equally competent.

In another recent study that compared the use of cardiac procedures in the United States versus Ontario, Canada, 224,258 Medicare patients were compared to 9,444 Canadian patients of a similar age.[45] In the U.S., 34.9% of the patients underwent coronary angiograms versus 6.7% of the Canadian patients. For angioplasty, 11.7% of the U.S. patients had these procedure versus 1.5% of the Canadian patients. For coronary artery bypass surgery, 10.6% of the U.S. patients underwent this treatment versus only 1.4% of the Canadian patients. The 30-day mortality for the U.S. patients was 21.4%, versus 22.3% for the Canadian patients. At one year, the mortality was 34.3% in the United States and 34.4% in Canada. Thus, there was a strikingly higher use of cardiac procedures in the United States without any significant benefit.

A similar comparison study between the United States, Hungary and Poland followed 8,000 patients with an acute myocardial infarction. Sixty percent of the American patients had an angiogram before discharge from the hospital, versus 20% in Hungary and 7% in Poland. Angioplasty was done three times more often and bypass surgery seven times more often in the United States than in Hungary and Poland. There was no difference in mortality in the different countries.[46]

Even in the United States, there is wide variation in the frequency with which cardiac procedures are done after a heart attack. For example, a patient in the south central United States is nearly twice as likely to have bypass surgery as a similar patient from New England, and 1.5 times more likely to have angioplasty. Yet there is no difference in mortality at one year.[47]

The studies quoted above are just a small sample of many similar reports showing a wide range in the frequency with which patients with heart attacks and coronary artery disease are made to undergo costly but unnecessary procedures that not only do not benefit the patient, they also often increase morbidity and mortality. It's hard to escape the conclusion that these profitable procedures are done more for the benefit of the doctor and the medical institution than they are for the patient. Patients are reassured that these procedures will improve the quality of life. Unfortunately, they are not told whose quality of life will be improved. When the surgeon or cardiologist appears at the patient's bedside after surgery and exclaims, "Boy, we got to you just in time!" what he or she really means is that if they had waited any longer, the patient would have improved on his or her own.

Where does all of this leave us? According to major authorities in the field, most patients with coronary artery disease can be safely treated medically.[48,49] The practice of doing immediate angiograms followed by either angioplasty or bypass surgery as the first treatment is unwarranted, and does not follow ethical practice guidelines. I have come up with the following list of recommendations, based on 18 years of experience in treating patients. During that time, only eight of approximately 500 patients have had to undergo angioplasty or bypass surgery because they no longer would respond to medical treatment. In that same period of time, both mortality from coronary artery disease and the incidence of heart attacks have been less than 1% per year. Indeed, in the two years prior to the writing of this book, in a practice devoted solely to the care of heart patients, there have been no admissions to the hospital for chest pain or heart attacks, no patient has required angioplasty or coronary artery bypass surgery, and no patient has died. These patients have had an excellent quality of life, and have remained symptom-free.

My personal guidelines are as follows:

1. Urgent or emergency angioplasty or coronary artery bypass surgery is almost never necessary in ambulatory patients, particularly not in patients who are rushed to an emergency room with chest pain. The mortality rate of patients treated this way is several times higher than those who are treated conservatively with medication. Nor is bypass surgery or angioplasty indicated for patients who are doing well shortly after a heart attack, merely because a routine angiogram shows blockage of one or more arteries. Patients who are having intractable chest pain not relieved by *adequate* medication would be an exception. Unfortunately, the risk of doing bypass surgery within 6 months of a heart attack is much greater than average. It is important to understand that *neither surgery nor angioplasty prevent heart attacks or premature death in most patients.*

2. Patients with coronary artery disease who do not have symptoms and have an acceptable quality of life almost never need surgery or angioplasty, no matter which tests are abnormal. The same holds true

for those with only occasional symptoms, or with symptoms that occur only with extremes of exertion. *Symptoms alone are not an indication for surgery— only if those symptoms interfere with day-to-day activities, and if they cannot be adequately relieved with medication in adequate doses.*

3. An abnormal test, be it an electrocardiogram, stress test, radioactive imaging or echocardiogram, is not a good reason for recommending an angiogram, as long as these noninvasive tests show reasonably good overall cardiac function. *Nor is the presence of blockage in one or more coronary arteries on an angiogram an adequate reason for angioplasty or bypass surgery.* The reason is, the heart muscle may be getting plenty of blood through the microcirculation which is not visible on an angiogram. Also, during strenuous exercise, the microcirculation may not be able to carry an adequate volume of blood, although it may be perfectly capable of doing so at rest or with mild exercise. The patient should be treated, not the test.

4. If a patient shows symptoms and is found to have evidence of coronary artery disease, that coronary artery disease may be coincidental. In other words, there may be some other reason for the symptoms. There are over 50 different reasons why someone may have chest pain! It often takes weeks and sometimes months to determine the cause of that pain. Furthermore, without a prior angiogram to compare to, the cardiologist has no way of knowing whether the coronary artery disease found has recently become worse, or if it is no different than it was 5 years ago. The same holds true for other tests that are done, such as echocardiograms and radioactive imaging tests.

5. If symptoms (i.e., chest pain) due to coronary artery disease are present, the patient must be treated with aspirin, beta blockers, nitrates, ACE inhibitors and diuretics, and sometimes even with calcium channel blockers, all in *adequate* doses. Failure to do so amounts to negligence on the part of the doctor. A program that is composed only of a cholesterol-lowering drug, aspirin and nitroglycerin for pain relief is not considered to be an adequate medical program. The beta blocker must be given in amounts sufficient to bring the heart rate down to the 50 to 60 beats per minute. Usually this means 120-160 mg of Inderal

(propranolol) every day, or 100-200 mg of Tenormin (atenolol) every day, or 150-200 mg of metoprolol every day. Of the nitrates, Isordil (isosorbide dinitrate) should be given in amounts of 90-180 mg per day. The recommended dose for diuretics such as hydrochlorothiazide is 50-100 mg per day; for Bumex it is 2-4 mg every day, and for Lasix 80-160 mg per day. The recommended dose of Monopril, an ACE inhibitor, is 10-20 mg per day. I make sure my patients understand that a normal blood pressure is too high for someone with coronary artery disease, unless their aortic valve is obstructed as well. Blood pressure during stress, e.g., during hand grip stress, should not rise higher than 125-130/80. If it does, and the patient is having chest pain during exertion, the pain may be caused by his or her elevated blood pressure.

6. Doctors who fail to prescribe medication that will relieve symptoms and protect the heart, or who say medical treatment is not an option, are either uninformed or are recommending angioplasty or coronary artery bypass surgery for economic reasons. It is unethical for a cardiologist not to inform a patient of his or her options. If the cardiologist says medication will not work, that's just his or her opinion. Don't hesitate to get another cardiologist's opinion, it might be different. Make sure, however, that the second opinion does not come from a colleague who will simply "rubber stamp" the first doctor's recommendation.

7. The vast majority of patients who have coronary artery disease will dramatically improve on an *adequate* medical program that consists of the drugs described in item 5. The reason is, if you eliminate the conditions that accelerate the progression of the disease— such as hypertension, smoking, and stress, and if you reduce the amount of work the heart has to do and increase the blood flow to the heart muscle with medication, then, over time, new blood vessels will grow into the area where there is blockage. In other words, the heart will revascularize itself without help from the surgeon.

8. While there is a possibility a patient may have a heart attack or die on a good medical program, in my opinion, this is far more likely to occur with angioplasty or coronary artery bypass surgery. The results of surgery are unpredictable, are accompanied by far more serious side effects, including heart attack, stroke and death, than patients are told,

and are much higher in older patients. Cardiologists and surgeons quote low mortality figures in order to lure patients into the operating room, but these often have little to do with reality.

Thus, the treatment may be considerably more dangerous than the disease. If you must gamble, do so in Las Vegas, not on the operating table where you will bet everything you own— and everything you are. After all, if medical treatment does fail after one or two months, then surgery can always be tried. But the patients I have treated almost never need to undergo surgery.

The wonders of modern technology are so great that it is very easy for an incompetent doctor to masquerade behind them. Choose wisely, for the doctor you select to treat your heart disease may be more dangerous than your disease.

REFERENCES

1. Grambow DW, Topol EJ. Effect of maximal medical therapy on refractoriness of unstable angina pectoris. Am J Cardiol 1992; 70:577-581.
2. Eisenberg MJ, Califf RM, Cohen EA, *et al.* Use of evidence-based medical therapy in patients undergoing percutaneous coronary revascularization in the United States, Europe and Canada. Am J Cardiol 1997; 79:867-872.
3. Viskin, Barron HV. Beta blockers prevent cardiac death following a myocardial infarction: So why are so many infarction survivors discharged without beta blockers? Am J Cardiol 1996; 78:821-822.
4. Knatterud GL, Bourassa MG, Pepine CJ, *et al.* Effect of treatment strategies to suppress ischemia in patients with coronary artery disease: 12-week results of the Asymptomatic Cardiac Ischemia Pilot (ACIP) Study. J Am Coll Cardiol 1994; 24:11-20.
5. Chaitman BR, Stone PH, Knatterud GL, *et al.* Asymptomatic Cardiac Ischemia Pilot (ACIP) Study: Impact of anti-ischemia therapy on 12 week rest electrocardiogram and exercise test outcomes. J Am Coll Cardiol 1995; 26:585-593.

6. Deedwania PC. Is there evidence in support of the ischemia suppression hypothesis? J Am Coll Cardiol 1994; 24:21-24.

7. Parisi AF, Hartigan PM, Folland ED, *et al.* Evaluation of exercise thallium scintigraphy versus exercise electrocardiography in predicting survival outcomes and morbid cardiac events in patients with single and double vessel disease. J Am Coll Cardiol 1997; 30:1256-1263.

8. Wayne HH. *How to Protect Your Heart from Your Doctor.* Santa Barbara, CA: Capra Press, 1995, page 121.

9. Podrid PJ, Graboys TB, Lown B. Prognosis of medically-treated patients with coronary artery disease with profound ST segment depression during exercising testing. N Engl J Med 1981; 305:1111-1116.

10. Graboys, TB, Headley A, Lown B, *et al.* Results of a second opinion program for coronary bypass graft surgery. JAMA 1987; 258: 1611-1614.

11. Hueb WA, Bellotti G, Almeida de Oliveira S, *et al.* The medicine, angioplasty, or surgery study (MASS): a prospective , randomized trial of medical therapy, balloon angioplasty, or bypass surgery for single proximal left anterior descending artery stenosis. J. Am Coll Cardiol 1995; 26:1600-1605.

12. Graboys TB, Ostrander RL, Blatt CM *et al.* Maximal medical therapy reduced referral for cardiovascular interventions for patients with coronary artery disease. J Am Coll Cardiol 1996; 27:132A

13. Conti CR. Treatment of ischemic heart disease: Role of drugs, surgery, and angioplasty in unstable angina patients. Clin Cardiol 1995; 18: 4-6.

14. Jamrozik K, Broadhurst RW, Parsons MST, *et al.* Ten year trends in medical management and case fatality in acute myocardial infarction. J Am Coll Cardiol Feb. 1996; 773-1, 278A.

15. Stock E. Preventive management of myocardial infarction mortality reduction outside coronary care unit. Med J Austral Feb. 14, 1970; 309-319.

16. Levine TB, Levine AB, Goldberg AD, *et al.* Clinical status of patients removed from a transplant waiting list rivals that of transplant recipients at significant cost savings. Am Heart J 1996; 132:1189-1194.

17. Kern MJ, Donohue TJ, Aguirre FV, *et al.* Clinical outcome of deferring angioplasty in patients with normal translesional pressure-flow velocity measurements. J Am Coll Cardiol 1995; 25:178-187.

18. Stone GW, Grines CL, Browne KF, *et al.* Predictors of in-hospital and 6-month outcome after acute myocardial infarction in the reperfusion era: The primary angioplasty in myocardial infarction (PAMI) trial. J Am Coll Cardiol 1995; 25:370-377.

19. Gersh BJ, Chesebro JH, Braunwald E, *et al.* Coronary artery bypass graft surgery after thrombolytic therapy in the thrombolysis in myocardial infarction trial, Phase II (TIMI II). J Am Coll Cardiol 1995; 25:395-402.

20. Yusif S, Zucker D, Peduzzi P, *et al.* Effect of coronary artery bypass surgery on survival: overview of 10-year results from randomized trials by the coronary artery bypass surgery trialists collaboration. Lancet 1994; 344:563-570.

21. King SB III, Lembo NJ, Weintraub WS, *et al.* A randomized trial comparing coronary angioplasty with coronary bypass surgery. N Engl J Med 1994; 331:1044-1045.

22. Peterson ED, Jollis JG, Bebchuk JD, *et al.* Changes in mortality after myocardial revascularization in the elderly. Ann Intern Med 1994; 121:919-927.

23. Wolfe MW, Roubin GS, Schweiger M, *et al.* Length of hospital stay and complications after percutaneous transluminal coronary angioplasty. Clinical and procedural predictors. Circulation 1995; 92:311.

24. Davis KB, Chaitman B, Ryan T, *et al.* Comparison of 15 year survival for men and women after initial medical or surgical treatment for coronary artery disease: a CASS registry study. J Am Coll Cardiol 1995; 25:1000-1009.

25. Harrington RA, Lincoff M, Califf RM, *et al.* Characteristics and consequences after myocardial infarction after percutaneous coronary intervention: Insights from the coronary angioplasty versus excisional atherectomy trial (CAVEAT). J Am Coll Cardiol 1995. 25:1693-1699.

26. Tsai TP, Chaux A, Matloff JM, *et al.* Ten-year experience of cardiac surgery in patients aged 80 years and over. Ann Thorac Surg 1994; 58: 445-451.

27. Peigh PS, Swartz MT, Vaca KJ, *et al.* Effect of advancing age on cost and outcome of coronary artery bypass grafting. Ann Thorac Surg 1994; 58:1362-1367.

28. Cannon C, Lambre CT, Tiefenbrunn AJ, *et al.* Influence of door-to-balloon time on mortality in primary angioplasty results in 3,648 patients in the second national registry of myocardial infarction (NRMI-2). J Am Coll Cardiol 1996; 717-3:61A.

29. VANQWISH Trial Research Investigators. Veteran Affairs Non-Q Wave Infarction Strategies In-Hospital. J Am Coll Cardiol 1997; 30:3.

30. VANQWISH Trial Research Investigators. Design and baseline characteristics of the Veteran Affairs Non-Q Wave Infarction Strategies In-Hospital Trial. J Am Coll Cardiol 1998; 31:312-320.

31. Rodriguez, A, Mele E, Peyregne E. *et al.* Three year follow up of the Argentine randomized trial percutaneous transluminal coronary angioplasty versus coronary artery bypass surgery in multivessel disease (ERACI). J Am Coll Cardiol 1996; 27:1178-1184.

32. Ruygrok PN, de Jaegere P, van Domburg RT, et al Clinical outcome 10 years after percutaneous transluminal coronary angioplasty in 856 patients. J Am Coll Cardiol 1996; 27:1669-1677.

33. Simoons ML. Myocardial revascularization—bypass surgery or angioplasty? N Eng J Med 1996; 335:275-276.

34. Berg JM, Gin MTJ, Ernest, S. *et al.* Ten year follow-up of percutaneous transluminal coronary angioplasty for proximal left anterior descending coronary artery stenosis in 351 patients. J Am Coll Cardiol 1996; 28:22-28.

35. Brodie BR, Stuckey TD, Kissling G, *et al.* Importance of infarct-related artery patency for recovery of left ventricular function and late survival after primary angioplasty for acute myocardial infarction. J Am Coll Cardiol 1996; 28:319-325.

36. Fitzgibbon GM, Kafka HP, Leach AJ, *et al.* Coronary bypass graft fate and patient outcome: Angiographic follow-up in 5,065 grafts related to

survival and reoperation in 1,388 patients during 25 years. J Am Coll Cardiol 1996; 28:616-626.

37. Morrison DA, Bies RD, Sacks J. Coronary angioplasty for elderly patients with "high risk" unstable angina: Short-term outcomes and long-term survival. J Am Coll Cardiol 1997; 29:339-344.

38. RITA-2 Trial Participants. Angioplasty or medical treatment for stable angina? Lancet 1997; 350: 461-468.

39. Laham RJ, Carrozza JP, Berger C, *et al.* Long-term (4- to 6-year) outcome of Palmaz-Schatz stenting: Paucity of late clinical stent-related problems. J Am Coll Cardiol 1996; 28:820-826.

40. Klugherz BD, DeAngelo DL, Kim BK, *et al.* Three-year clinical follow-up after Palmaz-Schatz stenting. J Am Coll Cardiol 1996; 27:1185-1191.

41. Waldecker D, Wass W, Haberbosch W. *et al.* Long-term follow-up (2.5 years) of 300 consecutive patients with primary angioplasty for acute myocardial infarction. Circulation 1995; 92: I-461.

42. Bax JJ, Wijns W, Cornel JH, *et al.* Accuracy of currently available techniques for prediction of functional recovery after revascularization in patients with left ventricular dysfunction due to chronic coronary artery disease: Comparison of pooled data. J Am Coll Cardiol 1997; 30:1451-1460.

43. Ryan TJ, Bauman WB, Kennedy JW *et al.* Guidelines for percutaneous transluminal coronary angioplasty. A report of the American College of Cardiology/American Heart Association Task Force on Assessment of Diagnostic and Therapeutic Cardiovascular Procedures. J Am Coll Cardiol 1993; 22:2033-2054.

44. McGovern PG, Herlitz J, Pankow JS, *et al.* Comparison of medical care and one- and 12-month mortality of hospitalized patients with acute myocardial infarction in Minneapolis-St. Paul, Minnesota, United States of America and Göteborg, Sweden. Am J Cardiol 1997; 80:557-562.

45. Tu JV, Pashos CL, Naylor CD, *et al.* Use of cardiac procedures and outcomes in elderly patients with myocardial infarction in the United States and Canada. N Engl J Med 1997 336; 1500-1505.

46. Yusuf, S. Organization to assess strategies for ischemic syndromes (OASIS registry). J Am Coll Cardiol 1997; 30:3.

47. Pilote L, Califf RM, Sapp S, *et al.* Regional variation across the United States in the management of acute myocardial infarction. N Engl J Med 1995; 333:565-572.

484.Pepine CJ. Management of myocardial ischemia: A time to reevaluate? J Myocard Ischemia 1995; 5:7-8.

49. Braunwald E, Antman EM, Evidence-based coronary care. Ann Intern Med 1997; 126:551-553.

14

EXERCISE AND HEART DISEASE

P hysical inactivity is a major cause of cardiovascular morbidity and mortality. Individuals who are sedentary are more likely to develop hypertension, or to have a heart attack at an earlier age and die prematurely. In contrast, even moderate physical activity reduces the likelihood of having a heart attack or dying from heart disease. More than 50 studies in the last 50 years confirm these observations. Here are just a few examples:

- In a study of 9,777 patients from the Cooper Clinic, the patients were classified into three categories— unfit, moderately fit or highly fit— and followed for 5.1 years. Of the 223 patients who died during the period of observation, the death rate for the unfit subjects was 122 out of 10,000 man-years, for the moderately fit it was 48.6 out of 10,000 man-years and for the highly fit subjects it was 34.4 out of 10,000 man-years. Thus, degree of fitness was directly related to survival.[1]

- In a study from Göteborg, Sweden, 7,142 patients were followed for 20 years. The most active subjects were only three-quarters less likely to die of coronary heart disease.

- A combined analysis of 22 clinical trial called a meta-analysis evaluated data on 4,554 patients who underwent a rehabilitation exercise program after a heart attack. The rehabilitation group was only 75% as likely to die as the control group.[2]

DANGERS OF EXERCISE

All of the studies that have been done indicate that exercise will not increase the risk of a heart attack. In a very large study based upon observations from 40 exercise facilities over a five year period, only 38 cardiovascular complications occurred in 33,726,000 participant hours of exercise. This translates to one death for every 887,526 hours of participation, or one death in 3,400 adults if they exercised five hours every week.

GENERAL BENEFITS OF EXERCISE

Although only moderate amounts of exercise are needed to provide important health benefits, the more exercise that is done, the less likely one is to have a heart attack or die of heart disease. If you do have a heart attack, it will occur at a later age and it will be less severe. Regular exercise after a heart attack can help speed up recovery and will reduce the risk of a second heart attack. The greatest reduction in mortality occurs among sedentary individuals who begin an exercise program versus those who go from a moderate exercise program to an intense one. Thirty to sixty minutes of exercise daily is enough to achieve moderate health benefits.

EFFECTS ON THE HEART WITH AGING SIMILAR TO DISEASE

Cardiovascular disease increases as we get older. Many studies have shown that a lack of exercise as we age has a major impact upon the development of heart disease. The changes from aging that take place in the structure and function of the heart are similar to those caused by heart disease. Thus, the damage that may occur as a result of disease may have twice the impact in an aged heart as it would in a healthy heart. Since only a limited amount of heart muscle is available, the loss of muscle reserve due to aging may mean the difference between life and death. Even a major heart attack is extremely well tolerated in younger victims while a small heart attack may be fatal in an elderly subject. *In other words, the effects of coronary artery disease may be due more to aging and to the lack of exercise than they are due to the effects of the disease.* Yet, there is hope. A number of studies have shown that adequate amounts of exercise can modify the aging pattern by maintaining the better function usually seen in younger individuals. In short, aging can be delayed.

The changes that occur in the cardiovascular system as we age, independent of disease, include the following: blood vessels become stiffer due to changes in the muscle cells of the arterial wall, in the fibrous tissue that surround these muscle cells, and in the endothelial lining on the inside of the blood vessel. This, in turn, causes the blood pressure to rise, because the stiffer vascular system can no longer easily expand to accommodate the input of blood with each heart beat. This causes the heart to work harder and its muscle cells to enlarge. Such enlargement alters both the function and the metabolism of the heart muscle. It, too, will become stiffer and less able to accommodate the inflow of blood from the lungs in the short time it has to fill. Thus, the heart fills slower, which causes an increase in the filling pressure. The increase in pressure is transmitted directly to the muscle walls, which compress the small arteries and veins of the coronary microcirculation and reduce the flow of blood to the muscle cells. The reduction in blood supply interferes with the muscle's ability to contract, and with the function of the whole heart.

Because the heart's microcirculation is already compressed, new blood flow entering the coronary circulation will be in the same predicament as is a car trying to enter a crowded freeway. The number of cars that can enter a crowded freeway is reduced, and so is the speed with which the cars can travel. In the same way, if the heart is called upon to work harder, it will need an increase in blood and blood flow to its muscle, but it will be unable to provide the increased flow of blood for the reasons described above. It should be evident that these effects of aging are, for all practical purposes, similar to the effects of obstructive coronary artery disease. A combination of the two can literally be deadly.

BENEFICIAL EFFECTS OF EXERCISE

As described at the beginning of this chapter, exercise reduces mortality from heart disease. it does so by slowing or preventing the effects of both aging and disease. These effects are translated into improved cardiac function, as demonstrated by an increase in the maximal amount of oxygen that can be taken up by the heart and lungs, an increase in the output of the heart and its ejection fraction, a decrease in the stiffness of the arteries, a lowering of blood pressure both at rest and during exercise, an increase in the maximal heart rate, a decrease in the maximal volume of the heart during contraction, a reduction in the stiffness of the heart, improved filling of the heart, a decrease in catecholamines that affect the heart, and a reduced tendency to sudden cardiac death.

Some of these benefits of exercise are due to the slowing of the progression of coronary artery disease or its actual regression. This is demonstrated in experimental as well as epidemiological studies. In other instances, there may be actual enlargement of the coronary arteries. Autopsies on marathon runners have shown that the diameter of their coronary arteries is two to three times more than normal. A study of vigorously active Masai tribesmen in Africa who died of noncardiac causes and had no clinical evidence of coronary artery disease showed that they had just as much coronary arteriosclerosis as American men, but had no obstructive coronary artery disease because of the large size of their coronary arteries. Intense exercise also has been shown to promote the formation of collateral vessels and the microcirculation in animals. Finally, in an angiographic study of marathon runners and sedentary subjects, the administration of nitroglycerin resulted in a 200% increase in coronary blood flow to the runners as compared to the sedentary subjects.

The benefits of exercise are not limited to the heart. There is a decreased tendency for blood platelets to clump and form blood clots, and insulin sensitivity and carbohydrate metabolism are improved, resulting in a reduced incidence of diabetes. Fat tissue is lost while lean muscle mass is protected, and there is a lower incidence of cancer, particularly cancer of the colon, a reduced incidence of depression, and an increase in bone density with less osteoporosis.

All of this means that older patients with heart disease who exercise will remain more physically active, will be healthier and will profit from a host of spin-off benefits. For example, exercising patients will be less deconditioned, will have less demineralization of bones and less fractures, and will be less impaired if their heart disease does affect their life-style. Indeed, physically active people are less likely to experience symptoms of heart disease. In short, regular exercise will not only allow you to live longer but it will improve the quality of your life.

WHO SHOULD EXERCISE?

The effects of exercise are indisputable. The questions to ask are who should exercise, how much and when? It may seem obvious that everyone without heart disease and who does not have some form of disability should be on a regular exercise program to prevent the effects of aging and to minimize the impact of heart disease when it does occur. There should be no dispute about this. For patients who do have heart disease, however, it is a different story. Such patients can be divided into two broad groups: those who have symptomatic or asymptomatic evidence of ischemic heart disease, and those who have recently had a heart attack and who need to be rehabilitated. Ischemic heart disease here means the patient has obstructive coronary artery disease and his or her heart muscle receives an inadequate amount of blood, either at rest or with physical activity.

There is actually a third group— those who have stable coronary artery disease that has recently become unstable; that is, those with unstable angina. This group should not be on an exercise program at all and we do not need to consider them here. Although the occurrence of chest pain during exercise is a limiting factor and should not be allowed to happen, most patients with ischemic heart disease do not have chest pain when they exercise. Accordingly, the absence of pain should not be used as a guide to how much exercise can be carried out. Fatigue and shortness of breath are far more common in patients with ischemic heart disease. The problem is that these symptoms are more often due to physical deconditioning, obesity and hypertension than they are to coronary artery disease. In addition, these same symptoms may be due to poor cardiac function from a prior heart attack, or from ischemic heart disease resulting from a severely narrowed coronary artery. Damaged heart muscle from a prior heart attack will not become ischemic. Indeed, the muscle is scarred and no blood is going to it at all. While it can't become ischemic, it can impair overall cardiac function, causing shortness of breath and fatigue, thereby limiting the amount of exercise that can be done.

FACTORS AFFECTING BENEFITS FROM EXERCISE

How well a patient with coronary artery disease does on an exercise program will depend upon a number of factors, including whether there has been a prior heart attack, how much irreversible damage occurred, and how much healthy, functioning heart muscle is left. It also will depend upon the presence or absence of ischemia during exercise, the patient's age, the patient's physical condition other than his or her heart disease, whether there is coincident lung disease, whether the patient smokes and/or drinks alcohol, the condition of the circulation in the patient's legs, his or her blood pressure and response to medication. It also depends a great deal upon the degree of physical deconditioning that is present as a result of the cardiovascular disease. Frequently, the degree of deconditioning is more limiting to the patient than is the patient's cardiovascular disease. A large amount of ischemic or irreversibly damaged heart muscle, or the presence of congestive heart failure may severely limit the amount of exercise that can be safely undertaken.

FREQUENCY OF EXERCISE

The minimum frequency of an exercise program should be 30-60 minutes three times weekly. The degree or intensity of exercise that can be attained will depend on overall conditioning and the functional capability of the heart. Ordinarily, exercises that increase the heart rate significantly should be utilized. While heart rate usually can be used as a guide, for patients with coronary artery disease it may not be reliable. For example, if a subject is deconditioned, even mild exercise will cause an inappropriate increase in heart rate. On the other hand, if an individual is on a beta blocker, even strenuous exercise will not increase the heart rate very much. More important than the actual heart rate is the change in heart rate with the continuation of the exercise program.

As the patient becomes less deconditioned with his exercise program, his heart rate will not become so rapid with exercise. In effect, it slows down. For example, if at the beginning of an exercise program, exercising on a treadmill at 3.5 miles per hour produced a heart rate of 120, after two months the same exercise may produce a heart rate of only 100. In contrast, if a patient is on a beta blocker, maximal exercise may produce a heart rate of only 80. After two months of exercise, the patient usually is capable of a higher level of exercise. Now he may be able to get his heart rate up to 90 or 100. This is a desireable effect.

The guidelines I use focus on whether or not a given activity produces symptoms. Chest pain is not a reliable guide because most patients with ischemic heart disease will not have chest pain with their ischemia. Fatigue and shortness of breath are more reliable. If an exercise program produces these symptoms, it is excessive. Another marker of excessive exercise are arrhythmias, or irregular heart beats. In the majority of cases, the patient who develops an arrhythmia is unaware of it, unless it is so great that it reduces the blood flow to the brain by causing a profound drop in blood pressure. Usually the victim will feel like he or she is going to faint. Faintness will be the warning sign, not the sensation of the arrhythmia itself. Whether or not an arrhythmia occurs is best determined by the prior performance of either a electrocardiogram monitored stress test or a Holter monitor. The presence of any significant arrhythmia should be a contraindication to the exercise activity that produced it.

There is no hurry to increase level and duration of exercise. Ultimately, if the patient is able, exercising one hour five times a week is a good goal. However, even 15 to 30 minutes each day may be acceptable for individuals who are somewhat limited in their ability to exercise. While my patients follow an exercise program, I adjust their medications to optimize the function of their heart. In the final analysis, each patient should be his or her own guide to what can be attempted comfortably. While formal rehabilitation programs have some merit, they aren't generally recommended because the patient usually feels compelled to achieve a predefined goal that may be unrealistic for the functional capacity of his or her heart. The exercise program of each patient must be individualized and constantly monitored. This helps to avoid the danger that a patient will try to do too much because the guy on the next exercise bike is doing better than he or she is.

Acceptable types of moderate exercise include walking, jogging, hiking, biking, swimming, tennis, rowing, racquetball, handball, lifting and carrying light objects, gardening, and home maintenance. Of the greatest benefit are activities involving large muscle groups. Resistance exercises such as weight-lifting are not recommended because they increase blood pressure. All exercising should be preceded by a 10 minute period of stretching and warm up, and should be followed by a 10 minute cooling-off period. The more strenuous the exercise, the more slowly one should build up to it. Remember, the occurrence of any symptoms is a signal that the exercise was too strenuous. Fatigue may not be immediate but it can be delayed. Remember, too, that exercise lowers the blood sugar and hypoglycemia may also cause fatigue.

REFERENCES

1. Blair SN, Kampert JB, Kohl HW, *et al.* Influences of cardiorespiratory fitness and other precursors of cardiovascular disease and all-cause mortality in men and women. JAMA 1996; 276:205-210.
2. O'Conner GT, Buring JE, Yusuf S, *et al.* An overview of randomized trials of rehabilitation with exercise after myocardial infarction. Circulation 1989; 80:234-244.

15

CHOLESTEROL AND OTHER MYTHS

The Truth About Cholesterol, Low Fat Diets, Vitamins & Antioxidants

In the past few years, a major media blitz has been orchestrated by the pharmaceutical industry to sell the newest group of cholesterol-lowering agents, the so-called statin drugs. These include pravastatin, lovastatin and simvastatin. The brand names for these drugs are respectively Pravachol, Mevacor, and Zocor. Media blitzes no longer appear only in medical journals. The FDA now allows pharmaceutical companies to advertise in all forms of communication, including the daily newspaper, magazines, radio, and television. Given the American public's penchant for buying what is advertised the most, sales of these drugs are tied directly to the advertising budget. The more that a product is advertised, the higher are its sales. It does not matter if the medication has to be prescribed by a doctor, for doctors are just as gullible as the public— or perhaps even more so. While it costs a bundle to market a drug (maybe $50 to $100 million), all that the pharmaceutical company has to do to finance this is increase the price of a cholesterol-lowering pill from fifty cents to $3.00. The result: billions of dollars in sales for a single drug. When you sell $5 billion worth of a drug a year, an advertising budget of $100 million is pennies.

But, are the claims you are reading, hearing and seeing accurate? The FDA wouldn't allow deceptive advertising, would they? You bet they would— and they do, every day. Let's examine the evidence to see for ourselves.

A total of 16 trials between 1985 and 1995 involving approximately 29,000 patients studied the effects of cholesterol-lowering statin drugs.[1] Total deaths for patients treated with the statin (16,988) over an average of 3.3 years were 3.1%, versus 5.3% in the control patients (11,995). This is a difference of 2.3% over the 3.3 year period, or about 0.7% per year. Cardiovascular mortality in the statin patients was 2.0% versus 3.7% in the controls, for a difference of less than 0.6% per year. Although this is statistically significant because of the large number of patients studied, it is hardly clinically significant, particularly in view of the expense of the statin drugs and their high incidence of side effects.

One of the largest of the trials involving statin drugs was the well advertised 4 S Trial, or Randomized Trial of Cholesterol Lowering in 4444 Patients with Coronary Heart Disease: the Scandinavian Simvastatin Survival Study.[2] Approximately half of the patients received the cholesterol-lowering agent simvastatin and the remainder received a placebo. Mortality in the patients treated with simvastatin was 8.2% over the 5.4 year study period, and 11.5% in the placebo group, for a difference of 0.6% per year. Interestingly, there was no difference in the mortality of females of participated in the study. The secondary endpoint was a major cardiac event. Twenty-eight percent of the placebo group and 19.4% of the simvastatin group experienced a major cardiac event, for a total difference of 8.6% or a per-year difference of 1.6%. The authors of this study stated that if 100 patients were to take simvastatin for 6 years, four lives would be saved. The cost of doing this for each patient would be $7,200. This amount of money is more than twice what a patient would pay for all other cardiac medications for a 6 year period, if they are taking all of the cardiac medications they should be taking. It is worth noting that, as a group, these patients were grossly undertreated with cardiac medications. Only 37% were taking aspirin, 57% beta blockers, 30% calcium channel blockers, 33% nitrates, and only 6% diuretics. The pharmaceutical manufacturer of simvastatin would like nothing better than for you to believe this is cost effective. Finally, the small differences between the placebo-treated and simvastatin-treated patients noted over the five years of treatment may have been more apparent than real. As pointed out by other medical scientists,[3,4] the placebo group had more severe coronary heart disease than the simvastatin treated group, as is indicated by the fact that there were 58 more patients in the placebo group with a history of heart attacks than in the simvastatin group. While this is only 2.6% more coronary heart disease patients in the placebo group compared to the simvastatin group, recall that there was only a 3.3% difference in total mortality between the two groups to begin with. In other words, the lower mortality in the group of patients treated with simvastatin may not have been due to the cholesterol-lowering effects of the simvastatin, but due to the higher mortality in the placebo group, simply because they had more heart disease to begin with. In support of this, there was no difference in the mortality between the women in the two groups— and for women, heart disease is usually less severe.

Why am I making such a fuss over such small differences? The answer is because the manufacturers of these cholesterol-lowering agents have taken these small percentages and, through statistical distortion, have made these small differences seem very much larger than they really are. The West of Scotland Study illustrates this deception.

The West of Scotland Study attempted to prevent coronary heart disease in men with hypercholesterolemia through the use of the drug pravastatin.[5] In this 5-year study carried out by the West of Scotland Coronary Prevention Study Group, 6,595 men with hypercholesterolemia were randomly assigned to be treated with the cholesterol-lowering agent pravastatin, or to be treated with a placebo. The men ranged from 45 to 64 years old. Although the presence of angina pectoris was allowed, no patient had a history of previous heart attack. Accordingly, this has been called a "primary prevention trial." There were 3,293 subjects in the placebo group and 3,302 subjects in the pravastatin group. At the end of the study period, 52 (1.6%) of the placebo-treated subjects had died from a coronary event versus 38 (1.2%) of the pravastatin-treated subjects for a difference of only 0.4% over five years. The effects on total cardiovascular mortality were similar: 2.2% for placebo and 1.5% for the pravastatin-treated subjects, for a difference of 0.7% over a five year period. Finally, 204 (6.2%) of the placebo-treated patients sustained a nonfatal heart attack during the study period, versus 143 (4.3%) of the pravastatin-treated patients, for a difference of only 1.9%.

These results can be discussed in terms of the total cardiovascular mortality, which is in fact the statistic the pharmaceutical company is using in its advertisements. There was an absolute reduction in cardiac mortality of 0.7% after 5 years of pravastatin treatment at a cost of $100 per month. Thus, 143 men with hypercholesterolemia must spend $858,000 to possibly save one person.

I find it hard to justify administering a drug with potentially serious side effects and an extremely high cost of $1,200/year, to 143 patients for five years on the chance that one individual may be saved from death, or one out of 53 may not have a nonfatal heart attack. There are other effective drugs for the treatment of heart disease that work 90-95% of the time, and save the lives of most patients who use them appropriately. Prescribing an expensive drug that might work in only one patient out of 143, but not until he or she took it for five years, does not seem like the logical alternative. However, this hasn't stopped the pharmaceutical company from carrying out a massive publicity campaign that is made worse by the distortion of the statistics. Colorful full-page advertisements in newspapers and medical journals proclaim, in large, bold-faced type, that pravastatin reduced the "risk" of a first myocardial infarction by 31%. Where in the world did they get the 31%?

It's simple: the difference between the mortality in the placebo group (2.2%) and the pravastatin group (1.5%) was 0.7%. By dividing this difference by 2.2 (2.2% minus 1.5% divided by 2.2%), one comes up with a 31% difference *between the two percentages*. Thus, this number is merely a percentage of a percent. If the interest rate for a loan at my bank is 5% but they decide to increase it to 6%, that's a 1% increase. However, using the pharmaceutical company's mathematics, it's a 20% increase.

This is not the first time the pharmaceutical companies have been deceptive with their inflated claims as to the effectiveness of cholesterol-lowering drugs. In 1987, the Helsinki Heart Study was published in the New England Journal of Medicine.[6] The study was well known because of the media blitz put on by the company that manufactured the drug gemfibrozil. Every medical journal every month for several years had large advertisements claiming a 34% reduction in mortality in heart attack victims if gemfibrozil were taken. If a doctor took the time to read the fine print of the medical report, he or she would have learned that there were 2,030 hypercholesterolemic subjects in the placebo-treated group and 2,051 hypercholesterolemic subjects in the gemfibrozil-treated group. At the end of five years, the mortality rate in the placebo-treated patients was 4.1%, while it was 2.7% in the gemfibrozil-treated patients. Thus, there was only a 1.4% difference between the two groups. What the researchers tried to minimize was that total mortality in the gemfibrozil-treated patients was actually higher because of the increased incidence of various forms of cancer, gastrointestinal disorders requiring surgery, e.g., gallstones, depression, suicide, and accidental death. This didn't prevent the pharmaceutical company from claiming there was a 34% reduction in mortality between the two treatment groups. How did they come up with a 34% difference from an absolute difference of only 1.4%? They subtracted 2.7% from 4.1% and divided the 1.4% difference by 4.1% to come up with a 34% difference between the two percentages. This is distortion, pure and simple. Unfortunately, busy doctors often have time to read just the headlines of an advertisement and will remember only the 34% difference.

It didn't take long for the marketing people at the pharmaceutical company to figure out that if they could get away with this fraudulent sales pitch, they could probably do the same thing in patients with a normal cholesterol. After all, more people have normal cholesterol levels than have elevated ones. This statistic was already known from the first cholesterol-lowering study in the early 1980s in which 3,806 subjects with elevated cholesterol levels were treated with a cholesterol-lowering agent known as cholestyramine for 7.4 years.[7] The researchers of that study used the same trick of using a percentage of a percentage to amplify the minuscule differences that were present. To obtain 3,806 subjects, the researchers of that study screened 480,000 people. Thus, only one out of every 126 people had elevated cholesterol in this study. No matter what the results, they could hardly have been representative.

With this data from the 1980s in mind, the manufacturers of pravastatin undertook a study in people with normal cholesterol. They knew at the start that there would be only small differences. Nevertheless, that didn't matter as long as there was a difference. If the difference was unfavorable to the cholesterol theory of heart disease, they didn't have to publish the results.

If the difference was in their favor, no matter how small, with statistical manipulation in a large enough group of patients and a heavy advertising budget, they could convince doctors, and the public as well, that their drug would "protect" them from having a heart attack or dying.

Thus, the effect of pravastatin in patients with average cholesterol levels was studied in 4,159 individuals who previously had a heart attack.[8] They were treated with pravastatin for an average of 5 years between 1991 and 1996. At the end of the five year period, there was only a 1.1% difference in mortality, a 1.8% difference in nonfatal heart attacks, and 0.6% difference in fatal heart attacks between the placebo-treated and the pravastatin-treated patients, with the differences favoring the pravastatin. Nevertheless, the authors of the study claimed there was a 24% reduction in risk by using the same statistical manipulation described previously. As an aside, it is worth noting that while 83% of those studied were taking aspirin, only 40% were taking beta blockers, and 33% nitrates, 39% calcium channel blockers, 15% ACE inhibitors, and only 11% diuretics— in other words, most were treated with inadequate amounts of medication. Another important observation is that the the women in this study developed breast cancer at a rate twelve times greater than usual. This was not mentioned in the abstract accompanying the article, nor was it in any of the press releases that I saw.

The article mentioned above claimed that there was a significant reduction in coronary events with pravastatin. Once again, we see the attempts to magnify small differences to make them appear more important than they really are. For, in fact, these results are hardly clinically significant.

The latest attempt to convince both the medical community and the public that cholesterol-reducing drugs prevent heart disease are a series of studies in which angiograms are obtained before and after the use of a cholesterol-lowering drug. In all of these studies, the researchers have claimed a "significant" reduction in the degree of narrowing of an obstructed coronary artery in the treated patients. This "significant" reduction was in the order of magnitude of from 0.035 mm to 0.38 mm. Such claims are preposterous and scientifically ludicrous. If I picked up an object, say a book, and without measuring it claimed it was 10.654 inches

CHOLESTEROL AND OTHER MYTHS

long, 8.432 inches wide and 2.657 inches deep, you simply would not believe me. Intuitively, you know that the human eye is incapable of measurements that precise. It is doubtful that one can come within an inch or two, no less one-tenth, one hundredth or one-thousandth of a *millimeter*. But that is exactly what these researchers claim to be able to do on an angiogram. The various factors controlling the diameter of a coronary artery, such as angle of view of the imaging device, the settings on the imaging equipment, when in the expansion and relaxation of a blood vessel the picture was taken, and a host of other details, ensure that there must be a change of two or more millimeters before one can presume it is due to treatment with a drug. This has been described superbly in greater details in an article in the *Annals of Internal Medicine* called "Limitations of Angiography for Analyzing Coronary Atherosclerosis Progression or Regression."[9]

Why, then, are there only small differences in heart attack rates and mortality between patients treated with cholesterol-lowering drugs and those who are not? Is the cholesterol theory of heart disease true, or is the whole thing just a giant hoax in order for researchers and pharmaceutical companies to make money? Not exactly. Like many successful frauds, there is always an element of truth in what is being sold. In the case of cholesterol, there is no denying the fact that there is a relationship between cholesterol and heart disease. *But*, that relationship exists only in a very small percentage of people who are of a certain age group and sex, and it is a very weak relationship. That was why 480,000 subjects had to be screened to find 3,806 with an elevated cholesterol in the study mentioned earlier.[7] Other observations illustrate this point.

A 25-year study of the frequency of heart attacks in relation to cholesterol levels was undertaken in 829 middle-aged men.[10] One hundred and seventy-nine subjects had a myocardial infarction. Men with low serum cholesterol had a 14% incidence of myocardial infarction at 25 years, while those with high cholesterol levels had a 23% incidence. Thus, there was only a 9% difference after 25 years— approximately one-third of a percent per year. One can also summarize the results this way: for over 90% of the subjects, there was no relationship between cholesterol and myocardial infarction rate.

Elevated serum cholesterol, low HDL (high density lipoprotein) and high total serum cholesterol to HDL ratio were not associated with a significantly higher all-cause mortality, coronary heart disease mortality, or myocardial infarction in patients above the age of 70.[11] In other words, it is irrelevant whether the cholesterol level or any of its fractions are increased in anyone above the age of 70 because they are not predictive of coronary heart disease. Nor does it make sense to recommend any form of treatment to lower cholesterol in this age group.

There are other reasons why the benefits of lowering one's cholesterol, if they exist, are confined to only a small fraction of the subjects in which it is attempted. All forms of treatment have side effects. When doctors recommend a treatment, they hope that the benefits will be greater than the side effects. A treatment may be considered effective when the benefit/risk ratio is large. When money is to be made, however, companies and people (researchers) are apt to change the rules. In this case, benefits are small, but the risk is small, too. Besides, with a good marketing program, the benefits can be amplified while the side effects can be minimized, even when those side effects counteract the beneficial effects.

In older patients, there is actually an inverse relationship between cholesterol levels and total mortality.[12] The lower your cholesterol level, the more likely you are to die. Another study in the *British Medical Journal*[13] found that a low cholesterol level was linked to depression and suicide. A study at the National Institute of Health and Medical Research in Paris followed 6,728 men over a 17-year period, and 32 of the men committed suicide. Men with low cholesterol levels were three times more likely to kill themselves than men with average levels. Another study at the University of Vienna in Austria found that there was a relationship between the mood swings occurring in women after birth and their cholesterol levels, which fall rapidly after delivering a baby. This rapid fall was thought to account for the depression that often occurs post-partum.

I well recall losing a physician patient who had been taking a cholesterol-lowering drug for several years before he came under my care. This particular drug has since been taken off the market because of the side effects it caused after it was released to the general public. In this case, the drug caused the formation of gallstones. After having his gallbladder removed, scars formed around the bile and pancreatic ducts of of the patient, causing extensive damage to the liver and pancreas, that resulted in his death.

Part of the explanation for the discordance between what researchers find in experimental animals in the development of an arteriosclerotic plaque, and the lack of clinical success in lowering cholesterol in humans, are the side effects associated with treatment. This also may explain why low cholesterol diets have failed. In the past 30 years, there have been more than 20 trials involving at least 50,000 patients with heart disease. It would be redundant and wearisome to list all these reports claiming a reduction in morbidity and mortality. If there truly is a benefit, it is minuscule and does not warrant a change in diet, other than what is necessary to lose weight, nor does it sanction treatment with an expensive cholesterol-lowering drug that may have serious side effects.

What about the beneficial effects claimed by the Pritikin and Ornish programs of the low cholesterol diets in patients with symptoms due to coronary artery disease? These claims are probably true. However, the benefits occur too quickly, i.e., within days or weeks, to be due to the lowering of cholesterol. All of these diets are accompanied by profound weight loss. This has an enormous impact on the heart's work load and can be very effective in lowering blood pressure. Both of these changes will effectively increase blood flow to heart muscle. It is because low-cholesterol diets are low in *calories* that they are helpful, not because they cause cholesterol levels to fall significantly.

Although almost all cholesterol-lowering studies involve only men and have excluded subjects above the age of 65 as well as children, this hasn't stopped the pharmaceutical companies from attempting to push the sale of these drugs in older men *and* women. Even worse are the attempts to frighten the public into believing that cholesterol control should extend to children. It is certainly not justifiable to place children on a low fat, low cholesterol diet. The harm it may cause to their growing brains may be incalculable.

A number of facts make it wise to question the credibility of the claims of the cholesterol researchers and the drug companies: e.g., the elaborate ruses used by cholesterol researchers to oversell their claims that lowering cholesterol will decrease heart attacks, the way the data are manipulated to "prove" preexisting theories, the failure to report the true incidence of side effects with these cholesterol-lowering drugs, the deceptive practices used in marketing of these medications, the inflated claims as to efficacy, the way cholesterol researchers are funded by the pharmaceutical manufacturers who sell the drugs being researched, their well known control of the researchers' rights to publish their findings, their failure to publish information that is negative to their cholesterol cause, the media blitzes used by cholesterol advertisers whenever a positive study is published, and the way public and even medical opinions can be influenced and even controlled by advertisements.

Why, then, do doctors continue to recommend these expensive, cholesterol-lowering drugs along with a low fat, low cholesterol diet to their patients? Most doctors try to remain up-to-date by following the results of studies in current medical journals. Articles continue to appear regularly from an army of cholesterol researchers who receive grant support money from cash-rich pharmaceutical companies. These researchers have a long history of outrageously inflating minuscule differences between a treatment claimed to lower cholesterol versus those subjects without treatment. In the process, many other facts are concealed, such as the side effects of the medication. Thus, the average physician, as well as the public, is being misled because the cholesterol drug advertisements have saturated medical journals, newspapers and magazines. If you don't think advertisements have an impact, think about the 3,000 teenagers who start smoking every day in this country alone. Unfortunately, many doctors are so ill-informed that they readily believe these advertisements, and whatever else they read about cholesterol in so-called "scientific articles" that recommend aggressive treatment. Both the experimental evidence and the statistics of such articles have been so manipulated that the "scientific paper" has been transformed into a medical advertisement. Sadly, these ill-informed doctors fail to recognize they are being manipulated by a pharmaceutical industry that is intent on selling their cholesterol-lowering drugs, even if it means lying to the public. Of course, they don't do the lying. They entice researchers into prostituting themselves in return for grant support for their research.

If one is going to be aggressive about treating patients with coronary artery disease, it makes much better sense to do so either in patients with symptoms of their disease, or in those with poor cardiac function. We know modern medications— including beta blockers, nitrates, ACE inhibitors, calcium channel blockers, aspirin and diuretics— are effective in almost all patients, not just a few percent after five years of treatment. It does not make sense to force an elderly patient who is underweight and undernourished to follow a low fat, low cholesterol diet, and to avoid excellent sources of protein such as eggs, merely because they also happen to have some cholesterol in them. Nor is it logical to have this patient take a drug at $3.50 per day, which is more than the cost of all of his or her other medications put together, when lowering the patient's cholesterol will *increase* his or her risk of death. Elderly patients simply don't have this kind of money. Nevertheless, the decision made by the patient's doctor frequently is made based on what the medical advertisements endorse, and not on scientific evidence.

Many of the recommendations I have made in this chapter on cholesterol screening and treatment are supported by the American College of Physicians Guidelines. These guidelines were published in the March 1, 1996 issue of the *Annals of Internal Medicine*. It is worth noting that they are hotly disputed by cholesterol researchers, all of whom receive grant support from the pharmaceutical companies, either directly or indirectly. They are also disputed by the American Heart Association, which has pushed the cholesterol theory of heart disease for decades. Keep in mind that not long ago the American Heart Association attempted to offer their seal of approval for low cholesterol foods, for a price— in some cases, over $100,000.

The views I have expressed in this chapter are shared by other physicians and groups, and have been expressed in published papers.[14,15]

ANTIOXIDANTS AND VITAMINS

In recent years, a number of epidemiological studies have noted that people who consume relatively large amounts of fruits and vegetables have a lower risk of cardiovascular disease. It was believed that the antioxidant vitamins in these foods hinder the development of the arteriosclerotic plaque by interfering with the oxidative damage to lipoproteins, the substances thought to be incorporated into the endothelial lining of the wall of an artery. The subsequent cellular and inflammatory reaction contribute to the formation of the plaque. The antioxidant vitamins involved include vitamins A, C, E and beta carotene. In addition, vitamins B6, B12 and folic acid have been found to play an important role in the breakdown of homocysteine which, as discussed earlier, is one of the important risk factors recently found to associated with the occurrence of coronary heart disease. Individuals with elevated levels of homocysteine have a much higher incidence of heart disease than those who do not.[16, 17]

The antioxidant vitamins are known to preserve the function of the endothelium, which is the smooth cellular lining along the walls of all blood vessels that allows blood to circulate freely without clotting. Numerous chemical substances secreted by endothelial cells interact with substances found in plasma and secreted by the platelets in the blood stream to maintain equilibrium. When that equilibrium is disrupted, blood begins to clot. If the clot that forms is minute, it may be layered upon the vessel wall, gradually building up to form the arteriosclerotic plaque. Alternatively, it may be carried downstream until it can go no further and blocks off a tiny artery. If the clot that forms is large enough, it will obstruct the blood flow in a large artery causing a heart attack or stroke, depending upon its location. Antioxidants also inhibit the ability of the platelets in the blood stream to agglutinate or clump. This, in turn, retards the progression of the arteriosclerotic plaque.

While these mechanisms have been established in animals, it is not known whether they also hold true in humans. The epidemiological studies that have been done only establish whether there is a relationship between intake of a vitamin and the incidence of disease, but not whether the vitamin plays a role in causing the disease. There are relatively few studies dealing with this question. One of the most recent and best was the Physicians' Health Study which was a double-blind, placebo-controlled trial of beta carotene in 22,071 male physicians from 40 to 84 years of age over an average of 12 years.[18] The 11,036 physicians assigned to receive beta carotene, showed virtually no differences in the incidence of cardiovascular disease or in overall mortality when compared to the 11,035 physicians who took the placebo. There were also no differences in deaths from cardiovascular disease, or the number of men with a heart attack or stroke. The authors conclude that supplementation with beta carotene for 12 years produced neither benefit nor harm.

In the Beta-Carotene and Retinol Efficacy Trial, 18,314 smokers, former smokers, and workers exposed to asbestos were the subjects of a randomized, placebo-controlled, double-blind study. A combination of 30 mg of beta carotene per day and 25,000 IU of retinol (vitamin A) were compared to placebo taken over an average of four years. The trial was stopped 21 months earlier than planned because of the apparent adverse effect on the incidence of lung cancer and cardiovascular disease. There was no benefit from either vitamin A or beta carotene.[19]

In a study of 34,486 postmenopausal women with no cardiovascular disease, the dietary intake of vitamins A, C, and E from food and supplements were related to the risk of death from coronary heart disease over a seven-year period.[20] During that period of time, 242 women died of coronary heart disease. Thus, while vitamins A and C were not shown to have any effect on coronary disease, the consumption of vitamin E from food (but not from supplements) was associated with a decrease in the incidence of coronary artery disease.

In a study of healthy Finnish men and women, ages 30-69 years, 5,133 subjects were followed for a period of 14 years. During this time, there were 244 fatal heart attacks. The subjects that had a higher vitamin E consumption had a lower mortality from coronary heart disease.[21]

What can we conclude at this time about the use of antioxidant vitamins to protect ourselves from coronary heart disease? Only vitamin E appears to be effective; however, the studies that are available at this time are hardly definitive. It is not known whether a high intake of vitamin E is responsible, or some as yet undiscovered substance in the food is the cause. Or it may be some characteristic about the people who ingest the food. Until such studies are forthcoming, it might be wise to consume an adequate intake of green leafy vegetables and fruits, which contain plenty of vitamins, including E.

Homocysteine

Homocysteine is another matter. The evidence of its influence on the development of the arteriosclerotic plaque is far more conclusive.[22,23,24] Elevated concentrations of homocysteine damage arteries, cause the clumping of platelets and promote clot formation. It has been estimated that up to 40% of patients with cardiovascular disease have elevated homocysteine blood levels. Accordingly, it has emerged as a strong risk factor for the development of coronary heart disease; perhaps a far stronger risk factor than cholesterol.

Homocysteine results from the normal breakdown of an essential amino acid known as methionine, which is abundant in red meat and milk products. Vitamins B6, B12 and folic acid are necessary for the metabolic conversion of homocysteine into its breakdown products. Many years ago, it was found that children who had abnormally high levels of homocysteine developed cardiovascular disease at a very early age.[25,26] Subsequently it was found that adults who had elevated homocysteine levels also had an increased incidence of arterial disease. In one study of 5,000 Canadians who had their blood folic acid measured as part of a nutritional survey between 1970 and 1972, re-contact 15 years later found that those with the lowest folic acid levels were 70% more likely to develop cardiovascular disease.

Although the focus of this chapter is on the nutritional aspects of cardiovascular disease, it is appropriate to mention that elevated homocysteine levels are not confined to the reduced intake of vitamins. Genetic defects also may result in elevated homocysteine levels. Elevated levels of this molecule are also found in individuals with chronic kidney disease, hypothyroidism, cancer of the breast, ovaries and pancreas, and following the ingestion of certain drugs such as methotrexate, anticonvulsants (such as phenytoin), and bronchodilators (such as theophylline).

Levels of homocysteine can be reduced by eating only moderate amounts of folic acid along with vitamins B6 and B12. Unfortunately, most of us do not get adequate amounts of these substances in our diets because we do not consume enough fruits, beans and leafy vegetables. Individuals who have high homocysteine levels can be brought back to normal by giving folic acid supplements either alone or in combination with other B vitamins.[27] In most cases, 5 mg of folate and 5 mg of B6 each day will suffice, but the actual amount depends upon your diet.

No doubt other substances will be found in foods that protect the heart from the development of coronary heart disease. Testimonials abound stating the beneficial effects of a wide variety of foods, additives and herbs. Some of these claims may be true. It is important for the reader to remember that whatever form of therapy is offered, whether vitamins, chelation therapy, acupuncture, bypass surgery, angioplasty, stents and even medical treatment, 75% of the subjects will have an improvement in their symptoms, as was explained in Chapter 12 under the section on placebos. Even placebos work. To determine if a treatment is successful, one must see not only whether there is improvement in symptoms and physical capabilities, but also whether the improvement is significantly better in enough subjects when compared to any spontaneous improvement that might occur. Beware of articles appearing in newspapers or prestigious medical journals that only talk about *percent improvement* without providing absolute numbers. A reduction in mortality from two out of 1,000 to one out of 1,000 is a 50% reduction, but is meaningless in terms of clinical effect. On the other hand, a reduction from 500 out of a 1,000 to 400 out of a 1,000 is only a 20% reduction but is enormously significant in terms of lives saved.

REFERENCES

1. Hebert P, Gaziano M, Chan KS, *et al.* Cholesterol lowering with statin drugs, risk of stroke and total mortality. JAMA 1997; 278:313-321.
2. Scandinavian Simvastatin Survival Study Group. Randomized trial of cholesterol lowering in 4,444 patients with coronary heart disease: The Scandinavian Simvastatin Survival Study (4S). Lancet 1994; 344:1383-1389.
3. Stehbens WE. Validity of the 4S, simvastatin trial. Lancet 1995; 345:264.
4. Grossman CM. Cholesterol reduction heart disease, and mortality. Ann Intern Med 1997; 126:661.

5. Shepherd J, Cobbe SM, Ford A, *et al.* Prevention of coronary heart disease with pravastatin in men with hypercholesterolemia. N Engl J Med 1995; 333:1301-1307.

6. Frick MH, Elo O, Haapa K, *et al.* Helsinki heart study: Primary prevention trial with gemfibrozil in middle-aged men with dyslipidemia. N Engl J Med 1987; 317:1238-1245.

7. Lipid Research Clinics Program. The lipid research clinics coronary primary prevention trial results. JAMA 1984; 251:351-363.

8. Sacks FM, Pfeffer MA, Moye LA, *et al.* The effect of pravastatin on primary events after myocardial infarction in patients with average cholesterol levels. N Engl J Med 1996; 335:1001-1009.

9. Hong MK, Mintz GS, Popma JJ, *et al.* Limitation of angiography for analyzing coronary atherosclerosis progression or regression. Ann Intern Med 1994; 121:348-354.

10. Kromhout D, *et al.* Serum cholesterol and 25-year incidence of and mortality from myocardial infarction and cancer: The Zutphen Study. Arch Intern Med 1988; 148:1051-1055.

11. Krumholz H, Seeman S, Merrill S *et al.* Lack of association between cholesterol and coronary heart disease mortality and morbidity and all-cause mortality in persons older than 70 years. JAMA 1994; 272:1235-1240.

12. Cardiovascular Disease. *Medical Tribune,* Nov. 27, 1997, page 6.

13. Zureik, M. Depression and suicide in 6,728 men followed for 17 years. Brit Med J 1996; 313:3-19.

14. Swan HJ. Primary prevention— have we gone too far? Amer Coll Cardiol Current Journal Review Sept./Oct. 1996:15-19.

15. Chalmers,T. Science 1985; 227: 40.

16. Nygard O, Nordrehaug JE, Refsum H, *et al.* The role of homocysteine in arteriosclerosis. N Engl J Med 1997; 337:230-236.

17. Moghadasian MH, McManus BM, Frohlich JJ. Homocysteine and coronary artery disease. Arch Int Med 1997; 157:2299-2308.

18. Hennekens C, Buring JE, Manson JE, *et al.* Lack of effect of long-term-supplementation with beta carotene on the incidence of malignant neoplasms and cardiovascular disease. N Engl J Med 1996; 334:1145-1149.

19. Omenn GS, Goodman GE, Thornquist MD, *et al.* Effects of a combination of beta carotene and vitamin A on lung cancer and cardiovascular disease. N Eng J Med 1996 334:1150-1155.

20. Kushi LH, Folsom AR, Prineas RJ, *et al.* Dietary antioxidant vitamins and death from coronary heart disease in postmenopausal women. N Engl J Med 1996; 334:1156-1162.

21. Knekt, P, Reunanen A, Jarvinen R, *et al.* Antioxidant vitamin intake and coronary mortality in a longitudinal population study. Am J Epidemiol 1994; 139:1180-1189.

22. Graham IM, Daly LE, Refsum HM, *et al.* Plasma homocysteine as a risk factor for vascular disease: the European concerted action project. JAMA 1997; 277;1775-1781.

23. Boushey CJ, Beresford SAA, Omenn GS, *et al.* A quantitative assessment of homocysteine as a risk factor for vascular disease: probable benefits of increasing folic acid intakes. JAMA 1995; 274;1049-1057.

24. Clarke R, Daly LE, Robinson K, *et al.* Hyperhomocysteinemia: an independent risk factor for vascular disease. N Engl J Med 1991; 324:1149-1155.

25. McCully KS. Vascular pathology of homocysteinemia: implications for pathogenesis of arteriosclerosis. Am J Pathol 1969; 56:111-128.

26. Mudd SH, Finkelstein JD, Irreverre F, *et al.* Homocysteinuria: an enzymatic defect. Science 1964; 143:1443-1445.

27. Rimm EB, Willett WC, Hu FB, *et al.* Folate and vitamin B6 from diet and supplements in relation to risk of coronary heart disease among women. JAMA 1998; 279:359-364.

16

NONCARDIAC SURGERY

J B was a 65-year-old retired real estate appraiser who had been under my care for about 15 years. Before he became my patient, he had sustained two previous heart attacks from which he had recovered only partially. In spite of the damage he had incurred, he was able to function reasonably well, although he required several medications to keep his symptoms to a minimum. He remained stable for many years and needed to be seen infrequently. Whenever he did come in, he always had a few jokes for me that he had collected between visits. In spite of his limitations of easy fatiguability and shortness of breath with walking on anything other than level ground, he was always cheerful and rarely complained.

One weekend I received a phone call from JB. He told me he was having abdominal pain and since he had no other doctor, he called me. I told him I would meet him in the emergency room of the hospital I used, would try to find out what was wrong, and then would call the appropriate specialist. When I did see him a short time later, it was obvious he was in distress. It seemed as if he were having an attack of appendicitis. The surgeon I called in agreed with me. Within the next hour, JB was undergoing an appendectomy. Unfortunately, by this time the appendix had already ruptured. Peritonitis, a dreaded complication, was sure to follow.

For the next few days, everyone's attention was on focused on JB's abdominal problem. Then, four nights after his surgery I received a call that he was in shock. I quickly hurried to the hospital to find him cold, pale, a blood pressure of 80/50, a rapid heart rate, and barely conscious. We managed to bring his blood pressure up, stabilize him, and get him out of congestive heart failure. His electrocardiogram revealed that he had developed a heart attack.

Over the next few days JB's condition was touch-and-go. Thinking that we were on the verge of losing him, I reluctantly had him undergo angiograms and coronary artery bypass surgery. "Save" him we did. I don't think we saved his life, however; more likely, we merely postponed his death. He was discharged from the hospital in one week only to be readmitted a few days later, suffering again from congestive heart failure. Over the next two years he was barely able to function, was constantly short of breath, tired, depressed, and failed to respond to all of my attempts to improve his condition. He had suffered too much damage to his heart and finally JB died, two years after the attack of appendicitis.

Could JB's heart attack have been prevented? I think so. Unfortunately, his story is a common one. The patient is well-controlled on several medications, usually with no symptoms, and consequently appears to be in no danger when he or she enters the hospital for surgery. Indeed, it would be better if the patient were having chest pain or were short of breath. The surgeon and nurses responsible for postoperative care would recognize the patient's need for medication, and would continue to administer those medicines. Unfortunately, no surgeon would operate on such a patient unless it were a true emergency. Even then, the patient is heavily sedated after surgery for a period of time, is restricted to bed rest, and is often confused, particularly if he or she is elderly. In other words, the patient is not complaining, and no one recognizes the patient's needs. The result: because the policy of most hospitals is to discontinue all medications preoperatively, necessary and even essential medications often do not get restarted. By the second or third day after surgery, the patient is on the verge of getting into trouble. Usually, he or she is receiving IV fluid since he or she is not ready to eat. If the patient had been taking a diuretic but has not had any in the postoperative period, all that fluid is building up. Then, all at once, it finally spills over, overloads the heart, floods the lungs, and sets the patient up for a stroke, heart attack, or pulmonary embolism (fatal blood clot to the lung).

There are many variations on this theme. Not long ago, one of my patients with long-standing coronary artery disease broke a hip and was hospitalized at a facility at which I did not have privileges. She underwent surgery to repair her hip and seemed to be doing well. Although she had angina in the past, on her current medical program she never had chest pain. Unfortunately, all preoperative medications were discontinued before surgery, and new orders were written postoperatively that failed to include any of her preoperative medications. This should not surprise anyone, for one would not expect an orthopedic surgeon to write cardiac orders. Since she was not having chest pain at the time of surgery, no one thought she needed a cardiologist; at least, that is, until she began having chest pain postoperatively. At that time, a cardiologist was called and, like most aggressive cardiologists, he immediately decided she needed angiograms and emergency coronary artery bypass surgery. Fortunately, the patient's husband stumbled onto this scenario and demanded his wife be placed back on her medications and that the angiograms and surgery be canceled. To top it off, the nursing staff had asked the patient to sign the release and consent form while the husband was at home. She was too groggy to know what was going on, and readily signed the form. It was sheer luck that allowed her husband to find out *before* she went to surgery. Incidentally, when she was placed back on her medications, her chest pain immediately disappeared.

Patients commonly experience heart attacks, strokes, congestive heart failure, embolism to the lungs, or cardiac arrest a few days after surgery, particularly if they are elderly. The postoperative period is far more dangerous than the surgery itself. It is not just because their medications may have been discontinued. Many have unsuspected heart or lung disease, borderline kidney function, arteriosclerotic plaques in their aorta or carotid arteries, diabetes and a host of other conditions just waiting to surface at the first opportunity— and surgery provides that opportunity. Typically, patients need to undergo only a brief examination before surgery. To be cleared, they usually have a simple electrocardiogram and some blood tests. Only the most advanced form of disease can be detected after such a cursory examination. Serious, asymptomatic illnesses of which the patient is unaware are often missed.

Prior to surgery, an intravenous infusion of saline is started. This is necessary so that the anesthesiologist may inject a variety of medications into the patient, including the intravenous anesthesia. When medication is not being administered, the saline is infused so that a clot will not form where the needle enters the vein and block the access to the blood stream. If the surgery is brief, there may not be a problem. If, however, surgery lasts over several hours, a fair amount of intravenous saline may enter the blood stream. This would not be a problem for a healthy patient, but those who have underlying heart disease often will not be able to handle the extra load, and will have a heart attack or die not long after surgery.

The recovery room is another area where problems can occur. The same intravenous saline that was started in the operating room is continued in the recovery room. Unless someone is watching very carefully to see that the patient does not become volume overloaded, the patient can get into trouble. In the recovery room the patient is usually still unconscious. Even if conscious, he or she may be heavily sedated. In either case, that patient is not in a position to complain about shortness of breath or chest pain. As a result, it may be some period of time before anyone is aware the patient is in trouble. The longer the delay, the more difficult it becomes to treat the problem. Usually these problems can be avoided with skilled nursing where one nurse handles only one or two patients. With the increasing spread of managed health care, however, hospitals have been forced to reduce their expenses to attract managed care contracts. In the process, they have cut back on expensive nursing care, hiring fewer and less skilled nurses. In so doing, the quality of postoperative care has declined noticeably. Consequently more patients are getting into trouble.

Even when patients are returned to their rooms, they are still dazed and not fully aware of what is transpiring. Most are unable to eat for one or two days; indeed, a common postoperative order is NPO, which means nothing *per os*, or nothing by mouth. Consequently, oral medications the patient was taking before the surgery are not restarted until the patient is able to eat. That is, if no catastrophe has occurred first.

Other problems may arise. The strain on the heart may cause cardiac arrhythmias. That is, it may cause the heart to beat irregularly and inefficiently. In turn, this may result in the formation of a blood clot within the left atrium. If the clot breaks lose it could lodge itself in an artery that goes to the lung or brain. Alternatively, the kidneys may not function normally after surgery. Retention of fluid may occur, causing the heart to be overloaded. If the patient has had abdominal surgery, normal bowel function may not return for several days. The result will be abdominal bloating, gas, abdominal pain, distension of the diaphragm and interference with the function of the heart.

Even if there was blood lost during the surgery, the surgeon may decide that giving a blood transfusion is too risky. Too many diseases can be transmitted with the transfusion of blood, and some of them can be fatal. Accordingly, the patient is left mildly to moderately anemic, putting another burden on the heart until a new blood supply can be regenerated. This may take one to three months depending upon the amount of blood that was lost during surgery. Finally, the patient can develop an infection that further complicates the recovery process and places an additional burden on the cardiovascular system.

These are just a few of the many problems that may surface in all patients undergoing any kind of surgery. It is not hard to understand why a relatively high incidence of cardiovascular problems occur. What can you do to avoid such problems if you have cardiac disease? The first thing to do is see your cardiologist a week or two before you are to undergo such surgery. Inform him or her that the surgery is coming up and ask for a careful and complete cardiac evaluation. This does not mean simply listening to your heart and taking an electrocardiogram, but preferably should include an echocardiogram and perhaps a low level, submaximal exercise test. If significant ischemia is present or cardiac function is impaired, postpone your surgery until the function of your heart has been improved and the ischemia has been eliminated, if possible.

Another caution involves the recommendation that you undergo prophylactic coronary artery bypass surgery or angioplasty before your surgery. If you are so advised, do not follow this suggestion. The so-called rationale your doctor will argue is that this surgery prevents a cardiac complication in patients, like yourself, who are at risk. However, there is no evidence to support this belief. The combined risk of the cardiac and noncardiac surgery is much greater than the the risk for noncardiac surgery alone. Make it clear that a noninvasive evaluation of your cardiovascular system is all you will allow. If there is evidence from these studies that you are at risk, then you should expect your cardiologist to minimize that risk by adjusting your medication. If he or she urges you to undergo prophylactic surgery because your risk will be less, tell your cardiologist to show you the scientific evidence supporting this opinion. He or she will not be able to do that. Make it clear that you will only allow an adjustment or intensification of your medical program. If you stand your ground, the cardiologist and the surgeon will back off. If your cardiologist or surgeon wishes to know why you feel the way you do, or tells you that you are not qualified to make such decisions, you can explain it is the official position of the American College of Physicians. The ACP has researched the subject, and has not found evidence to support having prophylactic bypass surgery before noncardiac surgery.

Perhaps the most valuable preventive measure you can take is to ask your cardiologist to notify the surgeon and to request that special precautions be taken to minimize the intravenous fluids you receive during and after surgery. Then ask your cardiologist to follow you closely throughout the postoperative period by visiting you daily. Tell him or her that you are perfectly willing to pay for their time and services. It may be the best investment you will ever make. In most cases, the complications that may accompany or follow any kind of surgery can easily be avoided by insisting that your cardiac medications be continued after surgery, and that volume overload be avoided.

Another wise move is to designate one or more members of your family to ask the nurses daily, if necessary, what medications you are receiving. Make it clear to this family member (be sure to pick one who is vocal) that if you are not receiving those medications, then he or she is to insist upon knowing why your medications have been stopped. The usual answer will be the doctor hasn't written the order yet. If this is the case, the relative you ask to do this must understand that his or her next step is to speak to the doctor directly, not a staff employee or nurse, and to ask the doctor why your medications have not been restarted. Frequently it will turn out that it has simply been overlooked, although no one will want to admit this. The only acceptable reason for failure to restart medications is that your blood pressure is too low, and restarting the medications will lower it further. If this happens, it shows that the doctor is aware that your medications have not been restarted, and has made a deliberate decision to delay restarting them. But, if your doctor has merely forgotten to restart them, something must be done. Sometimes a family member will be told that because you have not yet started eating, you cannot take your medication. However, this answer is not acceptable, medications can be administered with sips of water and will be absorbed.

Most hospitals do not have enough nurses to adequately supervise the postoperative care of all the patients undergoing surgery. An intelligent family member must assume this responsibility in order to minimize the risk of an avoidable postoperative complication. That individual must know the names of the medicines the person to be operated upon is taking, how often each drug is to be administered, and when. Such information can be written down on a piece of paper, with a copy given to whoever is to assume this responsibility. It would also be wise to bring your medications with you to the hospital before the surgery. Waiting for a doctor to write presecriptions and for the hospital pharmacy fill them can result in dangerous delays. Besides, bringing your own medication from home is a lot cheaper.

Preventing cardiac as well as other complications of surgery does not require much effort. It is well within the abilities of the average individual and a little effort can be highly effective in preventing the devastating and costly complications that often accompany relatively simple and safe surgeries. Indeed, it is not the surgery that you should fear, but the post-operative complications that are dangerous— but only if you let them be.

17

MISCONCEPTIONS ABOUT TREATMENT

There is so much misinformation about heart disease that this topic alone could be the subject of a whole book. Some of the material included in this chapter has already been mentioned in previous chapters but will be briefly discussed again for emphasis.

MISINFORMATION ABOUT RISK FACTORS

Misconception: If your parents or other family member had heart disease, you will get it, too.

Since cardiovascular disease is responsible for more than 50% of all deaths, the likelihood is that most of us will develop some form of heart disease if we live long enough. "Long enough" in this instance means we live into age 70 and beyond. If your parents died of heart disease in their seventies or later, and you have no other risk factor, there is no reason to believe that you, too, will also get heart disease. Chapter 3 describes many risk factors that will cause coronary heart disease to arise prematurely. It is when one or more of the risk factors are shared that heart disease usually results. For example, if Mom and Dad smoked, it is likely the children will smoke, too. If the parents are grossly overweight, the children are apt to be overweight as well.

Another frequent finding is the presence of hypertension, which can cause the early appearance of heart disease. Hypertension is an inherited characteristic, and if the children have it, they, too, may develop heart disease early in life. However, if their hypertension is treated, then the onset of heart disease can be delayed or prevented entirely. Similarly, diabetes is also inherited. If this disease appears early in life, then early heart disease is likely to be present as well. In this case, the heart disease is secondary to the diabetes.

When heart disease appears in individuals who are around fifty or sixty years of age, it is likely to be precipitated by the presence of one or more of the risk factors just mentioned, such as hypertension or cigarette smoking. On the other hand, when heart disease appears in individuals who are in their twenties, thirties, or forties, it is probably due to some inherited metabolic defect. For example, hypercholesterolemia, or marked cholesterol elevations of 500 and beyond, is one such genetic order. Hypercholesterolemia is rare and is not likely to be found in more than one out of 500 cases. It is one instance where the use of cholesterol-lowering drugs is justified. It would not be profitable for drug companies to market a cholesterol-lowering drug to such a small percentage of the population, and this is the reason why they have pushed their drugs onto patients who have only mildly elevated cholesterol levels and do not really need it.

Misconception: You will not have a heart attack if you do not have any risk factors.

Anywhere from 25-50% of heart attack victims do not have any of the well known risk factors for heart disease. That means there is no family history, they do not smoke, they do not have elevated blood pressure, they exercise, they are not overweight, etc. Often there is no apparent rational explanation for their heart attack. Close questioning may reveal there may be hidden precipitating causes that aren't recognized by the victim, such as the use of birth control pills and working in a smoke-filled office; or a highly stressful job. In addition, these individuals probably do possess one or more risk factors that we haven't yet identified. Homocysteinemia is one such example. Only recently have we recognized that levels of homocysteine in the blood that were thought to be normal were, in fact, high.

Misconception: If your are obese then you are at high risk of dying prematurely from a heart attack.

Obesity is a relative term. If you are 20 pounds overweight and have a big frame, it will probably not be noticed. On a small frame you might be considered plump with 20 extra pounds. With thirty to forty extra pounds, you may be considered fat, while with 50 extra pounds you would be considered obese. Individuals who are 100 pounds or more above their normal weight would fall into the morbidly obese category, and they do have an increased risk of death. Fortunately, relatively few people fall into this category. If you are merely obese or simply fat, your greatest danger is from lack of exercise and an increased likelihood of developing hypertension.

The connection of excess weight and heart disease mostly seems to hinge first on the fact that fat people tend not to exercise. Indeed, the very reason they are fat is because they fail to do regular physical activity. To achieve weight loss, a regular exercise program is far more effective than a diet. In addition, hypertension is frequently associated with being overweight. The combination of elevated blood pressure and the lack of adequate physical activity are the real reasons why obese people are more likely to have a heart attack. If high blood pressure is effectively treated with medication and an exercise program is undertaken on a regular basis (such as five times per week), then the risk of developing heart disease is no greater than it is for anyone else. To repeat, obesity itself does not predispose to heart disease, unless it is morbid obesity.

Misconception: Stress has no effect on the development of heart disease.

This subject was extensively discussed in Chapter 5 and need not be repeated, except to emphasize that stress has been shown to have a profound effect upon the heart and may result in a heart attack and even sudden death. Those who claim that stress is not harmful to the heart might as well claim that cigarette smoking is not harmful to the heart, either. Also, remember that one of the reasons that beta blockers are outstandingly successful for the treatment of heart disease is because these medications block the effects of stress on the heart.

MISINFORMATION ABOUT FOOD AND THE HEART

Misconception: To stay healthy you must drink eight glasses of water each day.

Patients often tell me that they try to drink eight glasses of water each day. The belief is that this amount of water is good for the body and, in particular, the cardiovascular system. It is nonsense, the body has its own feedback mechanism for determining how much water we need: it is called thirst. The problem with the "eight glasses of water" rule is that if you follow it, you may find yourself filling up on water even when you're not thirsty. If you happen to be on a diuretic for your blood pressure or heart, then an excess intake of water can cause overhydration, neutralizing the effects of the diuretic. I recommend to patients that if they are thirsty, they simply have a swallow of water and not necessarily a whole glassful. The less water the heart has to transport in the circulatory system to the kidney, the better.

Misconception: Eggs, meat and butter are bad for your heart.

The idea that a low cholesterol diet will protect you from heart disease has been pushed by the pharmaceutical industry for decades. In the 1970s and 1980s, a great deal of studies on low cholesterol diets were carried out on tens of thousands of people, and none of these studies showed any benefit in reducing mortality. Butter was replaced by margarine with the claim that it would protect the heart, but we now know that margarine is actually harmful. Also, the way meat is processed during this period of time has changed. Meat now has less fat in it, and if I might say so, steak never tastes as good as the way it used to, years ago!

Eggs have received the worst publicity of all. Frequently, patients tell me their doctors have told them to avoid eggs. The tragedy here is that many underweight elderly people who are on a fixed income are deprived of an excellent source of inexpensive protein. Again, there is really no evidence that a low cholesterol diet will reduce the risk of heart disease. The pharmaceutical companies who sell cholesterol-lowering drugs would love to have you believe this myth, for it means they sell more of their product. It is worth repeating that any benefit from such a diet comes from its low calorie content, not its low cholesterol content.

MISINFORMATION ABOUT SYMPTOMS

Misconception: If you experience shortness of breath, it must be a heart problem.

There is more than one kind of shortness of breath. In fact, shortness of breath is remarkably common in younger individuals and in people under stress or who suffer from asthma. Shortness of breath due to heart disease is always brought on by exertion, unless the disease is so far advanced that it also will be present at rest. The one exception to this is shortness of breath due to asthma, in which case it is usually accompanied by wheezing that can be heard by placing one's ear on the victim's chest or back, near the lung area. Patients with shortness of breath due to heart disease are so used to their impairment that they are often unaware it is present. Consequently, they don't usually complain about it.

On the other hand, the people who complain about shortness of breath the most are the ones who are hyperventilating. Typically, such individuals are short of breath at rest and describe their symptom as not being able to get enough air. This requires them to take deeps breaths throughout the day. Instead of making their symptom worse, exercise actually makes these patients feel better. Sometimes their hyperventilation is accompanied by chest pain which is usually confined to an area over the left chest. While this intensifies their fear that they really have a heart condition, the pain is actually caused by the fact that because they are constantly taking deep breaths, their chest muscles are overused and sore. The shortness of breath can be eliminated in these patients by simply explaining the poor breathing pattern and how it often accompanies stress.

Misconception: If you have chest pain, it must be due to your heart.

Chapter 6 presented many reasons why someone may get chest pain. The majority of those reasons have nothing to do with the heart. Even if the pain is true cardiac pain, its cause may be due to a disorder of another organ system that has a secondary effect upon the heart, causing chest pain to appear.

Consider, for example, an enlarged prostate. This can interfere with the flow of urine to such a degree that the urinary bladder will become enlarged, and this inhibits the formation of urine by the kidney. In turn, this will increase the volume of fluid within the circulatory system, elevate the blood pressure, and finally cause chest pain in patients who already have obstructive coronary artery disease. In such cases, the treatment should not be directed to the symptom (chest pain), but to the cause (enlarged prostate). That is, if surgery were to be done to correct the problem, it should be on the prostate and not on the heart. Removing the cause of the obstruction to the urine flow will cause the chest pain to disappear. Often the cause of such obstruction of the prostate is prostatitis. In this case, only antibiotics are required.

It takes time to determine why chest pain is present. A variety of diagnostic procedures that have nothing to do with the heart often have to be undertaken in the attempt to uncover the cause of a patient's chest pain. And even if a diagnostic procedure uncovers an abnormality, it doesn't mean it is responsible for the chest pain. The abnormality may have been there for years and its presence is simply coincidental.

For example, gallstones may cause indigestion and actual chest pain if the victim has a gallbladder attack. The detection of gallstones is accomplished by an abdominal ultrasound study. This usually takes a few days to schedule and accomplish. If the patient with gallstones has never had a gallbladder attack before and only rarely has had indigestion, then an appropriate form of treatment for the gallstones (and the chest pain) would be to have the patient merely avoid fatty foods. It may take a patient a minimum of a month or two to test out such a program. Unfortunately, too often aggressive cardiologists rush uninformed and helpless patients into the hospital for immediate angiograms and coronary artery bypass surgery or angioplasty the next day, instead of intelligently eliminating other possible sources of the chest pain.

Misconception: If you are having angina, you are at increased risk of having a heart attack.

Most individuals who have coronary artery disease do not have angina the majority of the time. When they do, it is almost always provoked by exertion, especially if the exertion closely follows a meal. In some patients angina is provoked by stress. Usually, the patient is quite familiar with the circumstances under which the chest pain appears, and attempts to avoid those situations. That may not always be possible. Typically, angina is promptly relieved with rest or with the sublingual administration of nitroglycerin. There is no evidence to indicate that there is an increased incidence of heart attacks in patients who have angina. Indeed, heart attacks are far more likely to occur in individuals who are unaware that they have coronary artery disease.

The patient with coronary artery disease and angina is not likely to be at increased risk of having a heart attack until the pattern of their symptoms change. For example, if a patient's chest pain occurs with far less exertion than before and lasts longer, or if the pain is not promptly relieved by nitroglycerin, or if it appears and stays while the patient is resting, or if it begins to occur during the night for the first time, *then* that patient has reason to be concerned. However, even if this does occur, the increased risk is relatively small, and it does not mean a massive heart attack is about to occur.

There are many reasons why patients with angina and coronary artery disease may have a change in their symptoms, and often those reasons have nothing directly to do with the heart. The same conditions that cause the appearance of pain may cause a change in the pattern of pain in those patients who already have it. A common example is in patients with both coronary artery disease and hypertension. Patients whose symptoms were under control and who then have a change in their symptoms, will frequently demonstrate a blood pressure that is considerably higher than was present in the past. Sometimes the reason is merely because they have developed an injury or have arthritic pain. Either on their own or because another doctor has proscribed a pain medication, they start taking NSAIDs (nonsteroidal anti-inflammatory drugs). These drugs interfere with kidney function, cause fluid retention, increase the volume of fluid within the circulatory system, and elevate the blood pressure. The result is chest pain. Treatment consists merely of stopping the NSAID.

Thus, the sudden occurrence of angina or an increase in preexisting angina should not be a cause for alarm. Instead, it should invite thoughtful analysis from the patient and his or her doctor about the possible reasons the change may have occurred. There are many noninvasive tests available that will help solve the problem.

Misconception: If you have a heart attack, it means "your days are numbered," or that you will die prematurely.

It is not uncommon for someone to have a heart attack at a relatively early age— e.g., when they are in the forties or fifties— and then never to have another problem after that. Often, obvious risk factors such as a marked increase in weight, hypertension, cigarette smoking or lack of exercise, can be eliminated. When a young heart attack victim starts an exercise program, loses 50 pounds, stops smoking, tries to avoid stress and gets his or her blood pressure under control, then he or she is no longer at increased risk of another heart attack and usually lives a normal life span. The heart has a tremendous amount of reserve and recovery powers. Give it a chance, and it will provide you with a long life.

Misconception: A doctor can tell if you have a heart problem merely by listening to your heart with a stethoscope and taking an electro-cardiogram. Likewise, if you have known heart disease, he or she can tell if it is progressing or getting better with the same instruments.

If you have a heart murmur or if you are in congestive heart failure, a doctor usually will be able to diagnosis the problem if your disease is fairly well advanced. However, most patients with ordinary obstructive coronary artery disease are neither in congestive heart failure, nor do they have significant murmurs. In these situations, the stethoscope and electro-cardiogram are nearly useless. One cannot diagnose coronary artery disease or its progression simply by listening to the heart. Nor will the electrocardiogram become abnormal until the patient's disease is advanced. Even if the patient's disease recently has become worse, it is unlikely that this information will show up on a simple electrocardiogram.

An experienced doctor can gain far more information merely by talking with the patient and getting a detailed history than he or she can by listening to the patient's heart and taking an electrogram. Tests that will diagnosis heart disease at an early stage and detect its progression were discussed in Chapter 9. Unfortunately, these tests are not being used by the average doctor. Thus, you should be aware that if you think you could have heart disease, examination with only a stethoscope and electrocardiogram is not adequate. It will not detect heart disease until it is far advanced. If you suspect that you have heart disease, you should insist that your doctor have you undergo extensive testing.

Misconception: A doctor can predict if you are about to have a heart attack.

Doctors like to believe they can predict if you are about to have a heart attack, but this is just wishful thinking. Of course, if you are having recurring episodes of typical cardiac chest pain which are becoming more frequent and more severe, you could easily recognize that something is about to happen. However, if you are merely having exertional angina and if the tests you have undergone are abnormal, there is no evidence to indicate that a major heart attack or death will occur soon. What abnormal tests do indicate is that you are at increased risk of having a cardiovascular event. But that does not mean in any way that you will have such an attack. A comparison can be made with an automobile traveling at 75 miles per hour compared to 60 miles per hour. At a higher speed you are more likely to have an accident, but that does not mean that you will.

Misconception: Irregular heart beats are dangerous.

All hearts miss a beat now and then. Each of us have approximately 30 million heart beats every year. The wonder is not that hearts beat irregularly at times, but that almost all of those beats are regular. Strangely, when an irregular heart beat is due to heart disease, rarely is the patient aware that his or her heart is beating irregularly. In my practice, it is my custom to hook a patient up to a cardiac monitor during the 20-30 minutes they are being examined. The monitor is being watched constantly. During this period of time, irregular beats often appear. In some cases there may be as many as 5 to 10 irregular beats a minute. Yet, rarely is the patient aware that they occur. Probably 99% of the time, such irregular beats are harmless. When the patient is aware they occur, it is usually secondary to stress. In some individuals an irregular heart beat is due to excessive alcohol consumption and occasionally to too much coffee. While the sensation of an irregular or premature heart beat is quite disturbing, be assured that if you can sense them, they are harmless. It's the ones that you are not aware of that are more likely to be a sign of poor cardiac function.

Misconception: If you have heart disease, the absence of symptoms means your disease is not getting worse.

This is a dangerous assumption, of which both doctor and patient are guilty. I like to think of a heart attack as like an earthquake: it can occur without warning, and may have devastating effects. Also, like an earthquake, the forces responsible for it have been building up for many years.

Congestive heart failure is the end result of most forms of heart disease and takes years to develop. However, the symptoms of congestive heart failure often come on quite rapidly. Sometimes those symptoms develop over a period of weeks, sometimes days, sometimes hours, and sometimes even minutes. Treating heart disease would be far simpler and more successful if everyone had warning symptoms that gradually developed over months and years. Unfortunately, while progressive impairment of cardiac function may take years to develop, the symptoms that result do not make an appearance until very late, often too late to do much about.

Modern day diagnostic exams are capable of detecting heart disease years before the appearance of symptoms. They also are able to detect improvement in cardiac function due to drug therapy and follow the progression of a patient's disease. But this requires an understanding on the part of the patient that drug therapy is necessary for almost everyone with obstructive coronary artery disease, even if symptoms are absent. This form of treatment is called preventive cardiology, and is vastly more successful than heroic treatments like angioplasty and coronary artery bypass surgery. It is also far less costly.

Misconception: A normal electrocardiogram means you do not have heart disease.

Briefly, the reason an electrocardiogram fails to detect disease is because it is insensitive, and also because it reflects only the electrical activity of the heart, not its mechanical function. Heart muscle must be extensively damaged before its electrical activity will be altered. Mild damage and impairment of function simply does not register. Consequently, don't put too much faith in a normal electrocardiograph tracing.

Misconception: An abnormal electrocardiogram means you have heart disease.

I receive many calls from spouses who tell me, "They said my husband had an abnormal electrocardiogram, and that he has to undergo an angiogram." Often the individual in question has already undergone an angiogram and now has been told he needs angioplasty or coronary artery bypass surgery. However, when asked whether the subject has symptoms, the answer is usually "no."In fact, typically the victim is vigorously active.

There are dozens of reasons why the electrocardiogram may be abnormal without there being any form of heart disease. As a general rule, abnormalities involving the EKG spike (the depolarization and contraction phase of the cardiac cycle) reflect disease, but relate poorly to function, whereas abnormalities of the repolarization of the heart are referred to as nonspecific abnormalities. Repolarization refers to the relaxation phase of the heart's cycle, during which the heart cells regain their electrical charge. There is a poor correlation between the appearance of an electrocardiogram and a patient's functional capacity. Many patients with quite abnormal tracings have normal cardiac functional capacity in every way. Some are even marathon runners. Indeed, as described in Chapter 2, athletes commonly have "abnormal" electrocardiograms, the "worst" being basketball players. Thus, interpretation as to the significance of an abnormal electrocardiogram depends primarily on the functional capacity of the heart. This can best be determined with a stress test or an echocardiogram.

Misconception: A doctor can tell how healthy your heart is from an electrocardiogram.

Here is the flip side of the previous misconception. How healthy the heart is depends upon its functional capability, which cannot be determined from an electrocardiogram. Any doctor who looks at your electrocardiogram and tells you your heart is fine is either deceiving you or is misinformed.

Misconception: Having a positive stress test or radioactive imaging procedure means you are in immediate danger of having a heart attack.

Doctors are not prophets. Many patients have had a normal stress test, and were told their hearts were fine, and then went on to have a heart attack a short time later. Conversely, far more patients with an abnormal test have never had a heart attack. It is fair to say that those who have an abnormal test are at increased risk of having a heart attack in the future, and that the more abnormal the test, the greater the risk. However, being at increased risk is not the same as being told you *will* have a heart attack. For example, in a group of 100 subjects who have a normal stress test, only 10 are likely to have a heart attack over a period of the next 10 years. In a sampling of 100 subjects who have an abnormal stress test, the number might be 30. And in a sampling of 100 subjects who have a markedly positive test, the number might be 45 over a 10 year period. Thus, the test does not identify who is going to be the victim, but is used only to determine the severity of risk. This allows them to identify subjects who should be treated most intensively. This approach is acceptable as long as treatment is confined to drugs. Accordingly, a patient with a mildly abnormal test might be treated with only two medications, whereas someone with a more positive test would be treated with three to four drugs.

It should be obvious that if surgery were to be used as a routine treatment for everyone with a positive test (a practice that is widely employed), then most of these people would be undergoing unnecessary surgery.

MISINFORMATION ABOUT ANGIOGRAMS

Misconception: Angiograms are routine x-rays of the coronary arteries and are perfectly safe.

Cardiologists commonly state this to patients with a cardiac problem. If the cardiologist is trying to allay a patient's fears, it is a poor choice of words. Furthermore, it is certainly not true. Angiograms are neither routine, nor are they without risk. They involve a surgical incision over an artery in the groin, and the insertion of a plastic tube or catheter into the artery. The catheter is pushed until it reaches the coronary arteries on the surface of the heart, where it is inserted into the coronary artery, and an x-ray opaque dye is injected at high pressure to image the lumen of the arteries. The catheter itself can and does traumatize any arteriosclerotic plaque along the way. If the trauma is great enough, pieces of plaque can break off and get carried downstream, occluding the blood supply to the tissues. If the plaque breaks off in a coronary artery, it can cause a heart attack. If a piece of a plaque breaks off in the aorta as it is exiting from the heart, it can cause a stroke.

If the catheter is pushed a little too hard, it may perforate the wall of an artery or cause a dissection where the walls of the artery separate. Sometimes the dissection will involve the aorta, interrupting the blood supply to the brain. In a number of instances, particularly in older patients who have rigid and even calcified arteries, extensive bleeding will occur when the catheter is removed, with devastating complications ranging from paralysis of the lower extremities to death.

Many thousands of patients of the two million who undergo angiograms each year suffer from complications. The worst of these include death, heart attack and stroke. Angiograms are *not* routine x-rays, nor are they always safe.

Misconception: Angiograms allow a cardiologist to determine the cause of your chest pain.

An angiogram only tells us whether an artery is narrowed or obstructed. It does not tell us whether the blood flow to the heart muscle is reduced. The reason is the angiogram is unable to image the microcirculation of the heart that often provides all the blood that the heart muscle needs. It is the lack of blood flow that causes coronary heart disease, not obstruction in a coronary artery. Such an obstruction can cause coronary heart disease but often does not. Reduced blood flow to the heart muscle always causes coronary heart disease.

Misconception: Doctors who order a lot of high-tech procedures are good doctors.

It's easy to fall into the trap of believing that more and more high-tech tests are good. Modern diagnostic procedures such as echocardiography, radioactive imaging and angiography are indeed impressive. But subjecting a patient to a variety of diagnostic tests makes it easy to neglect collecting a careful history and physical examination. Face-to-face time with a patient or his or her family is time-consuming. It's also not financially rewarding for physicians, because insurance companies and Medicare pay very little for such time. However, it happens to be the most rewarding time spent in terms of understanding the patient's disease, and in interpreting those high-tech tests. An angiogram might show severe coronary artery disease for which the cardiologist will recommend immediate surgery. While talking with the patient, the physician might uncover the significant fact that he or she is a marathon runner.

Overuse and inappropriate use of high-tech tests do not make one a good doctor any more than driving a high performance automobile makes one a good driver.

Misconception: Severe narrowing of a coronary artery means you are about to have a heart attack.

This misconception has been around ever since angiograms started to be used nearly 40 years ago, and is still used to frighten patients into having immediate surgery. Countless patients have been wheeled into the operating room from the catheterization laboratory, or not allowed to leave the hospital until surgery was performed. We now know that such obstructive lesions may have been present for years, largely unchanged, without being a threat. Because new collateral blood vessels have already taken over the job of supplying blood to the heart muscle, the patient is in no danger of a heart attack. The heart has put in its own bypasses. Consequently, even if the artery closes off completely, it is not likely to have any significant adverse effects.

Misconception: A cardiologist can determine your prognosis and how you should be treated from an angiogram.

This is simply not true. Both how you should be treated and what your prognosis is depends mostly on how well the heart functions, and not the degree of anatomical narrowing of a coronary artery. The former cannot be determined from the angiogram. Such information usually can be obtained from one or more noninvasive tests— in which case, why undergo an angiogram?

Misconception: If you have coronary heart disease and need to undergo noncardiac surgery, you need to have angiograms and possibly prophylactic angioplasty or coronary artery bypass surgery before the noncardiac surgery to prevent a heart attack or death during such surgery.

This was discussed in part in the previous chapter. My own view is that it's just another way for the surgeon to make more money or to escape the increased risk of operating upon someone with coronary heart disease. There is no evidence that such surgery reduces the patient's risk of having a heart attack or dying from noncardiac surgery. Indeed, a recent policy statement by the American College of Physicians pointed out that the combined morbidity and mortality from both surgeries is greater than the noncardiac surgery alone.[1] If you need to have noncardiac surgery, I would urge you to refuse if asked to undergo possible prophylactic cardiac surgery first. It is true that there is a chance you can have a heart attack or die with noncardiac surgery, but that possibility existed whether or not heart disease was known to be present. But to undergo two such surgeries doubles the risk, or perhaps more than doubles it, because cardiac surgery has far more complications than other forms of surgery. This is especially true in older patients who are the very ones most likely to need noncardiac surgery. I would suggest that if the surgeon who makes this request will not respect your wishes, then you should find another surgeon.

MISINFORMATION ABOUT CORONARY ARTERY BYPASS SURGERY

Misconception: You will have a massive heart attack and probably die if you don't have immediate surgery.

Having coronary artery disease means that there is an increased risk of having a heart attack or dying; however, we do not yet have the ability to predict in whom it will occur, or when it might occur. The implication of this misconception is that surgery will protect you from a heart attack or dying. But there is no evidence that this is so, although both the cardiologist and surgeon would like to have you believe it is true. In fact, there is considerable evidence to show that for most people with coronary artery disease, undergoing surgery or angioplasty is considerably more dangerous than receiving medical treatment. Thus, if you are going to sustain a heart attack or die because of your coronary artery disease, it is more likely to occur if you submit to one of these procedures. For further information on this subject please refer back to Chapter 13.

Misconception: The mortality risk of angioplasty and coronary artery bypass surgery is low.

This is another myth the cardiologist and surgeon would like you to believe but is not true. The mortality risk of angioplasty and coronary artery bypass surgery is much higher than many cardiologists and surgeons claim. This subject was discussed in detail in Chapter 13.

Misconception: If you have bypass surgery and your symptoms disappear, then it was the surgery that was responsible.

It is true that angina will disappear in 80-90% of patients after surgery. Often this is due to the surgery itself. In my opinion, however, most of the symptom relief is due to other factors, and the surgery is just coincidental.

Revascularization of the heart is not a new concept. Since the 1930s, pioneers like Dr. Claude Beck in Cleveland have been attempting to reach this goal. The techniques of intravascular surgery on individual blood vessels had not yet been discovered. Nor were the heart protection techniques during cardiac surgery known. Revascularization was accomplished by placing asbestos on the surface of the heart, or attaching the tissue covering from the intestine onto the heart. Although mortality from surgery was relatively high, those patients who survived did get relief from their chest pain. Similarly, placebo operations have been performed with the patient undergoing merely a skin incision after having been anesthetized. These patients also had pain relief.

What follows is a list of reasons why pain relief may occur after coronary artery bypass surgery that has nothing to do with the fact that an obstructed coronary artery was bypassed.

1. By far, the most important cause of pain relief that occurs after bypass surgery is due to the formation of new blood vessels in and around the obstructed coronary artery through the process of angiogenesis. Their primary limitation is that they cannot carry the large volume of blood that the main coronary arteries can. Thus, under extremes of exertion, such as stress test, a patient may have chest pain. These collateral vessels take time to develop. Accordingly, they may not be present in adequate amounts when chest pain initially occurs. However, the recovery period after bypass surgery is long enough for such vessels to grow and function causing pain relief.

2. Pain fibers going to the heart may be cut during surgery. If this happens, then the brain never receives the message that there is injury. Patients who undergo a cardiac transplant all develop a form of accelerated coronary artery disease for reasons we do not understand. Other than rejection, such coronary artery disease is the most common form of transplant failure and short survival. Yet these patients never have angina from their coronary artery disease because no pain fibers from the transplanted heart go to the brain.

3. The patient has a heart attack during or immediately after surgery. The very heart attack the cardiologist and surgeon had hoped to avoid with their surgery, may have occurred anyway. Thus, the cause of the patient's chest pain; that is, the nerve fibers coming from the ischemic heart muscle, no longer is a factor.

4. The pericardium— a thick, tough, protective membrane that surrounds the heart and prevents it from expanding— is cut during surgery in order to reach the obstructed vessels. It is allowed to remain open after surgery. Much like wearing tight clothes and then eating a big meal, we feel stuffed. Loosening one's clothes helps. In the case of the heart, as it enlarges to compensate for its limitations, the pericardium enhances the tension or pressure within the heart muscle because it fails to stretch as the heart is enlarging. This pressure helps to compress the very small blood vessels of the heart, and reduces the blood flow to the heart muscle. By opening the pericardium, the increased pressure within the muscle is reduced, allowing blood to flow more freely in the heart's microcirculation. This will eliminate the pain.

5. Many patients who undergo bypass surgery have hypertension. As was mentioned previously, hypertension is one cause of chest pain. It is a well known fact that if you put a patient with an elevated blood pressure to bed, his blood pressure will come down to normal. Sometimes this will occur within just a few days; sometimes it takes a week or two. If hypertension is the cause of a patient's angina, then bed rest will result in its disappearance. It might take months before the hypertension returns. Although postoperatively the patient who has had bypass surgery is not at bed rest very long, he or she usually spends 1 to 2 months in convalescence and does not have to deal with the day-to-day stresses of living that were the cause of the hypertension.

6. Weight loss often develops after undergoing heart surgery. Surgery causes loss of appetite and results in weight loss. It is well known that significant weight loss will result in the disappearance of angina. This is the basis of the Ornish and Pritikin diet programs. Thus, weight loss is an important reason why angina disappears after having bypass surgery.

7. Many patients will "get religion" after major cardiac surgery. That is, after years of inactivity and deconditioning, they finally decide to undertake an exercise program. Clearly, as discussed in Chapter 14, exercise is beneficial, and will help eliminate chest pain and keep it from returning.

8. Most patients have the sense to stop smoking if they have had to undergo coronary artery bypass surgery. At the very least, the forced hiatus from smoking during and after surgery is a major factor in their being able to break the habit. Smoking contributes to the development of chest pain, and stopping the habit will help to eliminate the pain.

9. I have already pointed out the many reasons why chest pain may appear that have nothing to do with the heart. Often these noncardiac causes of chest pain will disappear spontaneously. We have no way of knowing how many patients undergo unnecessary bypass surgery for chest pain that was noncardiac in origin. In these patients, the disappearance of their chest pain is merely coincidental.

10. The placebo effect of surgery can be a very powerful factor in the relief of symptoms.

11. Stress is an important cause of chest pain, and it contributes significantly to the progression of the arteriosclerotic plaque as well as hypertension. What better way to eliminate stress than to undergo a surgical procedure with a 2 to 3 month recovery period? Elimination of stress is bound to help in the relief of chest pain.
12. Finally, the enormous cost of bypass surgery has considerable psychological impact. This cannot be ignored in considering why patients get relief of their chest pain after bypass surgery.

Misconception: Bypass surgery will relieve chest pain in all patients and it will not come back.

About 10% to 20% of patients who undergo surgery continue to have pain afterwards. Another 10% have a return of their symptoms after the first year. Fifty percent have a return of their symptoms within 3 to 5 years. The reasons why symptoms return are multiple. In some cases, the diagnosis of coronary artery disease as a cause of chest pain was wrong, and the coronary artery disease was merely coincidental. I have previously discussed how hypertension may cause chest pain. The presence of an elevated blood pressure usually disappears in the hospital and convalescence. For example, hypertension may be the cause of the chest pain initially. The patient's blood pressure may have decreased after surgery and convalescence. Accordingly, medication for hypertension is not likely to be prescribed. When the patient becomes active again, however, and returns to the stresses of work, his or her hypertension returns, and along with it, the chest pains.

Another reason for the return of chest pain after bypass surgery is that putting in a bypass does not solve the problem of reduced blood flow to the heart muscle. Many studies have shown that ischemia continues after bypass surgery. The reason is that the area of impaired blood flow is downstream from the bypass. I have discussed this concept previously.

The current belief is that chest pain is caused by obstructive coronary artery disease. It is equally possible that the obstructive coronary artery disease is the result of impaired blood flow in the heart's microcirculation. If this is so, then bypassing the obstruction will not solve the problem.

Misconception: Having bypass surgery or angioplasty means you no longer need medications.

Patients often tell me that after they had a revascularization procedure, their cardiologist or surgeon said they no longer needed to take a handful of drugs every day. For those who maintain that an obstructive coronary artery is the sole cause of angina, this would be understandable. But neither bypass surgery nor angioplasty restores blood flow back to normal. In the majority of cases, impaired cardiac function can still be detected. Unless something is done to improve the blood supply to the heart muscle and to reduce the work load, the adaptive mechanisms that lead to enlargement of the heart will eventually lead to congestive heart failure. Because most patients who undergo bypass surgery are not placed on an adequate medical program, it is only a matter of time before the patient starts to experience the common symptoms of heart failure— shortness of breath and fatigue on exertion.

Misconception: Surgery is more effective than medical treatment.

Each year 800,000 victims of coronary artery disease are told this. Half undergo angioplasty, the remainder undergo coronary artery bypass surgery. But there are no modern studies that have compared adequate medical treatment with surgery. What few comparisons have been made are unacceptable because of the total inadequacy of drug therapy. Reports from the late 1970s and early 1980s concluded that patients with severely impaired cardiac function survived longer after surgery, but patients with good cardiac function were not effected. However, it is grossly unfair to compare the medical therapy of the 1970s with modern medical therapy. In my own experience, modern medical treatment of obstructive coronary artery disease is vastly superior to surgical treatment.

MISINFORMATION ABOUT DRUGS

Misconception: Taking a cholesterol-lowering drug will reduce your risk of a heart attack.

This myth was addressed in detail in Chapter 15. For more than 95% of the population, this claim is false.

Misconception: Diuretics are bad for you.

Incredibly, there are still doctors who believe this. This myth is based upon the fact that diuretics will lower blood potassium, and transiently elevate the cholesterol, uric acid and blood sugar levels. The transient elevations return to normal levels within a few months. Potassium loss continues but can be easily compensated for by adding a potassium-blocking drug to the patient's medical program. I have never seen a patient adequately control his or her hypertension who was not on a diuretic. The benefits of this medication, not only for patients with hypertension, but also for patients with coronary artery disease, far outweigh any theoretical disadvantage.

Misconception: You're taking too many drugs.

Many doctors seem to have a built-in resistance to using more than one or two drugs in patients with heart disease. The majority of such patients also have hypertension. In most of these individuals it usually takes *three* drugs to control their blood pressure: a beta blocker, a diuretic and an ACE inhibitor. Add coronary artery disease, and an additional drug is needed to increase the blood flow to the coronary arteries. Most of these patients also will need a potassium-blocking drug to prevent potassium loss, and some will need a drug to lower uric acid, which often rises as a result of coronary artery disease. Yes, these patients are taking a lot of medication, but each of the medications is needed for a specific purpose. Rarely are the side effects significant when doses are individualized. And the reward is great: the patient experiences no intereference with the quality of life, little or no limitation of activities because of symptoms, and almost no heart attacks, strokes or premature death. The alternative is surgery or angioplasty, often on a repeated basis, the complications that accompany these procedures, their horrendous costs and the continued need for medications. By every comparison, a normal life span and quality of life with multiple drug therapy is preferable to an abbreviated life with symptoms, multiple surgeries— but fewer drugs.

Misconception: Cardiac medications cause impotence.

Sometimes cardiac medication probably does cause impotence. However, they seem to do so in people who already have some impotence. Countless times, male patients have complained they have lost their sexual drive. Almost all of them are in the 60 to 70-year-old category. Typically, they have been taking their medications for several years and haven't had a problem. When impotence does occur, it is more acceptable to blame it on the medications rather than on simply getting older. Discontinuing the medication does not usually improve the problem. Thus, while some cardiac medications may interfere with sexual drive, it probably occurs only in a small minority.

Misconception: You don't need medication for your heart if you are not having any symptoms.

We used to believe this, but have learned it is not true. Heart disease can progress in the complete absence of symptoms. This was discussed at length earlier in this chapter.

Misconception: If you enter the hospital, it is all right if the nurses stop your medication.

Wrong! This was discussed in detail in the previous chapter. If you undergo noncardiac surgery, make sure you are back on your cardiac and hypertension medications as soon as possible.

Misconception: Your blood pressure is too low.

A normal blood pressure is too high for someone with coronary heart disease. The lower the blood pressure, the better the heart is able to function. Only if the blood pressure is associated with prolonged symptoms such as profound fatigue, dizziness and weakness can it be considered too low. Many patients can function quite nicely with pressures as low as 100/60. I recall one patient whose lower half of his heart was destroyed by a massive heart attack. I kept his pressure at about 90/50. He never complained of any symptoms, and he worked regularly as an accountant.

REFERENCES

1. American College of Physicians. Guidelines for assessing and managing the perioperative risk from coronary artery disease associated with major noncardiac surgery. Ann Int Med 1997; 127:309-312.

18

PUTTING IT ALL TOGETHER

Are you confused by what you have read so far? No doubt you grew up with the belief that if you felt healthy and had no symptoms, you didn't need the services of a doctor. But, if you had symptoms, you went to a doctor, he or she would treat you and you would get better. It was an unambiguous arrangement. There was no controversy about whether or not you had a disease, or how it should be diagnosed and treated. Back then, the practice of medicine was far simpler than it is today, and there were not enough choices to argue about. For instance, heart disease could be diagnosed only when it was far advanced. It had to be advanced in order for such primitive tools as the stethoscope, electrocardiogram and chest x-ray to detect it. Treatment for heart disease was also limited. There were either digitalis drugs or diuretics.

Doctors of that era were dedicated to the care of their patients. The money they received was enough to provide them with a comfortable living, but not much more. Other people and companies did not make money from doctors. That arrangement had not yet developed, and money was not the objective in health care. The satisfaction of saving lives and helping others compensated physicians for the long hours and hard work. The dedication and concerned care these doctors provided earned them the trust and love of their patients. Patients believed their doctor like they believed their parents. Anything less was unthinkable. Physicians were held in high esteem and were greatly respected.

This trust in the medical profession has endured for so long that it has prevented the American public from coming to grips with the enormous changes that have come about in the delivery of health care over the past

10 to 15 years. Those changes include the explosive development of technology for the diagnosis and treatment of disease, the vast increase in the number of specialists, the revolution in health care delivery, and above all, the industrialization of medicine. As a result, there are now many ways in which heart disease can be diagnosed and treated, as well as different ways to pay for that care. To make what you have read in this book more understandable and to help you to understand why there is so much variation and controversy in the practice of medicine, this chapter explains how medical care has changed, and why trust in doctors has eroded. If you wish to survive in the jungle of modern medicine, it will be necessary for you to change the way you think about doctors and the health care industry. Conversely, if medicine is to survive as a profession, doctors will have to alter the way they have been thinking about health care.

In present day United States, there is only one thing that is more important than saving lives, and that is making money. If anyone doubts the truth of this paradigm, they ought to reflect upon the tobacco industry and the managed health care industry —or, more precisely, the managed *lack* of health care by *reduced* provider associations. Saving and making money are more important to HMOs, pharmaceutical companies, hospitals, and even to some doctors than is saving lives.

Meanwhile, the spiraling costs of medical care due to the explosive use of ever more complex tests and treatment have led to a point where health care is no longer affordable by any one individual, company or even by the United States Government. I am not referring to the use of an expensive antibiotic to treat a serious infection, for such costs are relatively minuscule, such treatments are almost always effective and truly saves lives. Instead, I am referring to the widespread use of costly, complex surgical and technological procedures whose benefits are marginal, where the treatment may be worse than the disease, and where the result is to postpone death, rather than to prolong life. Both doctors and patients must be willing to accept the fact that treating a disease is like driving a car. Although we know there is a chance we may not reach our destination alive, we still drive. Doctors know (although they would be reluctant to admit it), and patients are often unaware that the treatment of disease is imperfect because medicine is an inexact science. Often, the outcome of medical care is unpredictable. Doctors understood this very well in the past, as did the patient and his or her family. When the doctors said, "We've done all we can," it was an acceptable response. However, such a response is no longer acceptable to either doctors or attorneys, and by default, to the patient and his or her family. "Do all you can," they demand instead. In fact, doing nothing will not be tolerated, even when "doing something" is more dangerous. After all, there is always a chance the patient will benefit, no matter how much it will cost.

The use of the new clot-dissolving drugs (thrombolytic agents) for heart attacks is a classic example of irrational thinking. A recent study of approximately 41,000 patients who were admitted to a hospital with a heart attack demonstrated that the mortality with the low cost thrombolytic agent streptokinase was 7.1%. This drug costs $300 per injection. In contrast, if the thrombolytic agent tPA was used at $2,200 per injection, the mortality rate was 6.1%. Not surprisingly, the manufacturer of tPA has undertaken an expensive advertising campaign in an attempt to convince all physicians that the drug is worth the extra cost. Yet, if all one million people who have heart attacks each year were to automatically receive tPA, the annual cost would be $2.2 billion, where as if streptokinase were used, the cost would be only $300 million. Only one life out of 100 might be saved with all that expense, and that might be by chance, and that's the chance we must not take. Besides, there are better ways of saving far more than one life out of 100 at a fraction of the cost of that $2.2 billion. For example, currently the Medicare program will not pay for the cost of an annual blood count, chemistry panel, chest x-ray, blood test for homocysteine, mammogram or PSA (prostate specific antigen) test. Consequently, these tests are no longer performed on older patients. Yet, the cost of doing all of these procedures would be no more than several hundred dollars and might save between 5 and 10 lives out of 100.

THE INDUSTRIALIZATION OF MEDICINE

In order to understand how the lives of each of us may be adversely influenced by doctors, hospitals, and other forces that control the practice of medicine, it would be best to acquaint you with how these interests came to control health care delivery. It wasn't always this way. Indeed, that is part of the problem. Most of us continue to remember things as they were, and behave accordingly —i.e., when a doctor recommended a test or a treatment, you knew it was for your benefit, and you agreed. Today it is different —the test or procedure may be more for the doctor's benefit than for the patient's. If you knew this to be true, you might not agree to have the test or procedure.

COMMERCIALISM IN MEDICINE

In 1980, Dr. Arnold S. Relman, editor of the *New England Journal of Medicine*, addressed the issue of commercialism in medical care in a series of brilliantly perceptive articles.[1-3] He coined the term "Medical-Industrial Complex" in reference to a new industry of health care delivery for a profit. He included proprietary hospitals, nursing homes, diagnostic laboratories, home care services, emergency room facilities, kidney dialysis units, and a wide variety of other medical services that had formerly been provided by nonprofit hospitals. Relman predicted, quite accurately, that this new Medical-Industrial Complex would become a huge new industry, and that its marketing and advertising strategies would lead to high costs and widespread overuse of medical resources. He forecast that it might overemphasize expensive technology, and neglect less profitable personal care. Finally, it also might influence national health policy, and change the attitude of physicians toward their profession.

It was Relman's belief that three forces set the stage for the development of the Medical-Industrial Complex. The first was the increase in the relative and absolute number of medical specialists. At the end of World War II, 70% of all doctors were primary care physicians. Now it was the other way around: 70% of all doctors are specialists. This has led to a fragmentation of medical care, and to less personal concern by doctors for their patients.

The second major force was the explosive development and use of medical technology. Not only did the new group of specialists catalyze that development, but the rapid growth of technology accelerated the increase in specialists.

The third major force was the development of medical insurance and third-party payers, the most important of whom was the federal government. The introduction of the Medicare program in 1965, and the manner in which reimbursement to physicians was set up, completely changed how medicine was practiced and set the stage for the rise of the Medical-Industrial Complex. It has been estimated that the revenues of the Medical-Industrial Complex, a system that did not even exist 30 years ago, exceeded $150 billion in 1990 out of a total national expenditure of $700 billion.3

HISTORICAL PERSPECTIVE

Prior to World War II, there were few specialists and a chronic shortage of doctors. All doctors were busy and had little time to devote to anything other than essential services for their patients, and these were not expensive. There were relatively few medical journals for doctors to read, so keeping abreast of the medical literature was not an overwhelming task. Progress in the medical sciences was relatively slow. It was carried out chiefly by researchers in medical schools, most of whom were laboratory people who did not see patients. Their pay was quite limited compared to their colleagues in private practice. This was because government funding was still in the future, and all funds had to come from a relatively few philanthropic agencies.

Consequently, only the most dedicated individuals opted for careers in medical research. If a researcher discovered a new diagnostic test or treatment, it would be presented at one of the few national medical meetings that were in existence at that time. If the new findings sounded promising, the treatment or procedure would be tried out by some of those physicians attending the meeting. In time, these physicians would present confirmatory evidence, and more and more doctors would use the new test or treatment. Progress, therefore, was slow— slow enough so that there was ample time for a new treatment to be tested in the vast laboratory of human experience. If the new treatment ultimately proved to be harmful, then relatively few patients would suffer.

IMPACT OF GOVERNMENT SPENDING ON THE GROWTH OF TECHNOLOGY AND PHYSICIAN SUPPLY

After World War II, the most significant development to take place was the federal government's funding of medical research with immense sums of money. At the same time, the government encouraged and made possible the education and training of more doctors to accomplish that research. These events ultimately led to the explosive increase in technology development, and to the increase in the numbers of medical specialists who could use this technology. These developments, along with the rapid dissemination of information that was possible after World War II and assisted by almost unlimited funding, changed the way research and medical progress were accomplished. Whereas once the tests available for the diagnosis of a disease were quite limited, as were the number of treatment options, now there were many different ways to diagnosis and treat most diseases. Together, these changes were ultimately responsible for the progressive increase in the cost of medical care that encouraged the growth of medical insurance, and led to the introduction of Medicare.

By 1970, while there was no longer a scarcity of physicians in the major population areas, there continued to be a shortage in less desirable locations such as inner cities and rural areas. At that time, there were 153 active physicians per 100,000 population. By 1993, the number exceeded 230 per 100,000 population. Thus, the total physician population was now 50% greater than the number of doctors seeing patients in 1970, and nearly three-quarters of them were specialists.

HOW THE INCREASE IN SPECIALISTS AFFECTS THE COST OF CARE

How this increase in the number of specialists affects the cost of medical care is reflected in what happens to the number of coronary bypass surgeries that are done in a community when the number of surgeons increases. It is not the same as what occurs in other markets. For example, if there were two supermarkets in the same community and a third competitor were added, the market share of each store would drop from 50% to 33%, assuming business were equally divided between the three.

However, this pattern does not hold up if there is a 50% increase in the number of cardiac surgeons from 20 to 30. Assuming each surgeon does 50 bypass procedures per year, 20 x 50 or 1000 surgeries were done annually before the influx of new doctors. Increasing the number of surgeons from 20 to 30 does not mean that each surgeon now will do only 33 such surgeries a year (1000/30). Instead, studies have shown that when the number of surgeons in an area increases, the total number of surgeries performed will also grow, although there might be a small decrease for each surgeon. Accordingly, each surgeon might do only 45 surgeries a year. This means there will be 30 x 45 or 1350 patients undergoing a bypass procedure annually. It also means the yearly cost of medical care in the community will increase by more than 20 million dollars.

THE EFFECTS OF MEDICAL INSURANCE ON SPECIALISTS, HOSPITALS AND PATIENTS

Effect on Specialists

The spread of medical insurance, third-party reimbursements and the introduction of the Medicare program has had an even greater impact on how medicine was practiced than has the increase in doctors. It changed the way specialists used technology, how hospitals were run, and even how patients behaved. Since there were more specialists using the new technology, it encouraged a different fee schedule for these physicians compared to nonspecialists. Specialists demanded reimbursement for their special skills and knowledge of the procedures they performed on patients. In many instances, costly equipment and trained personnel were required to operate that equipment, and higher fees were necessary to pay for those expenses. In contrast, the cognitive skills used by nonspecialists were not considered to be worthy of higher fees. Accordingly, being a specialist was far more lucrative and prestigious than being a family practitioner. Inevitably, this led American medicine to be procedure-oriented and technology-dependent.

Effect on Hospitals

When the Medicare program entered the picture in 1965, hospitals were still social entities that were nonprofit, and dedicated to the noble task of helping their staff physicians take care of patients. Quality of care was their priority. The doctors controlled the hospital; the hospital administrators and nursing staff were there to help them. Profit was not a motivating factor since, if there were any deficit, contributions by members of the community covered the losses. As we shall see, the Medicare reimbursement system changed all of that.

The original purpose of the Medicare Act in 1965 was to provide medical assistance to the elderly. The method of reimbursement was designed as payment for costs, plus an additional service fee. This meant that no matter how many tests were performed on an individual, the hospital always would be fully reimbursed. It was clear from the beginning that the more tests and procedures that were performed, the greater the hospital's profit. Fueling this was the rapid spread of technology, and the increase in specialists.

Effect on Patients

At the same time, "health" insurance began to be purchased on a wider scale, by both individuals and by companies for their employees, from such entities as Blue Cross and Blue Shield. Before long, 85% of the population had some form of insurance, including benefits for illness outside of the hospital. For the first time, a patient didn't have to pay for the complete costs of a medical visit, hospitalization or surgery. The insurance plan would pay after a certain deductible was met. Indeed, patients felt entitled to medical care because they had paid their premiums.

IMPACT OF CHANGES ON COST OF MEDICAL CARE

With the development of new ways to diagnose and treat disease, it was inevitable that the public would demand to be treated for their illness with the latest technology, and with little regard for the cost. The doctor did not worry about the expense because he or she knew the insurance company would pay for whatever tests or procedures were ordered. The insurance company wasn't concerned, either. They knew that premiums would simply have to rise to cover the increased costs, and this would mean greater profits. None could foresee that here were the seeds for the enormous increase in the cost of medical care.

In 1965, the total amount spent on health care was about 6% of our gross national product (GNP). At that time, the projected cost for Medicare was less than $10 billion a year. In 1992, the total amount spent on health care was nearly 14% of the GNP, or $838 billion, while Medicare costs reached $146 billion. The Commerce Department expects the total to grow by 12-15% a year —more than triple the current rate of inflation. By the end of the decade, health care costs are projected to reach 20% of the GNP, unless some kind of control is instituted. In addition, all that medical care needs administrators and bureaucracy. Remarkably, between 19 and 24 percent of the total spending on health care is consumed by administrative costs. For 1992 that figure was between $159 and $201 billion.

WITH ALL THAT MONEY, PROFIT ENTERS THE PICTURE

As indicated earlier, Medicare and third-party carriers changed the way hospitals were run. Most hospitals were nonprofit institutions when Medicare entered the picture. However, there was no law that said hospitals could not make a profit, or even be a for-profit institution. Not surprisingly, with all that Medicare and insurance money available, it didn't take long for the hospitals to realize that health care could be very profitable, when combined with in-house specialists who could order high technology tests and treatments.

There were others who recognized the financial rewards of health care. Corporations began to appear in the late 1960s like Humana, National Medical Enterprises, and Hospital Corporation of America. Their schemes all followed the same pattern: take advantage of the Medicare legislation, create a corporation, have a public issue of stock, and use the capital to acquire hospitals and health care facilities. The hospitals all would be for-profit places of service.

Accordingly, investor-owned chains of for-profit hospitals began to appear in ever increasing numbers. By 1980, there were over 1000. Today, nearly 30% of the 5000 hospitals in this country are for-profit hospitals. A number of studies in the past decade compared not-for-profit hospitals with investor-owned hospitals. The charges and profits of for-profit hospitals were 15-20% greater than the not-for-profit hospitals for the same type of cases. In addition, the for-profit hospitals tended to use aggressive marketing policies to increase both profits and growth.

TRANSFORMATION OF NOT-FOR-PROFIT HOSPITALS INTO CORPORATIONS

The lessons, the earnings, as well as the competition from the for-profit chains, did not go unobserved by the nonprofit hospitals. Soon they began to change. What was once a cottage industry with many individual hospitals began to grow into a corporation of multi-hospital systems. In this scenario, one large hospital takes control of several smaller hospitals.

As the not-for-profit hospitals expanded into multi-hospital systems, they became more like the for-profit hospitals by dramatically increasing their charges. In part this was due to the change in the way Medicare paid for hospital services. In 1983, in an attempt to put a cap on the ever increasing charges by hospitals, the government introduced the DRGs (diagnosis related group) system of payment. No longer could hospitals order as many tests as they wished with a substantial profit, and then pass on the bill to Medicare. Instead, payment was made according to diagnosis. Not only were the hospitals to be paid by diagnosis, it was a fixed payment. Now the hospitals had to keep their charges as low as possible. Indeed, the fewer the tests, and the earlier the patient was discharged, the greater were the profits.

This posed a problem, however, if there were any delay in patient recovery, or if there were complications of the illness. This was especially apt to happen with older patients, and those with multiple diseases. Since the hospital was allowed to charge only a certain amount for a given diagnosis, it lost money when the patient's recovery was delayed. Some hospitals began discharging Medicare patients before they had completely recovered from their illness or surgery. If a complication developed, the patient could be readmitted with that complication as a new diagnosis. This practice became known as dumping. It provided the hospital with a new diagnosis and additional reimbursement. Although Congress eventually put a stop to this, countless numbers of patients suffered from this practice.

By this time, the not-for-profit hospitals had undergone a metamorphosis into for-profit institutions. Since they could no longer depend upon charitable contributions to cover their losses, or upon a guaranteed profit from Medicare, they became more like corporations. Cost shifting entered the picture to cover their losses on Medicare patients, and those without insurance. Soon private paying patients and their insurance companies felt the impact. The prices these patients had to pay became obscene. Overnight observation of an elderly automobile accident victim with mild chest trauma and who required no surgery would be over $10,000! Minor surgery that did not even require an overnight stay could be $6,000 —and this did not include the surgeon's fee.

Not content with the profits they were making, hospitals began to look for other ways to make money. The aggressive ones already had expanded horizontally by taking over other hospitals. Soon they began to expand vertically to integrate with other forms of health care delivery, such as medical practices, nursing homes, diagnostic medical laboratories, and home health services. Some hospitals even went so far as to develop their own managed health care plans or HMO that would provide them with a constant source of patients. Soon hospitals were aggressively setting up their own satellite medical practices with either purchased practices or with hired young doctors. Before long, advertisements began to appear on television, on radio, in newspapers and even on billboards, extolling the benefits of using the hospital's health care network. It was all perfectly legal. While it was, and still is, considered to be poor taste for a physician to advertise, this was not so for hospitals.

EFFECT OF HOSPITAL EXPANSION ON PHYSICIANS

What was particularly galling to most physicians was the encroachment on the doctor's practice by the hospital's satellite medical practices, HMOs and managed health care plans. The result was that the doctor's own hospital captured a major share of the patient market. This was the same hospital he or she had donated time, services and money to, and the very one his or her efforts, as well as those of colleagues, had elevated to a prominent status in the community. Now that same hospital was "biting the hand that fed it" by taking away the physician's own patients.

The hospitals were now under the control of a CEO, and were run like corporations: profit had a higher priority than patient care. The medical staff, who once controlled the hospital, were under the total domination of the hospital administrators. The slaves had become the masters, and doctors were treated like pawns. In large measure this was due to a 1975 Supreme Court decision that said the activities of physicians relative to the delivery of health care were now subject to antitrust laws.[5] Accordingly, even when physicians acted in defense of their patients, they were unable to act collectively. This meant that the individual physician was powerless to stop the hospital from expanding its health care delivery system, and taking over patients by offering cheaper care.

HOW THE PROFIT MOTIVE DOMINATES THE MANAGEMENT OF PATIENTS

Doctors were not angry at hospitals merely because they represented competition for patients. There was a widespread feeling that hospitals had turned the practice of medicine from a humanitarian profession dedicated to quality patient care into a business in which the welfare of the patient was secondary to making a profit. In such a scenario, the patient is a helpless victim of the hospital health care system. For example, while a patient with chest pain once would have been placed in a medical intensive care unit and carefully watched by the nursing staff and the patient's doctor until he recovered, now he or she was rushed to the cardiac catheterization laboratory by a team of doctors. There the patient underwent angiograms, angioplasty or bypass surgery.

It didn't matter that the mortality associated with these aggressive interventions were often considerably greater than the mortality levels for simple medical treatment. Besides, the hospitals could justify what its doctors were doing. This new kind of treatment for heart attacks was being widely reported at medical meetings, and was now being carried out by most hospitals with cardiac surgery capabilities. In contrast, hospitals that did not have cardiac catheterization capabilities and cardiac surgery did not rush their patients into surgery but continued to treat them in the conventional way. There were wide discrepancies in the way patients were treated in different parts of the country. California and Texas, for example, both had much higher rates of interventional procedures than did New York and the New England states.

Ironically, the antitrust law which prevented doctors from collectively acting together, did not apply to hospitals' imitating each other. The patient —helpless, dependent, and intimidated— was the last one to recognize that he or she was a guinea pig for the latest in medical experimentation. It is worth adding that if the "new treatment" for heart attacks were not extremely profitable, it would not be in such widespread use.

There was good reason for hospitals all over the country to be rushing into aggressive forms of treatment for heart attacks. Since hospitals found themselves limited in how much they could recoup from a simple heart attack due to the introduction of DRGs, they changed the game. It was relatively easy to encourage their cardiologists to recommend routine angiograms and bypass surgery as a new treatment for heart attacks. The economic incentive was too irresistible to ignore for both. Thus, instead of receiving $4,000 to $6,000 for a plain heart attack, the hospital would be reimbursed with $20,000 to $25,000. The cardiologist would be amply rewarded as well. It was a simple matter of economics. Ironically, the very technology that had been responsible for the phenomenal changes in the practice of medicine, and that added years to our life expectancy, was now being overused, and making the treatment more hazardous than the disease. In the process, lives were being lost.

THE FAILURE OF MARKET FORCES TO CONTROL THE COST OF MEDICAL CARE

Unfortunately, these events were the direct result of the government's failure to recognize that the usual rules could not be applied to the practice of medicine. It was the policy of the Republican administration to have the government intervene as little as possible. It depended upon market forces and competition to keep the cost of medical care under control. The problem with this approach was twofold. First, most hospitals responded to the market forces in the same way. Those who didn't, quickly became aware of what the other hospitals were doing, and rapidly followed suit. Thus, all the competition did the same thing, and prices were not controlled. Secondly, medicine did not follow the rules of ordinary market forces. For example, in a department store, the purchase of a product depends upon the cost and the customer's needs. The final decision is always made by the customer. In contrast, with health care delivery, the purchase of a service is often independent of the customer's (patient's) need, is not influenced by price (a third party pays), and the final decision is not made by the buyer but the seller. Bypass surgery is an excellent example —the patient usually doesn't need it, the cost is astronomical, and the doctor tells the patient it must be done.

THE GROWTH OF FREE-STANDING HEALTH CARE CENTERS

Hospitals were not the only ones who recognized that great profits could be made from medical care. Soon it was apparent to entrepreneur doctors that there were vast sums of money to be made with health care. In the 1980s, a variety of health care services began to be offered on an ambulatory basis in free standing medical facilities. Most of these centers were owned by doctors. An example is the imaging center that does x-rays, computed tomography (CT) scans and magnetic resonance imaging (MRI). If a doctor, who is a part owner of one of these facilities, orders a simple x-ray of a patient's back, the imaging center will be reimbursed only $50 to $100. On the other hand, if an MRI is ordered, the facility can now charge $800.

The entrepreneur doctors or corporations who own these imaging centers can increase their profits by encouraging other doctors to use their facilities. Merely sending out advertising brochures may not be sufficient. A common technique used to encourage other doctors to use the more expensive procedures is to collect a series of cases in which there is a dramatic difference between the findings of the older technology as compared to the newer technology. There is no doubt there are many such instances. These selected cases are presented to a physician audience that can hardly fail to be impressed by the dramatic difference. What is not presented are the large number of cases where the new technology is not helpful, or where it provides misleading information. As a result of these biased presentations, more physicians are induced to use the newer technology, thereby increasing the centers' profits.

The growth of free-standing health care facilities was not limited to imaging centers, nor was their ownership limited to doctors. As indicated earlier, in the late seventies there was a marked growth of for-profit hospitals. After the introduction of the Medicare caps in 1983, the growth of these investor-owned hospitals slowed down considerably. Hospitals were no longer considered as profitable as they once were. Consequently, corporations began looking for other forms of health care facilities from which they could make a profit. A variety of such facilities were either purchased or built. They included sports medicine clinics, rehabilitation centers, surgical centers, medical equipment companies, imaging centers, diagnostic medical laboratories, emergency room services, kidney dialysis units, and home care services for the chronically or terminally ill. There has been a prolific increase in the use of such health care services. Many of these services were formerly available only in hospitals. For example, 10-15 years ago only minor surgery was performed in an office setting. Today, with the development of free-standing centers for ambulatory surgery, about half of all surgical procedures are performed in such centers, including those that require general anesthesia. Indeed, more than ever, hospital care is reserved only for the acutely ill who require skilled nursing care and complex high technology equipment that is not suited for home use. The availability of ambulatory centers has tended to reduce the cost of care for a major illness that lasts over a protracted period of time. This doesn't mean that such services are cheap, but only that they are not nearly as expensive as similar hospital services that are notorious for their exorbitant prices.

HOW THE MEDICAL-INDUSTRIAL COMPLEX INFLUENCES MEDICAL CARE

The vast complex of corporations that own chains of for-profit hospitals, nursing homes, and ambulatory health care facilities, all comprise the Medical-Industrial Complex described by Dr. Arnold Relman. That complex also includes the not-for-profit, multi-hospitals systems, pharmaceutical corporations, and manufacturers of medical equipment. It has had an enormous influence on every aspect of medicine and health care delivery. A typical scenario on how the Medical-Industrial Complex operates is illustrated by a medical corporation's purchase of a for-profit hospital in an affluent suburban community with an adjacent medical building. Advertisements are immediately placed in medical journals for new doctors, describing in glowing terms all the attributes of the community and the practice opportunities. Physicians who are looking for a place to set up a practice are lured to the new locations with enticing offers of low rent, and a promise by the hospital to refer them patients. There even may be a guarantee of the first year's income. The implied understanding is that the new doctor will admit his patients to the corporation's hospital. In reality, this is a form of fee splitting, but the gyrations are so convoluted and the relationship so vague that it is difficult to prove. Such hospitals and medical buildings are never in inner city areas where there is a shortage of medical facilities. Instead, these corporations make sure they are dealing with well-to-do patients, all of whom have insurance.

There are many people who feel that the Medical-Industrial Complex caters to over-zealous and over-trained specialists, and encourages them to over-utilize expensive equipment, and overtreat patients with a relatively benign disease. Its purpose is to fill the operating rooms, support the diagnostic laboratories, keep the surgeons, nurses, technicians and other support people busy, and fill the empty beds. This is an important reason why medicine has become technology-driven and profit-oriented. The result is that large numbers of patients are receiving expensive tests and costly treatments that are not needed.

The overuse of technology is a major reason for the high cost of medical care. Paradoxically, it is frequently not known whether a new technology is more effective, or even more cost-beneficial than that which it replaced. Furthermore, new technology often doesn't replace older technology, but is merely added on to it. For example, echocardiography provides so much information about a patient's heart that most of the time it is unnecessary to perform an angiogram. Similarly, a radioactive imaging study is often perfectly adequate to determine whether there is blood flow to the heart muscle. Yet, many cardiologists will order all three tests to obtain information. The reason is that many physicians are not secure with the results provided by only one of the new technologies. This is because none of them is 100% or even 90% accurate. Because of this uncertainty in diagnosis, there is the constant fear of malpractice suits should something go wrong. No doubt the following legal scenario has passed through the minds of all cardiologists when called upon to make a life and death decision.

Prosecuting attorney: *"Doctor, you knew that the test you ordered was not 100% accurate, and that in some studies it was only 80% reliable."*

"Yes," is the reply.

"Yet, you failed to get a confirmatory test, and instead recommended immediate bypass surgery, which the plaintiff patient did not need, and now her left arm and leg are useless and she is unable to talk!"

Because a malpractice suit can destroy a physician's career and his financial security, most of them take the easy way out by ordering as many tests as possible. While the threat of a malpractice suit would seem to support the practice of ordering as many high technology tests as possible, in reality, there are so many tests to choose from that it has become impractical and far too costly. An experienced cardiologist, who has the patient's best interests at heart, will order the minimum number of tests that are the safest for the patient while providing the information necessary to make a diagnosis and decide on the best form of treatment. In most instances, the combination of a stress test with either an echocardiogram or a radioactive imaging procedure is all that is required. If the patient's response to treatment is carefully monitored, and his or her symptoms disappear, the doctor cannot be faulted. If, however, improvement fails to occur, then additional diagnostic procedures are warranted. Unfortunately, that's not the way it's being done. Partly under the fear of legal action if something goes wrong, and mainly under the concealed goal of maximizing income, the patient is made to undergo costly and unnecessary tests and interventions.

LIVES VS. PROFIT

The industrialization of medicine as described here means that if a choice of testing or for treatment interferes with bottom line profit, then a decision will be made favoring profit, even if it means loss of lives. The automobile industry is a good example of this common problem. Many times cars are built with defects that are not recognized as defects before they leave the factory. Most of these are minor and are not a safety hazard. Others, however, are discovered to be dangerous if the vehicle is ever involved in an accident. If enough vehicles are involved, a pattern emerges that is eventually brought to the attention of the manufacturer. When this happens, most manufacturers will recall the vehicle and repair the defect at no charge to the owner. If, however, the repairs are costly, then the manufacturer is faced with the decision of not recalling the vehicles, and gambling that there will be no further injuries or deaths. Implicit in such a decision is the gamble that even if there are further accidents, and the manufacturer is sued, and has to settle, the cost will be far less than recalling and repairing a large number of defective cars.

A similar thing is now happening in medicine. Heart transplantation is a good example. It is well recognized that heart transplantation requires the ultimate in medical technology involving cardiologists, surgeons, biochemists, immunologists, microbiologists, and a host of other specialists and technical help. It is a complex task, and only a few can be accomplished in any given month, for it is difficult and expensive to acquire a donor heart. Accordingly, it is certainly not a volume operation, nor is it profitable. In fact, for years insurance companies refused reimbursement for the procedure on the grounds it was still considered as research.

Nevertheless, there is a need for a heart transplant center in a major metropolitan area. There are about 25 such major metropolitan areas in this country, yet there are over 100 heart transplant centers in the United States. The lion's share of transplants go to such major centers as Stanford, the

University of Pittsburgh, and others like them. Smaller centers may only carry out a relatively few procedures each year.

It is an acknowledged fact that the more you do something, the better you get at it. This is illustrated in the statistics from some hospitals that do only 50-100 coronary artery bypasses per year with an operative mortality of 15-20%. In contrast, institutions performing 400 or more such procedures per year have a mortality of only 2-3%. The point here is that those hospitals doing relatively few transplants a year are going to have a much higher mortality than the major transplant centers. Such information must have been known to the hospital administrators at the time a decision was made to offer transplant services. It was also known that one, and perhaps two to three other transplant centers, existed within a relatively few miles. The decision to start such a center is clearly not in the best interest of the patients. The existence of a second or third transplant center in the same community will certainly dilute the efforts of the others to obtain the highly skilled physicians and technical help needed to carry out such an effort. The mortality at the new center is bound to be higher, if for no other reason than there will be a learning curve for the entire team.

Why, then, go ahead? For business reasons. A hospital that claims to have a transplant center will be looked upon as a better hospital than one that is not. This will help to attract more and better doctors (and their patients), provide the hospital with more prestige, allow cost shifting and a host of other fringe benefits. In short, it is a marketing decision that will cost both lives and money, but eventually mean greater profits. It also is an administrative decision made with the willing cooperation of doctors. It is no different than urging a heart attack patient to undergo angioplasty or bypass surgery before noninvasive medical treatment is attempted, or for a managed health care plan to deny a patient admission to the hospital merely because his chest pain has temporarily subsided. In every case, a business decision that leads to more profits takes precedence over a patient's life.

A further example of how economics controls the practice of medicine can be gleaned from a story in the *Phoenix Gazette* which appeared several years ago. Prior to March 15, 1985 there were 10 hospitals in the Phoenix area that were eligible to perform open heart surgery —a more than adequate number. On this date, the hospital industry was deregulated. In spite of the fact that there were ten facilities capable of performing such surgery at an acceptable mortality rate, seven additional hospitals began performing bypass surgery, with a striking increase in mortality. At some hospitals the mortality rate was over 14% At the same time, hospital charges for bypass surgery increased 50% with some hospitals netting profits of over $1 million. The difference in death rate after deregulation was 60 per 1,000 patients in the hospitals already doing surgery compared to 117 per 1,000 in the seven hospitals that started open heart surgery after deregulation. Once again, this shows how decisions are made with a blatant disregard for need and result in the loss of life.

EFFECT OF INDUSTRIALIZATION ON PHYSICIANS AND THEIR PRACTICE

The industrialization of medicine has affected doctors profoundly. Its most important effect has been the marked increase in HMOs and managed health care plans. Anywhere from one-third to one-half of all patients are now being seen by managed care plans in some cities. Consequently, there has been a gradual decline in the number of patients seen by the average physician. An additional loss of patients has resulted from a doubling of the number of physicians in practice over the past 30-40 years, according to the Graduate Medical Education Advisory Committee. For example, by the end of the decade there will be 643,000 physicians, which will be about 145,000 more than the country needs. Further encroachment on the physician's turf can be expected by the increasing numbers of physician's assistants and nurse practitioners. The result will be intense competition for fewer patients.

Because of the progressive loss in the number of patients seen by solo physicians, many doctors have had to join HMOs, managed health care plans, or large groups of doctors. Inevitably this has resulted in a considerable loss of freedom by both doctor and patient. In fact, in many ways the physician functions more like an employee, in that managed care really means both managed doctors and managed patients for the purpose of controlling cost. Years ago, a physician decided what tests were needed to confirm his or her suspected diagnosis, what consultant the patient should see, what drugs should be prescribed, whether surgery should be performed, what hospital a patient should be admitted to, what surgeon would operate if surgery were needed, how long the patient would remain in the hospital, and when he or she should be discharged. Now the physician has little control over any of those decisions. The tests the physician is allowed to use, what treatment he or she can recommend, and even how much time he or she is allowed to spend with the patient, often may all compromise quality of care in favor of cost. You can be sure that the compromise favors the managed care plan and not the patient. It also has caused a tremendous amount of frustration and despair among physicians. These forces have transformed the practice of medicine from a humanitarian profession controlled solely by doctors, to a technology-driven, profit-oriented enterprise, heavily influenced by business interests. As a result, the welfare of the patient often seems to be secondary to the welfare of the managed health care plan.

Another factor adding to the frustration of doctors is advertising. Where once it was considered unethical for a physician to advertise, now it is common. It used to be that physicians could depend on the truism that if they practiced their craft well, their reputation would spread through word of mouth and they would prosper. This is no longer so. In many cases, incompetent doctors may become successful by using a public relations firm, aggressive marketing tactics, and by tasteless advertisements that frighten patients into believing a harmless problem is life threatening.

The concerned doctor is surrounded by examples of the industrialization of medicine. An example of the kind of commercialism that has evolved is witnessed in the fact that cardiologists receive hundreds, if not thousands of advertisements from medical equipment manufacturers during their careers. One might assume that these advertisements describe the benefits of the test device for the detection of disease, address how it compares with older equipment, discuss how accurate it is, its limitations, and all of the other information that would be necessary for its proper use. And while most of the time this is the information that appears, sadly, there are countless examples where none of these facts is addressed. Instead, the whole advertisement concerns itself with how much money can be made by the test, how many tests per month would be required to pay for the

315

equipment, and how to maximize reimbursement for the use of the test from third-party carriers. What was unthinkable and abhorrent a relatively few years ago; i.e., that a test should be used primarily for making money on sick, helpless patients, is now becoming commonplace.

Another grave by-product of the industrialization of medical care has been a loss of the personal touch by physicians, and along with it, an erosion of the patient-physician relationship. In the past, most doctors had long-term relationships with patients, patients' spouses and other members of their family. This is why they were called family physicians. When a family member became ill, the doctor took a personal interest because he or she cared. And if a patient died, the doctor grieved with the family. Even if there were some question as to whether the doctor might have contributed to the patient's demise through the wrong treatment, or failure to make a timely diagnosis, the family felt no ill-will to the doctor, simply because the doctor had meant well, and was doing his or her best. Litigation was rare. Today, it is a different story. An HMO or managed health care patient is assigned to a doctor with whom he or she is unfamiliar. Conversely, the doctor must deal with a patient who is a total stranger, and one whom he or she may never see again. These are hardly optimal conditions for a close patient-physician relationship. Accordingly, if a mishap or an unsatisfactory outcome results from the doctor's care, a malpractice suit can easily follow. Sometimes an honest, competent physician may be dragged into a malpractice suit because of an unsatisfactory outcome that was not his or her fault. This constant threat of litigation from malpractice suits has forced doctors to practice defensive medicine by ordering as many tests and procedures as possible. This has also had a major impact on the rising costs of medical care.

THE BOTTOM LINE

It is no wonder why doctors no longer seem to care. The profession they love is being destroyed by the forces described in this chapter, and they are helpless to stop them. On the one hand, they see patients whose health or life may be destroyed from denial of essential health care services. On the other hand, the same effect may occur from the overuse and abuse of technology. They are no longer held in the esteem they once were, and they are even no longer in control of their own patients. At the same time, their income has been drastically reduced. Many physicians are barely able to keep up with the expenses of just moderate living. Worst of all, they are frequently unable to maintain the sacred trust that they once had with every patient. As defined by Relman, "the physician is obligated to act as the trustee for the patient's interest, and whenever possible, with the patient's informed consent. The patient's interest takes precedence over all other considerations —certainly over any financial or other personal interests of the physician."[2]

PROTECT YOURSELF FROM THE INDUSTRIALIZATION OF MEDICINE AND LIVE LONGER WITH HEART DISEASE

How can you minimize the effects of the industrialization of medicine should you, or some member of your family become ill? The most important fact is for you to be aware that it has happened, that the profit motive is often more important than your welfare, and that you can be the innocent victim of overtreatment or undertreatment, depending upon the kind of doctor you are seeing, and the health plan to which you belong. Sometimes the doctor's advice is made merely to protect himself or herself; i.e., to prevent the possibility of a malpractice suit. It is, of course, not possible for you to have the same knowledge about the diagnosis and treatment of a disease as the doctor, particularly if he or she is a specialist. At the very least, though, you can ask questions as to the purpose of the doctor's recommendation, the dangers of not following his or her advice, and your options. Alternatively, if you are not sure whether enough is being done for your problem, ask if other doctors would treat you in the same way. Then you can make a more rational decision. If you still are not certain as to what you should or shouldn't do, ask for another doctor's opinion. When you feel comfortable with the information you have, then you can decide whether to follow the doctor's advice. Never blindly agree to whatever you are told to do. Ask for explanations. Your doctor has an obligation to provide that to you. If he or she refuses, then you refuse. If time permits, go to the library or book store. Read about your disease. The more you know, the safer you will be if major decisions have to be made. Take an active part in your own health.

Sadly, you can no longer afford to *totally* entrust your life to a strange doctor. I hope this book will teach you that. If, on the other hand, you have the good fortune to be under the care of the same doctor for many years, and he or she has demonstrated over and over he or she has your best interests at heart, hang on to that doctor! He or she may save your life. Never give such a doctor up simply because you can find somebody else who will provide medical care more inexpensively. There are some things, like trust, that you can't afford to cut back on.

REFERENCES

1. Relman AS. The new medical-industrial complex. N Engl J Med1980; 303:963-70.
2. Relman AS. The future of medical practice. Health Aff (Millwood) 1983; 2(2):5-19.
3. Relman AS. Shattuck Lecture. The health care industry: Where is it taking us? N Engl J Med 1991;325:854-59.
4. Woolhandler S, Himmelstein DU. The deteriorating administrative efficiency of the U.S. health care system. N Engl J Med 1991; 324:1253-8.
5. *Goldfarb v. Virginia State Bar*, 421 U.S. 773, 1975.

INDEX

abdominal causes of chest pain 91, 92, 108

Academic Hospital in Leiden 223

ACE inhibitors ix, 46, 109, 136, 140, 183-187, 191, 208, 211, 230, 250, 291

acebutolol 183

acetylcholine 199

acute stress 29, 30, 65

Adalat 192

adrenal glands ix, xiv, 45, 94, 179, 183, 185

adrenaline x, 59, 62

age, aging 25-28, 33, 36, 46, 50, 73, 113, 116, 117, 122, 148, 150, 151, 211, 212, 215, 219, 238-241, 251-253, 256, 271, 272, 278

alcohol 26, 37, 38, 48, 49, 84, 92, 97, 242

Aldactazide 189

Aldactone 189

Ambrose, Dr. John 7

American College of Cardiology (ACC) 225

American College of Physicians (ACP) 255, 268, 285

American Heart Association (AHA) 225, 255

amiloride 189

amino acids xvi, 39, 258

aminophylline ix, 109

amlodipine 192

anemia xviii, 94, 174

anesthesia 83, 266, 309

aneurysm 89, 142

anger 26, 29, 34, 35, 49, 73-75, 173

angina (*see also* chest pain) ix, xi, xvii, xviii, xxiii, 9, 11, 37, 46, 63, 64, 73, 74, 84, 117, 118, 120, 121, 136, 158, 159, 168, 169, 174, 179, 180, 187, 190, 194, 195, 200, 201, 204, 218, 219, 265, 276, 277, 279, 286-288, 290

pectoris ix, xi, xviii, 11, 37, 46, 74, 84, 117, 158, 159, 178, 180, 197, 247

angiogenesis ix, 9, 160, 287

angiogram(s) ix, xii, xviii, 7, 14, 52-54, 73, 81-84, 89, 93, 98, 99, 101, 115, 117, 118, 121, 129, 130, 136, 149, 151, 153-163, 204, 205, 207, 210, 212, 226-228, 229, 250, 251, 264, 265, 276, 281-285, 306, 307, 311

angioplasty v, xiii, xxi, 7, 34, 53, 56, 84, 93, 95, 98, 101, 102, 110, 111, 117, 121, 122, 136, 138, 139, 149, 150, 153, 156, 158, 161, 162, 186, 188, 205-230, 259, 267, 276, 280, 281, 285, 286, 290, 291, 306, 313, 329

angiotensin converting enzyme (ACE) inhibitors (*see* ACE inhibitors)

angiotensin II ix, 46, 183, 184, 186

Annals of Internal Medicine 251, 255

antacids 83, 84

antibiotics 83, 93, 276, 296

antidepressants 173

anti-inflammatory drugs (*see also* NSAIDs *and* ibuprofen) 174, 191, 277

antioxidants x, 26, 39, 179, 245, 255-258

anxiety (*see also* fear) 49, 90, 117, 178

aorta x, xi, xii, 3, 4, 6, 7, 20, 43, 44, 87, 89, 144, 265, 283

aortic valve 44, 55, 87, 144-146, 174, 230

apexcardiogram x, 141-144, 146

arrhythmia(s) x, xi, xii, xvi, 30, 35, 37, 49, 66, 173, 179, 180, 243, 266

arteries (*see also* coronary artery(ies)) x, xi, xii, xvii, xviii, xix, xxiii, 3, 15, 29, 37, 39, 43, 44, 46, 37, 49, 52, 54, 81, 86, 87, 94, 109, 115, 119, 121, 129, 130, 131, 134-136, 139, 140, 144, 150, 153, 155-161

arterioles 184, 187, 193

arteriosclerosis x, 14, 224, 240

arteriosclerotic plaque (*see also* plaque) x, xiii, xviii, xxiii, 3-7, 9-11, 13-15, 20, 29, 30, 37, 43, 48, 50, 53, 69, 75, 82, 120, 140, 184, 194, 199, 200, 216, 253, 256, 258, 265, 283, 289

arthritis vii, 93, 100, 154, 174

aspirin 5, 6, 93, 102, 109, 121, 128, 136, 194, 200, 201, 208, 209, 211, 229, 250, 255

atherectomy x, 53, 216, 233

atherosclerosis (*see also* arteriosclerosis) 69

athletes 20, 22, 281

atria 20, 144, 145

atrium x, xvii, xviii, xxi, xxii, xxiii, 12, 20, 21, 88, 103, 107, 134, 143-146, 266

autoimmune disease 85

Cedars-Sinai Medical Center 217
central nervous system 14
cervical disk 89
chest pain (*see also* angina) vi, xvii, xviii, xix,
    6, 9, 11, 17, 23, 31, 32, 34, 35, 37, 40, 52,
    53-55, 61-64, 81-99, 101, 102, 105, 114,
    115, 117-119, 121, 127-129, 132, 133,
    135, 149, 154, 155, 157-159, 161, 168,
    169, 171, 172, 180, 187, 190, 192, 193,
    195, 197, 201, 203-207, 209-211, 224,
    228, 229, 230, 241, 243, 264-266,
    275-277, 279, 283, 286-289, 306, 313
chest x-ray (*see also* x-ray) 295, 297
chlorothiazide 189
cholesterol xii, xvi, xxii, 5, 13, 14, 26, 32, 38,
    43, 44, 102, 121, 187, 191, 245-255, 291
cholesterol-lowering drug/medication xii,
    xxii, 5, 13, 14, 136, 201, 229, 245-254,
    290
chronic stress 29, 30, 65, 71
cigarette smoking 11, 25, 26, 28, 29, 31, 36,
    44, 154, 167, 278
cine magnetic resonance imaging 139
circulation xvii, xviii-xxi, xxiii, 4, 44, 46, 55,
    63, 130, 137, 143, 168, 193, 194, 199,
    239, 241
circulatory system 14, 36, 47, 55, 94, 109, 188,
    191, 195
cirrhosis 3, 154
Cleveland Clinic 129, 130, 208
clotting and clotting factor(s) xx, xxii, 5, 38,
    39, 173, 194, 256
coincidental coronary artery disease 54, 89,
    93, 130, 154, 162, 229
coincidental illness 96, 98, 242
collateral vessels xii, 8-11, 136, 150, 157, 160,
    194, 200, 224, 240
colon 92, 94, 174, 240
Commerce Department 303
complications 130, 138, 155, 162, 263,
    267-269, 283, 285, 291, 304
    of heart disease vi, 14, 28, 69, 105, 106
    of high blood pressure 46, 47, 51, 52, 104
computed tomography (CT) xii, 139, 308
congenital heart disease 26, 87, 151
congestive heart failure ix, xii, xiv, 28, 47,
    105, 108, 116, 121, 122, 143, 173, 178,
    181, 182, 195, 201, 209-211, 242, 264,
    265, 278, 280, 290
Conti, Dr. C. Richard 212

contraction phase xxii, 12, 30, 50, 67, 133,
    134, 136, 142, 143, 145, 146, 184, 191,
    240, 281
Cooper Clinic 33, 237
Coreg 183
Corgard 182, 183
coronary artery(ies) x, xi, xii, xiii, xiv, xvi,
    xviii, 4, 6, 9, 10-14, 87, 94, 98, 109, 115,
    121, 122, 128, 129, 131, 134, 136, 139,
    140, 154, 155, 157, 159, 160, 169, 179,
    184, 188, 190, 193, 194, 199, 200, 209,
    216, 218, 221, 224, 250, 251, 282-284,
    286, 287, 290, 291
coronary artery bypass surgery (*see* bypass
    surgery)
coronary artery disease v, xiii, xv, xix, xxi, 3,
    11, 14, 15, 24, 27, 28, 31, 34, 36, 37, 39,
    40, 43, 51, 54, 57, 63-65, 67-75, 84,
    87-89, 93-98, 104, 105, 107, 110, 117,
    119, 121, 127-129, 131, 134, 135, 137,
    148, 149, 151, 153-155, 157, 158, 161,
    167-169, 173, 174, 177, 179, 181, 186,
    188, 190-193, 195, 199, 201, 207-210,
    212, 214, 219, 220, 222, 227-230,
    238-242, 253, 257, 264, 276-278, 280,
    284-287, 289-291
Coronary Artery Surgery Study 8
coronary heart disease 28, 31, 39, 44, 44, 47,
    48, 70, 73-75, 120-122, 167-175, 177,
    178, 183, 186-188, 192, 195, 237, 246,
    247, 252, 256-259, 271, 283, 285, 292
cortisol xiv, 36, 119, 120
Covera-HS 192
Danchin, Dr. Nicolas 8
death rates xviii, 33, 34, 171, 213, 216, 237,
    238, 314
deconditioning 96, 97, 102, 168-170, 240-
    242, 288
Demadex 188, 189
depression 23, 35, 36, 38, 61, 70, 71, 74, 75,
    117, 173, 182, 183, 240, 249, 252
diabetes xiv, xviii, 3, 26, 27, 31, 32, 34, 36,
    44, 47, 48, 116, 121, 172, 173, 240, 265,
    272
diagnosis, heart disease 17-24, 127-152, 157,
    162, 06, 207, 210, 289, 296, 300, 311,
    314, 317
    angiogram(s) 129-139, 157-161
    echocardiography 132-137
    MRI 137
    PET 137-139
    radioactive imaging 130-132

ABOUT THE AUTHOR

Howard H. Wayne, M.D., F.A.C.C., F.A.C.P. obtained a combined M.D. and Masters degree in cardiovascular physiology at the Bowman Gray School of Medicine in Wake Forest and received his training at the Cleveland Clinic. While on the Faculty of the United States Air Force School of Aerospace Medicine, he became involved in discovering new ways of uncovering heart disease in pilots and future astronauts. This started him on a career-long quest to discover an early warning system for the diagnosis of heart disease. With grant support from the American Heart Association, Dr. Wayne was successful in applying new methods of studying heart function and using these procedures to uncover heart disease before its advanced stages. He wrote the first textbook on noninvasive cardiology in the early 1970s.

Dr. Wayne lectured throughout the United States, Europe and Asia, teaching other doctors about the new methods of examination. He was also able to discover more effective ways of treating coronary heart disease with medication. This combination of early detection and treatment has been so successful that only eight of his patients have had to undergo coronary artery bypass surgery or angioplasty in the past 15 years.

Currently Dr. Wayne is Director of the Noninvasive Heart Center based in San Diego, California. He also also author of *How to Protect Your Heart from Your Doctor*.